MCQs and EMQs in
HUMAN
PHYSIOLOGY

6th edition

MCQs and EMQs in

HUMAN
PHYSIOLOGY

with answers and
explanatory comments

6th edition

Ian C Roddie CBE, DSc, MD, FRCPI
Emeritus Professor of Physiology, The Queen's University of Belfast; former
Head of Medical Education, National Guard King Khalid Hospital, Jeddah,
Saudi Arabia

William FM Wallace BSc, MD, FRCP, FRCA, FCARCSI, FRCSEd
Emeritus Professor of Applied Physiology, The Queen's University of Belfast;
former Consultant in Physiology, Belfast City Hospital, Belfast, N. Ireland

ARNOLD

A member of the Hodder Headline Group
LONDON

First published in Great Britain in 1971
Second edition 1977
Third edition 1984
Fourth edition 1994
Fifth edition 1997
This sixth edition published in 2004 by
Arnold, a member of the Hodder Headline Group,
338 Euston Road, London NW1 3BH
http://www.arnoldpublishers.com

Distributed in the United States of America by
Oxford University Press Inc.,
198 Madison Avenue, New York, NY 10016
Oxford is a registered trademark of Oxford University Press

Whilst the advice and information in this book are believed to be true and
accurate at the date of going to press, neither the author[s] nor the publisher
can accept any legal responsibility or liability for any errors or omissions
that may be made. In particular (but without limiting the generality of the
preceding disclaimer) every effort has been made to check drug dosages;
however it is still possible that errors have been missed. Furthermore,
dosage schedules are constantly being revised and new side-effects
recognized. For these reasons the reader is strongly urged to consult the
drug companies' printed instructions before administering any of the drugs
recommended in this book.

British Library Cataloguing in Publication Data
A catalogue record for this book is available from the British Library

Library of Congress Cataloging-in-Publication Data
A catalog record for this book is available from the Library of Congress

ISBN 0 340 811919

1 2 3 4 5 6 7 8 9 10

Commissioning Editor: Georgina Bentliff
Project Editor: Heather Smith
Production Controller: Jane Lawrence
Cover Design: Amina Dudhia
Index: Dr Laurence Errington

Typeset in 9pt Rotis Serif by Servis Filmsetting Ltd, Manchester
Printed and bound in Malta

What do you think about this book? Or any other Arnold title?
Please send your comments to feedback.arnold@hodder.co.uk

CONTENTS

PREFACE

This book has now reached its sixth edition since it was first published over 30 years ago. Our aim to base the questions on generally accepted aspects of physiology most relevant to clinical practice seems to have been fulfilled – medical, dental and other health care students and doctors in specialty training in countries around the world have told us of the book's relevance and usefulness.

We have tried to cover most of the concepts and knowledge typically asked for in physiology examinations and to concentrate on the core knowledge that is essential to pass them. We believe that students who score consistently well in these questions know enough to face most examinations in physiology with confidence. By concentrating on the area where yes/no answers can be given to questions with reasonable certainty, we have had to exclude areas where knowledge is as yet conjectural and speculative. We have tried to avoid excessive detail in the way of facts and figures; those which are included are of value in medical practice. Both conventional and SI units are generally quoted. Comments on the answers are given on the reverse of each question. We hope that, with the comments, the book will provide a compact revision tutor, encouraging understanding rather than rote learning.

For most questions the common five-branch MCQ format has been used. The stem and a single branch constitute a statement to be judged True or False by the reader. Care has been taken that the statements in any question are not mutually exclusive, so five independent decisions are required to answer each question. This system has the advantage of simplicity and brevity over most other forms of multiple-choice question. In this edition, a further opportunity has been taken to prune and edit questions for greater compactness, clarity and precision and to bring in new areas of knowledge which have emerged since the last edition went to press. We have also tended to expand the comments in an effort to increase the clarity of our explanations and so add to the educational value of the self-assessment exercise.

The book is divided into sections, each section containing questions related to one of the main physiological systems of the body. They cover both basic and applied aspects of the subject. The applied questions are designed so that the answers may be deduced mainly by making use of basic physiological knowledge and should provide a link with clinical practice. There is also a section on sports and exercise physiology and one containing '*Interpretative*' questions to provide practice in the interpretation of data, diagrams and figures. A new feature in this edition is the addition of a number of *Extended Matching Questions* (EMQs) for each section of the book. EMQs are an alternative form of multiple-choice question where answers have to be selected from lists of options. They are becoming increasingly popular in undergraduate and postgraduate examinations.

We thank colleagues for suggesting questions and all who commented on previous editions. We continue to welcome such comments.

ICR
WFMW
September 2003

HOW TO USE THIS BOOK

1. A stimulus to fill gaps in your knowledge

This book is intended as a revision tutor and should help you to revise your physiology in preparation for examinations. It is particularly aimed at helping you to identify areas where your knowledge and understanding need to be improved. The statements in this book are presented so that you can commit yourself in written opinion and can then confirm correct information and identify errors. The comments should reinforce your knowledge when you are correct and indicate why you were mistaken if your answer is wrong.

2. Scoring your answers – multiple choice questions

A   Answer, say, 20 questions (100 decisions), aiming to complete them in about 50 minutes. In our experience of this type of question (one point tested in each Part), it is best for candidates to answer virtually all questions.

B   Score your answers by giving +1 for a correct response, −1 for an incorrect response and 0 for any omitted. It is suggested that this approach is in line with professional life when many true/false decisions must be taken – send the patient to hospital? Begin a certain treatment? Carry out surgery urgently? The penalties for a wrong decision can be considerable!

C   As a very approximate guide, the following scale would apply to candidates who have not spent time memorizing particular questions:

50–60	fair
60–70	good
70–90	excellent
90 100	outstanding

3. Scoring your answers – extended matching questions

For these questions it is usual not to subtract marks for wrong answers, since the chance of randomly getting the correct answer is much less than for multiple-choice questions, where it is 50%. The same stratification of results (above) can then be applied.

4. Range of options

Please note for the MCQs that all, some, or none of the branches in each question may be true. Also, for the EMQs a given option may be used more than once, or not at all.

MCQs

Questions 1–7

1. Extracellular fluid in adults differs from intracellular fluid in that its

A. Volume is greater.
B. Tonicity is lower.
C. Anions are mainly inorganic.
D. Sodium:potassium molar ratio is higher.
E. pH is lower.

2. Blood group antigens (agglutinogens) are

A. Carried on the haemoglobin molecule.
B. Beta globulins.
C. Equally immunogenic.
D. Not present in fetal blood.
E. Inherited as recessive Mendelian characteristics.

3. Total body water, expressed as a percentage of body weight

A. Can be measured with an indicator dilution technique using deuterium oxide.
B. Is smaller on average in women than in men.
C. Rises following injection of posterior pituitary extracts.
D. Falls during starvation.
E. Is less than 80 per cent in young adults.

4. Breakdown of erythrocytes in the body

A. Occurs when they are 6–8 weeks old.
B. Takes place in the reticulo-endothelial system.
C. Yields iron, most of which is excreted in the urine.
D. Yields bilirubin which is carried by plasma protein to the liver.
E. Is required for the synthesis of bile salts.

5. A person with group A blood

A. Has anti-B antibody in the plasma.
B. May have the genotype AB.
C. May have a parent with group O blood.
D. May have children with group A or group O blood only.
E. Whose partner is also A can only have children of groups A or O.

6. Blood platelets assist in arresting bleeding by

A. Releasing factors promoting blood clotting.
B. Adhering together to form plugs when exposed to collagen.
C. Liberating high concentrations of calcium.
D. Releasing factors causing vasoconstriction.
E. Inhibiting fibrinolysis by blocking the conversion of plasminogen to plasmin.

7. Plasma bilirubin

A. Is a steroid pigment.
B. Is converted to biliverdin in the liver.
C. Does not normally cross cerebral capillary walls.
D. Is freely filtered in the renal glomerulus.
E. Is sensitive to light.

MCQ

Answers

1.

A. False   Cells contain half to two-thirds of the total body fluid.
B. False   It is the same; if it were lower, osmosis would draw water into the cells.
C. True   Mainly Cl^- and HCO_3^-; inside, the main anions are protein and organic phosphates.
D. True   Around 30:1; the intracellular ratio is about 1:10.
E. False   Intracellular pH is lower due to cellular metabolism.

2.

A. False   They are part of the red cell membrane.
B. False   They are glycoproteins.
C. False   A, B and D antigens are more immunogenic than the others.
D. False   Fetal blood may elicit immune responses if it enters the maternal circulation.
E. False   They are Mendelian dominants.

3.

A. True D_2O (heavy water) exchanges with water in all body fluid compartments.
B. True   Women carry relatively more fat than men and fat has a low water content.
C. True   ADH in the extracts inhibits water excretion by the kidneys.
D. False   It rises as fat stores are metabolized to provide energy.
E. True   70 per cent, the percentage in the lean body mass, is about the maximum per cent possible.

4.

A. False   The normal erythrocyte lifespan is 16–18 weeks.
B. True   The RES removes effete RBCs from the circulation.
C. False   Most of the iron is retained for further use.
D. True   The protein makes the bilirubin relatively water-soluble.
E. False   Bile salts are synthesized from sterols in the liver.

5.

A. True   This appears about the time of birth.
B. False   This would make them blood group AB.
C. True   They could inherit an A gene from the other parent to give genotype AO.
D. False   B or AB are possible depending on the partner's genes.
E. True   In this case, neither parent has the B gene.

6.

A. True   e.g. Thromboplastin, part of the intrinsic pathway.
B. True   Vascular leaks are sealed by such platelet plugs.
C. False   High Ca^{2+} levels are not needed for haemostasis; normal levels are adequate.
D. True   e.g. Serotonin (5-hydroxytryptamine).
E. False   Serotonin from platelets can release vascular plasminogen activators.

7.

A. False   It is a porphyrin pigment derived from haem.
B. False   Bilirubin is derived from biliverdin formed from haem, not the other way about.
C. True   The 'blood–brain barrier' normally prevents bilirubin entering brain tissue.
D. False   The bilirubin-protein complex is too large to pass the glomerular filter.
E. True   Light converts bilirubin to lumirubin which is excreted more rapidly; phototherapy may be used in the treatment of haemolytic jaundice in children.

Questions 8–13

8. Monocytes

A.   Originate from precursor cells in lymph nodes.
B.   Can increase in number when their parent cells are stimulated by factors released from activated lymphocytes.
C.   Unlike granulocytes, do not migrate across capillary walls.
D.   Can transform into large multinucleated cells in certain chronic infections.
E.   Manufacture immunoglobulin M.

9. Erythrocytes

A.   Are responsible for the major part of blood viscosity.
B.   Contain the enzyme carbonic anhydrase.
C.   Metabolize glucose to produce CO_2 and H_2O.
D.   Swell to bursting point when suspended in 0.9 per cent (150 mmol/litre) saline.
E.   Have rigid walls.

10. Human plasma albumin

A.   Contributes more to plasma colloid osmotic pressure than globulin.
B.   Filters freely at the renal glomerulus.
C.   Is negatively charged at the normal pH of blood.
D.   Carries carbon dioxide in blood.
E.   Lacks the essential amino acids.

11. Neutrophil granulocytes

A.   Are the most common leukocyte in normal blood.
B.   Contain proteolytic enzymes.
C.   Have a lifespan in the circulation of 3–4 weeks.
D.   Contain actin and myosin microfilaments.
E.   Are present in high concentration in pus.

12. Bleeding from a small cut in the skin

A.   Is normally diminished by local vascular spasm.
B.   Ceases within about five minutes in normal people.
C.   Is prolonged in severe factor VIII (antihaemophilic globulin) deficiency.
D.   Is greater from warm skin than from cold skin.
E.   Is reduced if the affected limb is elevated.

13. Antibodies

A.   Are protein molecules.
B.   Are absent from the blood in early fetal life.
C.   Are produced at a greater rate after a first, than after a second, exposure to an antigen six weeks later.
D.   Circulating as free immunoglobulins are produced by B lymphocytes.
E.   With a 1 in 8 titre are more concentrated than ones with a 1 in 4 titre.

MCQ

Answers

8.

A. False   They originate from stem cells in bone marrow.
B. True   Activated T cells release GMCSF (granulocyte/macrophage colony stimulating factor) which stimulates monocyte stem cells to proliferate.
C. False   After 4–6 days in the circulation, monocytes migrate out to become tissue macrophages.
D. True   The 'giant cells' seen in tissues affected by tuberculosis and leprosy.
E. False   Immunoglobulins are made by ribosomes in lymphocytes.

9.

A. True   Blood viscosity rises exponentially with the haematocrit.
B. True   It catalyses the reaction $CO_2 + H_2O = H^+ + HCO_3^-$.
C. True   Glycolysis generates the energy needed to maintain electrochemical gradients across their membranes.
D. False   This is isotonic with their contents.
E. False   The walls deform easily to squeeze through capillaries.

10.

A. True   Its greater mass and lower molecular weight provide more osmotically active particles.
B. False   Only a small amount is filtered normally and this is reabsorbed by the tubules.
C. True   Blood pH is well above albumin's isoelectric point so negative charges (COO^-) predominate.
D. True   As carbamino protein ($R-NH_2 + CO_2 = R-NH\ COOH$).
E. False   It is a first class protein containing essential and non-essential amino acids.

11.

A. True   They comprise 60–70 per cent of circulating leukocytes.
B. True   Their granules contain such enzymes, which, with toxic oxygen metabolites, can kill and digest the bacteria they engulf.
C. False   Less than a day.
D. True   Responsible for their amoeboid motility.
E. True   Pus consists largely of dead neutrophils.

12.

A. True   Due to the effects of tissue damage and serotonin on vascular smooth muscle.
B. True   This is the upper limit of the normal 'bleeding time'.
C. False   Factor VIII increases clotting time, not bleeding time.
D. True   Warmth dilates skin blood vessels.
E. True   Intravascular pressure is reduced in an elevated limb.

13.

A. True   They are made by ribosomes in plasma cells.
B. True   Immunological tolerance prevents the fetus forming antibodies to its own proteins.
C. False   The response to the second exposure is greater since the immune system has been sensitized by the first exposure.
D. True   T lymphocytes are responsible for cell-mediated immunity.
E. True   Antibody with a 1 in 8 titre is detected at greater dilution than one with a 1 in 4 titre.

Questions 14–19

14. Circulating red blood cells
A. Are about 1 per cent nucleated.
B. May show an intracellular network pattern if appropriately stained.
C. Are distributed evenly across the blood stream in large blood vessels.
D. Travel at slower velocity in venules than in capillaries.
E. Deform as they pass through the capillaries.

15. Lymphocytes
A. Constitute 1–2 per cent of circulating white cells.
B. Are motile.
C. Can transform into plasma cells.
D. Decrease in number following removal of the adult thymus gland.
E. Decrease in number during immunosuppressive drug therapy.

16. The specific gravity (relative density) of
A. Red cells is less than that of plasma.
B. Plasma is due more to its protein than to its electrolyte content.
C. Plasma decreases as extracellular fluid and electrolytes are lost.
D. Blood is higher on average in women than in men.
E. Urine can fall below 1.000 in a water diuresis

17. Blood
A. Makes up about 7 per cent of body weight.
B. Forms a higher percentage of body weight in fat than in thin people.
C. Volume can be calculated by multiplying plasma volume by the haematocrit (expressed as a percentage).
D. Volume rises after water is drunk.
E. Expresses serum when it clots.

18. The cell membranes in skeletal muscle
A. Are impermeable to fat-soluble substances.
B. Are more permeable to sodium than to potassium ions.
C. Become more permeable to glucose in the presence of insulin.
D. Become less permeable to potassium in the presence of insulin.
E. Show invaginations which connect to a system of intracellular tubules involved in excitation contraction coupling.

19. The osmolality of
A. A solution determines its freezing point.
B. Intracellular fluid is about twice that of extracellular fluid.
C. 1.8 per cent sodium chloride is about twice that of normal plasma.
D. 5 per cent dextrose solution is about five times that of 0.9 per cent saline.
E. Plasma is due more to its protein than to its electrolyte content.

Answers

14.

A. **False** Nucleated red cells are not normally seen in peripheral blood.
B. **True** Reticulocytes, the most immature circulating RBCs, show this pattern when stained with certain dyes.
C. **False** They form an axial stream away from the vessel wall.
D. **False** The capillary bed has a greater total cross-sectional area than the venular bed.
E. **True** Normal cells, around 7 microns in diameter, become bullet-shaped as they pass through 5 micron diameter capillaries.

15.

A. **False** About 20 per cent of leukocytes are lymphocytes.
B. **True** They migrate by amoeboid movement to areas of chronic inflammation.
C. **True** As plasma cells they manufacture humoral antibodies.
D. **False** The thymus is atrophied and has little function in the adult.
E. **True** Lymphocytes and immune responses are closely linked.

16.

A. **False** Red cells are heavier and hence sediment on standing.
B. **True** The mass of plasma proteins (70–80 grams/litre) far exceeds that of plasma electrolytes (about 10 grams/litre).
C. **False** It increases; plasma specific gravity is an index of ECF volume if protein levels are normal.
D. **False** It is higher in men, who have a higher haematocrit.
E. **False** The specific gravity of pure water is 1.000; urine is water plus solutes.

17.

A. **True** For example, 5 kg (about 5 litres) in a 70 kg man.
B. **False** Since fat tissue is relatively avascular, the reverse is true.
C. **False** It can be calculated by multiplying plasma volume by 1/1 minus haematocrit (expressed as a decimal).
D. **True** The water is absorbed into the blood.
E. **True** Serum is plasma minus its clotting factors.

18.

A. **False** The membrane consists largely of lipid.
B. **False** The reverse is true; sodium ions, being more hydrated than potassium ions, are larger complexes.
C. **True** Thus glucose is stored as muscle glycogen after a meal.
D. **False** They become more permeable; injections of insulin and glucose lower the serum potassium level.
E. **True** These are called the T system of tubules.

19.

A. **True** Depression of the freezing point is an index of a solution's osmolality.
B. **False** Their osmolality is the same; osmotic water movements ensure that this is so.
C. **True** Plasma has the tonicity of a normal saline solution (0.9 per cent sodium chloride).
D. **False** They have the same number of particles.
E. **False** Proteins account for only 1 per cent of plasma osmolality.

Questions 20-25

20. The pH
A. Of arterial blood normally ranges from 7.2 to 7.6.
B. Units express [H^+] in moles/litre.
C. Of blood is directly proportional to the P_{CO_2}.
D. Of blood is directly proportional to [HCO_3^-].
E. Of urine is usually less than 7.

21. Cerebrospinal fluid
A. Is an ultrafiltrate of plasma.
B. Is the main source of the brain's nutrition.
C. Has the same pH as arterial blood.
D. Has a higher glucose concentration than has plasma.
E. Has a higher calcium concentration than has plasma.

22. Antigens
A. Are usually proteins or polypeptide molecules.
B. Can only be recognized by immune system cells previously exposed to that antigen.
C. Are normally absorbed from the gut via lymphatics and carried to mesenteric lymph nodes.
D. Induce a smaller immune response when protein synthesis is suppressed.
E. Are taken up by antigen-presenting macrophages which activate the immune system.

23. Blood eosinophils
A. Have agranular cytoplasm.
B. Are about a quarter of all leukocytes.
C. Are relatively abundant in the mucosa of the respiratory, urinary and alimentary tracts.
D. Release cytokines.
E. Increase in number in viral infections.

24. Normal blood clotting requires
A. Inactivation of heparin.
B. Inactivation of plasmin (fibrinolysin).
C. Calcium ions.
D. An adequate intake of vitamin K.
E. An adequate intake of vitamin C.

25. Antibodies (agglutinins) of the A and B red cell antigens (agglutinogens)
A. Are present in fetal plasma.
B. Cause haemolysis of RBCs containing the A and B antigens when added to a suspension of red cells in saline.
C. Do not normally cross the placental barrier.
D. Have a molecular weight in excess of 500 000.
E. Are monovalent.

Answers

20.

A.   False   The range is normally between 7.35 and 7.45.
B.   False   They express it as the negative logarithm of the [H$^+$] in moles/litre.
C.   False P_{CO_2} raises [H$^+$] and hence lowers pH.
D.   True   [HCO$_3^-$] lowers [H$^+$] by buffering and hence raises pH.
E.   True   The normal diet leaves acidic, rather than alkaline, residues.

21.

A.   False   It is secreted actively by the choroid plexuses.
B.   False   Brain nutrition is delivered mainly by cerebral blood flow.
C.   False   It is around 7.3 compared with 7.4 in blood.
D.   False   It is about two-thirds that of plasma.
E.   False   About half; protein-bound calcium is negligible in CSF.

22.

A.   True   Large carbohydrate molecules may also be antigenic.
B.   False   The ability to recognize foreign antigens is innate and does not depend on previous exposure to them.
C.   False   Antigens, being proteins or carbohydrates, are not normally absorbed; they are digested in the gut.
D.   True   Antibodies are proteins synthesized by ribosomes in activated lymphocytes.
E.   True   Antigens can also act directly on receptors on lymphocyte membranes.

23.

A.   False   They have eosinophilic granules (eosinophilic granulocytes).
B.   False   Only 1–4 per cent of white cells are eosinophils.
C.   True   They are involved in mucosal immunity.
D.   True   Interleukin 4 and platelet activating factor (PAF).
E.   False   Their number increases in parasitic infections and allergic conditions.

24.

A.   False   The anticoagulant effects of heparin are overwhelmed.
B.   False   Blood clots in spite of the fibrinolytic system.
C.   True   Removal of calcium ions prevents clotting.
D.   True   Vitamin K is needed by the liver for synthesis of prothrombin and other factors.
E.   False   The spontaneous bleeding from the gums etc. seen in scurvy is due to capillary abnormality, not a clotting defect.

25.

A.   False   They form shortly after birth, possibly in response to A and B antigens carried into the body by invading bacteria.
B.   False   They cause agglutination (clumping) of A, B and AB cells.
C.   True   Unlike Rh antibodies which have a smaller molecular size.
D.   True   Around 1 000 000.
E.   False   They are divalent and hence cause red cells to adhere to one another during agglutination.

Questions 26–31

26. Lymph
A. Contains plasma proteins.
B. Vessels are involved in the absorption of amino acids from the intestine.
C. Production increases during muscular activity.
D. Does not normally contain cells.
E. Flow is aided by contraction of adjacent skeletal muscles.

27. Blood platelets
A. Are formed in the bone marrow.
B. Are normally more numerous than white cells.
C. Have a small single-lobed nucleus.
D. Increase in number after injury and surgery.
E. Alter shape when in contact with collagen.

28. The conversion of fibrinogen to fibrin
A. Is effected by prothrombin.
B. Involves the disruption of certain peptide linkages by a proteolytic enzyme.
C. Is followed by polymerization of fibrin monomers.
D. Is inhibited by heparin.
E. Is reversed by plasmin (fibrinolysin).

29. An appropriate dilution indicator for measuring
A. Total body water is sucrose.
B. Plasma volume is radioactive sodium.
C. Extracellular fluid volume is inulin.
D. Intracellular fluid volume directly is heavy water (deuterium oxide).
E. Total body potassium is radioactive potassium.

30. Thirst can be
A. Produced by a rise in plasma tonicity.
B. Produced by stimulation of certain areas in the hypothalamus.
C. Produced by a fall in blood volume.
D. Associated with decreased secretion of ADH.
E. Relieved by water intake before the water has been absorbed from the gut.

31. Intravenous infusion of
A. Two litres of normal saline restores blood volume in a patient who suddenly lost two litres of blood.
B. Bicarbonate is appropriate for patients being treated for cardiac and respiratory arrest.
C. Potassium-free fluids are appropriate for a patient with severe vomiting.
D. Isotonic glucose will expand both intracellular and extracellular fluid compartments.
E. Hypertonic saline will raise intracellular osmolality.

Answers

26.

A.	True	Derived from plasma proteins leaked from capillaries into the tissues; it returns these to the blood.
B.	False	Lymph vessels are involved in the uptake and transport of absorbed fat.
C.	True	Increased capillary pressure due to muscle vasodilatation increases tissue fluid formation.
D.	False	It contains lymphocytes derived from lymph nodes.
E.	True	In addition, intrinsic rhythmic contractions in lymphatics help to propel lymph.

27.

A.	True	They are formed from megalokaryocytes.
B.	True	By a factor of 20 or more.
C.	False	No nucleus – but the cytoplasm contains electron dense granules, lysosomes and mitochondria.
D.	True	This increases the tendency of blood to clot.
E.	True	They put out pseudopodia and adhere to the collagen and to one another.

28.

A.	False	It is effected by thrombin; prothrombin is the inactive precursor of thrombin.
B.	True	Thrombin breaks off the solubilizing end groups.
C.	True	Polymerized fibrin monomers form the strands of the clot meshwork.
D.	True	This is a rapidly acting anticoagulant.
E.	False	Plasmin does not convert fibrin back to fibrinogen, it degrades both fibrin and fibrinogen to products which can inhibit thrombin.

29.

A.	False	Sucrose does not cross the cell membrane freely to equilibrate with ICF.
B.	False	Sodium ions migrate easily from plasma to equilibrate with interstitial fluid.
C.	True	Inulin crosses capillary walls freely but does not enter cells.
D.	False	ICF volume is not measured directly; it is calculated by measuring ECF volume and total body water and subtracting the former from the latter.
E.	True	Radioactive K^+ equilibrates with the body pool of non-radioactive K^+; both isotopes are treated similarly in the body.

30.

A.	True	Stimulation of osmoreceptors by the increased tonicity generates thirst sensation.
B.	True	The supraoptic nucleus of the hypothalamus contains osmoreceptors.
C.	True	This can happen, even though blood tonicity is unchanged; volume receptors may be involved.
D.	False	ADH secretion is increased.
E.	True	Flushing out the mouth with water can provide temporary relief from thirst.

31.

A.	False	Some of the saline escapes from the circulation to the interstitial fluid.
B.	True	It corrects the acidosis caused by accumulation of lactic acid and CO_2 in the tissues.
C.	False	Alimentary secretions are rich in potassium.
D.	True	Glucose is metabolized, leaving the water to be distributed in both compartments.
E.	True	Hypertonic extracellular fluid will draw water osmotically from the cells.

MCQ

Questions 32–37

32. Excessive tissue fluid (oedema) in the legs may

A. Be associated with a raised extracellular fluid volume.
B. Result from hepatic disease.
C. Result from blockage of pelvic lymphatics.
D. Increase local interstitial fluid pressure.
E. Result from a high arterial blood pressure in the absence of heart failure.

33. Haemolytic disease of the newborn

A. Affects mainly babies of Rh-positive mothers.
B. Occurs mainly in babies who lack D agglutinogen.
C. Causes jaundice which clears rapidly after birth.
D. Can be treated by transfusing the affected baby with Rh-positive blood.
E. Can be prevented by injecting the mother with anti-D agglutinins just after delivery.

34. The appearance of centrifuged blood may suggest that

A. Anaemia is present if there is more plasma than packed cells.
B. The plasma lipid level is high.
C. The patient has jaundice.
D. Haemolysis has occurred.
E. The patient has leukaemia.

35. Patients with moderate to severe anaemia have a reduced

A. Cardiac output.
B. Incidence of vascular bruits.
C. 2:3-diphosphoglycerate blood level.
D. Arterial P_{O2}.
E. Capacity to raise oxygen consumption in exercise.

36. Iron deficiency

A. Frequently follows persistent loss of blood from the body.
B. Is more common in men than in women.
C. May cause anaemia by inhibiting the rate of multiplication of RBC stem cells.
D. May cause large pale erythrocytes to appear in peripheral blood.
E. Anaemia should normally be treated by injections of iron

37. Severe reactions are likely after transfusion of blood group

A. A to a group B person.
B. O to a group AB person.
C. A to a group O person.
D. A to a group AB person.
E. O Rh- negative to a group AB Rh-positive person.

MCQ

Answers

32.

A. True   Oedema is an increase in the interstitial component of ECF.
B. True   Albumin deficiency reduces plasma colloid osmotic pressure.
C. True   Protein accumulates in interstitial fluid and reduces the colloid osmotic pressure gradient across the capillary wall.
D. True   This contributes to a new pressure equilibrium.
E. False   Arteriolar constriction in hypertension raises arterial, but not capillary, pressure.

33.

A. False   It affects babies of Rh-negative mothers when the child's red cell membranes carry the D antigen.
B. False   It occurs in Rh-positive babies.
C. False   The jaundice deepens rapidly after birth as bilirubin is no longer excreted by the maternal liver.
D. False   This would be attacked by maternal Rh antibodies in the infant's blood; Rh-negative blood is given.
E. True   These destroy fetal Rh-positive cells in the maternal circulation before such cells can sensitize her to D antigen.

34.

A. False   If the normal percentage of plasma in centrifuged blood is about 55 per cent.
B. True   If the plasma is cloudy or even milky.
C. True   If the plasma is yellow.
D. True   If the plasma is red.
E. True   If the buffy coat is greatly thickened.

35.

A. False   Output rises to compensate for the blood's reduced O_2 carrying capacity.
B. False   Bruits are common since increased flow velocity and decreased blood viscosity increase the likelihood of turbulent flow.
C. False   2:3-DPG is increased, shifting the dissociation curve to the right so that blood gives up its oxygen more easily.
D. False   Arterial P_{O_2} is normal; it is O_2 content which is reduced.
E. True   Due to the reduced capacity to deliver O_2 to the muscles.

36.

A. True   Especially if dietary intake of iron is limited.
B. False   It is more common in women due to menstrual blood loss.
C. False   It causes anaemia by limiting the rate of haemoglobin synthesis.
D. False   In iron deficiency anaemia, RBCs are small and pale due to lack of haemoglobin.
E. False   Oral iron is avidly absorbed in iron deficiency states.

37.

A. True   The recipients have anti-A antibody.
B. False   Group O people are 'universal donors'.
C. True   The recipients have anti-A antibody.
D. False   Group AB persons, 'universal recipients', lack anti-A and anti-B antibodies.
E. False   The recipients lack anti-A, anti-B and anti-Rh antibodies.

Questions 38–43

38. The haematocrit (packed cell volume)
A. May be obtained by centrifugation of blood.
B. May be calculated by multiplying the mean cell volume by the red cell count.
C. Rises in a patient who sustains widespread burns.
D. Rises following injections of aldosterone.
E. Rises in macrocytic megaloblastic anaemias such as pernicious (B_{12} deficiency) anaemia.

39. Red cell formation is increased
A. By giving vitamin B_{12} injections to healthy people on a normal diet.
B. In blood donors one week after a blood donation.
C. In patients with haemolytic anaemia.
D. By giving injections of erythropoietin to nephrectomized patients.
E. In patients who have a raised blood reticulocyte count.

40. Vitamin B_{12} deficiency may
A. Result from disease of the terminal part of the ileum.
B. Result in anaemia with small RBCs well filled with haemoglobin.
C. Cause wasting (atrophy) of the gastric mucosa.
D. Cause a reduction in the circulating platelet level.
E. Cause pathological changes in the central nervous system.

41. A raised blood pH and bicarbonate level is consistent with
A. Metabolic acidosis.
B. Partly compensated respiratory alkalosis.
C. A reduced P_{CO_2}.
D. Chronic renal failure with a raised P_{CO_2}.
E. A history of persistent vomiting of gastric contents.

42. A patient with partly compensated respiratory acidosis
A. Must have a raised P_{CO_2}.
B. May have a reduced hydrogen ion concentration [H^+].
C. Must have a raised bicarbonate concentration [HCO_3^-].
D. May have evidence of renal compensation.
E. May have respiratory failure due to hypoventilation

43. A patient with an uncompensated respiratory alkalosis may have
A. Been exposed to living at high altitudes.
B. A reduced [H_2CO_3]:[HCO_3^-] ratio.
C. Neuromuscular hyperexcitability.
D. An arterial pH of 7.3.
E. A blood [H^+] of 30 nmol/litre.

Answers

38.

A. True   Since red cells are heavier than plasma.
B. True   This gives a slightly lower value than centrifugation which traps a little plasma between cells.
C. True   Due to loss of plasma and interstitial fluid.
D. False   It falls as extracellular fluid and hence plasma volume increases.
E. False   Though individual RBCs are large, total red cell mass is decreased.

39.

A. False   Healthy normal people do not benefit from vitamin B_{12} supplements.
B. True   The RBC deficit is corrected by bone marrow stimulation by erythropoietin.
C. True   The reduced oxygen carrying capacity of the blood causes release of erythropoietin which stimulates RBC stem cells in the bone marrow.
D. True   The anaemia seen in nephrectomized patients is due largely to lack of erythropoietin.
E. True   A raised reticulocyte count is evidence of a hyperactive bone marrow.

40.

A. True   The B_{12}/intrinsic factor complex is absorbed in the terminal ileum.
B. False   Lack of B_{12} results in a macrocytic hyperchromic anaemia.
C. False   Gastric mucosa atrophy is a cause, not an effect, of B_{12} lack; gastric mucosa normally produces the 'intrinsic factor' required for B_{12} absorption.
D. True B_{12} is used in the DNA synthesis required by platelet precursor cells.
E. True   Maintenance of myelin in neural sheaths also depends on vitamin B_{12}.

41.

A. False   It is consistent with a metabolic alkalosis.
B. False   A partly compensated acidosis has a low pH.
C. False P_{CO_2} is normally raised in metabolic alkalosis as a compensatory mechanism.
D. False   All these values are reduced in chronic renal failure.
E. True   Pyloric obstruction causes a metabolic alkalosis.

42.

A. True   This is the hallmark of a respiratory acidosis.
B. False   [H^+] is raised in uncompensated acidosis.
C. True   The raised [HCO_3^-] is compensating partly for the raised P_{CO_2}.
D. True   The raised [HCO_3^-], compensating the raised P_{CO_2} is generated by the kidneys.
E. True   This leads to retention of carbon dioxide.

43.

A. False   Living at high altitudes induces partial compensation, i.e. fall in [HCO_3^-]
B. True   This is consistent with alkalosis.
C. True   Alkalosis favours the development of tetany by increasing the binding power of plasma protein for ionic calcium.
D. False   This is an acidotic pH.
E. True   The normal level is 40 nmol/litre.

Questions 44–49

44. In investigating a patient's acid–base status
A. Venous rather than arterial blood should be studied.
B. Blood samples may be stored for up to 12 hours at room temperature before analysis.
C. pH can be calculated if $[HCO_3^-]$ and P_{CO_2} are known.
D. Raised urinary ammonium salts suggest renal compensation for respiratory acidosis.
E. An early fall in $[HCO_3^-]$ suggests that the acid-base disturbance is respiratory in origin.

45. Respiratory alkalosis differs from metabolic alkalosis in that the
A. Likelihood of tetany is less.
B. Urine is alkaline.
C. Arterial blood $[HCO_3^-]$ is normal or low.
D. Arterial blood P_{CO_2} is reduced.
E. Reduction in cerebral blood flow is greater.

46. Rejection of a transplanted organ is made less likely by
A. Treatment which reduces the blood lymphocyte count.
B. Keeping the recipient in a germ-free environment.
C. Irradiation of the transplanted organ with X-rays.
D. Drugs which interfere with mitosis.
E. Transplanting between identical twins.

47. Reduction in the neutrophil granulocyte count may be
A. Caused by drugs suppressing bone marrow activity.
B. A consequence of tissue damage.
C. Associated with painful throat ulcers.
D. Associated with widespread purulent infections.
E. Caused by high levels of circulating glucocorticoids

48. A fall in plasma sodium concentration
A. May result from excessive production of ADH.
B. Decreases intracellular fluid volume.
C. May occur in people engaged in hard physical work in humid tropical climates.
D. Reduces plasma osmolality.
E. Is likely to cause thirst.

49. Sodium retention
A. Occurs for several days after major surgery.
B. Occurs in response to secretion of aldosterone, but not cortisol.
C. Expands the extracellular fluid volume.
D. Expands the blood volume.
E. Increases the severity of oedema.

Answers

44.

A. False   Only arterial blood is precisely regulated for $[H^+]$.
B. False   Analysis should be prompt; acid-base status is affected by blood cell metabolism.
C. True   pH is a function of their ratio.
D. True   Ammonia is secreted to buffer the hydrogen ions being excreted as the kidneys manufacture bicarbonate.
E. False   A primary respiratory acid–base problem leads initially to an altered P_{CO_2}.

45.

A. False   Both kinds of alkalosis may result in tetany.
B. False   It is likely to be alkaline in both.
C. True $[HCO_3^-]$ is raised in metabolic alkalosis but falls to compensate for the low P_{CO_2} in respiratory alkalosis.
D. True P_{CO_2} is reduced in respiratory alkalosis but rises to compensate for the high $[H_2CO_3^-]$ in metabolic alkalosis.
E. True   The greater fall in P_{CO_2} in respiratory alkalosis causes more cerebral vasoconstriction.

46.

A. True   T lymphocytes are responsible for tissue rejection.
B. False   This environment may be necessary because of suppression of the recipient's immune responses; it has no bearing on the rejection process.
C. False   This would not affect the transplant antigens.
D. True   These suppress the multiplication of lymphocytic stem cells.
E. True   Identical twins have identical antigens and do not reject each other's tissues.

47.

A. True   Granulocytes are formed in the bone marrow.
B. False   Production of neutrophils increases following tissue damage.
C. True   Neutrophils are not available to kill bacterial invaders.
D. False   There will not be much pus since pus consists mainly of dead neutrophils.
E. False   These suppress lymphocytes and eosinophils.

48.

A. True   Due to excessive reabsorption of water from the collecting ducts of the nephron.
B. False   Water is drawn into cells from the hypotonic extracellular fluid; water intoxication may occur.
C. True   People sweating heavily may replace their water, but not their salt, deficit; they tend to get muscle cramps unless they supplement their salt intake.
D. True   Sodium ions are responsible for nearly half of plasma osmolality.
E. False   The hypothalamic osmoreceptors responsible for thirst respond to hypertonicity, not hypotonicity of the ECF.

49.

A. True   This is part of the metabolic response to trauma.
B. False   Both have mineralocorticoid effects.
C. True   Sodium chloride is the 'skeleton' of the ECF; chloride and water are retained with the sodium.
D. True   Plasma is part of extracellular volume.
E. True   Oedema fluid is excess interstitial fluid.

MCQ

Questions 50-55

50. Sodium depletion differs from sodium retention in that it causes a reduction in

A. Central venous pressure.
B. Renin production.
C. The specific gravity of the blood.
D. Intracellular fluid volume.
E. Total body mass.

51. Sodium depletion differs from water depletion in that

A. Cardiovascular changes are less pronounced.
B. Intracellular fluid volume is less affected.
C. The haematocrit increases.
D. Thirst is more severe.
E. Antidiuretic hormone levels are higher.

52. Potassium depletion

A. Can be detected by analysis of a biopsied sample of muscle.
B. Can result from loss of gastrointestinal secretions.
C. Causes increased activity of intestinal smooth muscle.
D. Exacerbates pre-existing acidosis.
E. Increases T wave amplitude in the electrocardiogram.

53. A high blood potassium level (hyperkalaemia)

A. Occurs in acute renal failure.
B. Follows severe crush injuries to the limbs.
C. May diminish cardiac performance and cause death.
D. Increases skeletal muscle strength.
E. May be reduced by intravenous infusion of insulin and glucose.

54. Deficiency of factor VIII (antihaemophilic globulin)

A. Increases the bleeding time.
B. Is due to an abnormal gene on the Y chromosome.
C. To 75 per cent of its normal value results in excessive bleeding after tooth extraction.
D. Causes small (petechial) haemorrhages into the skin to cause purpura.
E. Affects the extrinsic, rather than the intrinsic, pathway for blood coagulation.

55. A raised level of calcium in the blood (hypercalcaemia)

A. May occur when parathyroid activity decreases.
B. May occur when the plasma protein level falls.
C. May occur in chronic renal failure.
D. Causes increased excitability of nerve and muscle.
E. Increases the risk of stone formation in the urinary tract.

Answers

50.

A. True   Blood volume parallels body sodium levels; it expands with sodium retention and shrinks with sodium depletion.
B. False A reduced blood volume stimulates release of renin.
C. False It is increased in sodium depletion due to an increased haematocrit.
D. False If anything, ICF volume expands osmotically in sodium depletion.
E. True   Due to the loss of extracellular fluid in sodium depletion.

51.

A. False Blood volume is more reduced with sodium depletion; cardiovascular changes are more pronounced.
B. True   Extracellular volume is a function of body sodium content.
C. False It increases in both cases.
D. False Hypertonicity is the main stimulus causing thirst.
E. False Here also, hypertonicity is the main stimulus for ADH secretion.

52.

A. True   Since most body potassium is intracellular.
B. True   Gastrointestinal secretions are rich in potassium.
C. False Activity decreases and intestinal paralysis (paralytic ileus) may occur.
D. False K^+ competes with H^+ for excretion in the renal tubules; a low $[K^+]$ favours renal excretion of H^+ ions and this would reduce the severity of acidosis.
E. False The amplitude of the T waves decreases.

53.

A. True   Due to inability to excrete K^+ ingested and released from cell breakdown in the body.
B. True   Potassium is released from the damaged muscle fibres.
C. True   Abnormal rhythms and heart failure may result.
D. False Both hypo- and hyperkalaemia cause skeletal muscle weakness.
E. True   This facilitates entry of potassium into cells.

54.

A. False Clotting time is increased, but bleeding time is determined by platelets and by vascular contraction.
B. False It is due to a recessive abnormality of the X chromosome.
C. False Abnormal bleeding does not occur until the level falls below 50 per cent.
D. False Purpura is caused by capillary or platelet disorders.
E. False It affects the intrinsic pathway.

55.

A. False This reduces blood calcium.
B. False This lowers the protein-bound, and hence the total, calcium level.
C. False In chronic renal failure PO_4 retention raises blood PO_4 levels; Ca^{2+} levels fall to maintain a constant $[Ca^{2+}]$ $[PO_4^-]$ product.
D. False It depresses excitability.
E. True   More calcium is filtered and this increases the urinary $[Ca^{2+}]$ $[PO_4^-]$ solubility product.

Questions 56–57

56. Intravenous infusion of one litre of

A. Normal (isotonic) saline increases the ECF more than the ICF volume.
B. 10 per cent dextrose provides sufficient energy for a sedentary adult for one day.
C. A suspension of lipids provides 2–3 times the energy of a suspension of carbohydrates with the same concentration.
D. Isotonic (5 per cent) dextrose raises total body water by 1–5 per cent in the average adult.
E. An amino acid solution provides between 3–4 times the energy of a carbohydrate solution with the same concentration.

57. In patients with the acquired immune deficiency syndrome (AIDS)

A. Neutrophils are more affected than lymphocytes.
B. Total white cell count is a better indicator of progression than any subset of white cells.
C. Host DNA is incorporated into the human immunodeficiency (HIV) virus.
D. Occurrence in infancy results from transmission of infection rather than inheritance.
E. There is increased risk of malignant tumours.

Answers

56.

A. True   Sodium and chloride remain mainly extracellular.
B. False   It provides less than a quarter of the daily energy requirement.
C. True   A gram of fat when oxidized liberates 2–3 times the energy liberated by a gram of carbohydrate.
D. True   Total body water (about 40 litres) increases to about 41 litres (2.5 per cent increase).
E. False   Amino acids and carbohydrates provide similar energy per unit weight but amino acids are useful for maintaining body tissue proteins.

57.

A. False   Lymphocytes are more involved than neutrophils with immunity.
B. False   The CD4 (or T_4) count is a major indicator and falls markedly as AIDS progresses.
C. False   Viral reverse transcriptase incorporates viral RNA into host DNA.
D. True   In contrast to genetic immune disorders such as X-linked hypogammaglobulinaemia.
E. True   The normal immune system suppresses such tumours.

EMQs

Questions 58–67

EMQ Question 58

For each case of disordered haemostasis A–E, select the most appropriate option from the following list of findings.

1. Capillary abnormality.
2. Deficiency of factor VIII.
3. Increased fibrinogen level.
4. Deficiency of prothrombin.
5. Deficiency of vitamin K.
6. Excessive heparin activity.
7. Massive blood transfusion.
8. Platelet count 90×10^9 per litre.
9. Platelet count 20×10^9 per litre.

A. A 15-year-old child is admitted to hospital with recent onset of widespread purpura (pin-head areas of haemorrhage into the skin). Laboratory investigations reveal an abnormality which accounts for the bleeding tendency.

B. A 50-year-old man is receiving anticoagulant therapy (warfarin, a vitamin K antagonist) after heart valve replacement. He is admitted to hospital with haematuria (blood in the urine) and his INR (international normalized ratio, a measure of the prothrombin clotting time in relation to the normal time) is found to be 4.2.

C. A 90-year-old women has blotchy purple areas about 5 cm diameter on her hands and arms. They are not uncomfortable and she has no health complaints.

D. A 70-year-old man is operated on for aneurysm (swelling) of his aorta. Severe bleeding requires infusion of forty units of blood. His recovery is complicated by a bleeding tendency and he is found to have a very low level of fibrinogen. His treatment includes administration of heparin.

E. A 10-year-old child with no known medical problems has been admitted to hospital for persistent bleeding after tooth extraction. Haemostasis had been achieved initially after the extraction but subsequently prolonged oozing from the tooth socket began.

Answers for 58

A.   **Option 9**   *Platelet count 20 × 10⁹ per litre.* Widespread purpura is due to failure of platelet plugging of capillaries and may be due to a low platelet count or to capillary abnormality. An abnormal laboratory test to account for this would be a low platelet count. Although both those given are below normal, only values below 20–40 $\times 10^9$ per litre account for serious bleeding.

B.   **Option 4**   *Deficiency of prothrombin.* The action of warfarin, a vitamin K antagonist, is to impair formation of several coagulation factors, notably prothrombin. There are a number of cardiological indications for the use of warfarin, including heart valve replacement. The value quoted is above the usual recommended range and the prolonged prothrombin time due to a low level of prothrombin would account for the bleeding.

C.   **Option 1**   *Capillary abnormality.* With advancing age, capillaries like tissues generally become less resilient in the face of stress such as a relatively high internal pressure. This leads randomly to patchy areas of bleeding such as those described. Apart from their appearance they cause no problems.

D.   **Option 7**   *Massive blood transfusion.* Massive blood transfusion may lead to widespread activation of the coagulation mechanism – diffuse intravascular coagulopathy. This in turn causes so much deposition of fibrin that the circulating fibrinogen level falls to levels which result in a bleeding tendency. Paradoxically heparin, by preventing the abnormal coagulation, allows the fibrinogen level to rise and can relieve the condition.

E.   **Option 2**   *Deficiency of factor VIII.* This condition (haemophilia) does not interfere with initial haemostasis due to vascular closure, so the bleeding time is normal as in this case. However, when the vascular spasm wears off, failure to clot is revealed as a persistent ooze of blood. Treatment is by supplying the missing factor VIII.

EMQ Question 59

For each case of disturbed acid–base balance A–E, select the most appropriate option from the following list of results of arterial blood analysis.

	pH	P_{O_2} (kPa)	P_{CO_2} (kPa)	HCO_3 (mmol/l.)
1	7.15	16	3	11
2	7.4	14	5	25
3	7.25	9	8	32
4	7.55	10	3	20
5	7.55	11	7	32
6	7.2	25	9	32

100 mmHg = 13.3 kPa

A. A 60-year-old woman who suffers from long standing chronic bronchitis has just been admitted to hospital because her condition deteriorated when she developed a chest infection. No treatment had been given before the blood sample was taken.
B. A 50-year-old man with long-standing chronic bronchitis has been in hospital for several days for treatment of an exacerbation. He is receiving oxygen therapy but his condition is deteriorating.
C. A 50-year-old woman with long-standing renal disease has been admitted with deterioration of her condition, including marked drowsiness. She is noticed to be hyperventilating.
D. A 25-year-old man is taking part in a mountain climbing expedition in the Himalayas and the medical officer of the team is carrying out physiological measurements. The subject has been through the usual protocol for acclimatization to high altitude.
E. A 30-year-old man has been admitted to hospital suffering from abdominal pain and general malaise. He has long-standing upper abdominal pain for which he has been treating himself for some years with quite large amounts of sodium bicarbonate which rapidly relieves the pain. He has begun to get muscle spasms in his hands and feet.

Answers for 59

A. **Option 3**   This patient has features suggesting respiratory failure – drowsiness and cyanosis in someone with chronic obstructive airways disease. So we are looking for signs of a respiratory acidosis – low pH due to high carbon dioxide levels and a reduced oxygen level to account for the cyanosis. Only Option 3 has these three features. In someone with a long-standing respiratory acidosis the bicarbonate is usually raised as in this case (for comparison, results in Option 2 are all average normal).

B. **Option 6**   This patient is very similar to the one above except that he has been receiving oxygen therapy for his hypoxic hypoxia. Deterioration on oxygen suggests the possibility that complete relief of the hypoxia has resulted in respiratory depression with a rising carbon dioxide level and worsening respiratory acidosis. Results in Option 6 confirm this with the very high oxygen pressure which can be produced by breathing oxygen together with a high carbon dioxide level and a dangerously low pH. Correct therapy is to give controlled oxygen at, for example, 24–28 per cent and monitor the blood gases so that the oxygen level is above dangerous levels but the carbon dioxide does not rise dangerously.

C. **Option 1**   This patient has the symptoms of severe renal failure, a condition which leads to a non-respiratory (or metabolic) acidosis. This is confirmed by the very low bicarbonate level and the very low pH. Such a condition leads to respiratory compensation by hyperventilation to lower the carbon dioxide level as shown. The hyperventilation also raises the oxygen level towards that in the atmosphere.

D. **Option 4**   High altitudes lead to hyperventilation triggered by the carotid bodies in response to hypoxic hypoxia. The hyperventilation improves the oxygen level (which is still below that at sea level) but produces a respiratory alkalosis due to washout of carbon dioxide. With acclimatization the kidney responds by lowering the bicarbonate level by reducing tubular secretion of the now scarce hydrogen ions.

E. **Option 5**   This is now a rather rare cause of metabolic alkalosis – ingestion of large amounts of sodium bicarbonate which relieves ulcer pain by temporarily buffering the gastric acid. However the bicarbonate is absorbed and can lead to a metabolic alkalosis. Alkalosis increases the binding of available calcium ions in the blood by plasma proteins and can lead to tetany, which usually starts in adults with 'carpo-pedal' spasm. Metabolic alkalosis is compensated by depression of respiration, allowing the carbon dioxide level to rise and balance the increased bicarbonate level. The oxygen pressure tends to fall with the hypoventilation.

EMQ Question 60

For each case of fluid balance disturbance A–E, select the most appropriate option from the following list.

1. Increased total body water.
2. Decreased total body water.
3. Increased extracellular fluid.
4. Decreased extracellular fluid.
5. Increased interstitial fluid.
6. Decreased interstitial fluid.
7. Increased blood volume.
8. Decreased blood volume.
9. Increased plasma volume.
10. Decreased plasma volume.

A. A 20-year-old mentally disturbed patient has refused all food and drink for several days. Urine volume has fallen to around 100 ml in five hours. Plasma osmolality has risen to 320 mosmol per litre (previously 290 mosmol per litre).

B. A 50-year-old man has suffered from vomiting and diarrhoea for several days. His peripheries are cold and he has a heart rate of 120 per minute and an arterial blood pressure of 90/65.

C. A 50-year-old woman is suffering from weakness and mild confusion. She is found to have a plasma sodium level of 125 mmol/litre (normal about 140 mmol/litre) and has a raised level of vasopressin (antidiuretic hormone).

D. An 80-year-old woman has been admitted to hospital after vomiting blood. Following transfusion of several pints of blood she has become breathless and is found to have an increased jugular venous pressure.

E. A 40-year-old man has been admitted to hospital with full thickness burns of 40 per cent of his body surface. Next day his blood pressure has fallen. A blood test shows a haematocrit of 54 per cent.

Answers for 60

A. **Option 2**   *Decreased total body water.* In the absence of any water intake, a person loses a minimum of around 1500 ml per day (500 ml insensible loss from the lungs, 500 ml insensible loss from the skin and 500 ml as the minimum amount of water which can dissolve excreted solid waste products in the urine). A urine volume of 100 ml in five hours confirms this condition. After several days there will be a water deficit of around four to five litres or 10 per cent of total body water, so the osmolality has risen by about 10 per cent. The water deficit is distributed between intracellular and extracellular fluid and oral water would correct the deficit.

B. **Option 4**   *Decreased extracellular fluid.* The patient has lost a considerable volume of intestinal secretions. This fluid is isotonic and rich in sodium and chloride, the main extra-cellular ions. His main depletion is of extracellular fluid and this is confirmed by signs of severe peripheral circulatory failure evidenced by a low arterial blood pressure despite vasoconstriction (cold peripheries) and a rapid heart rate. He urgently needs replenishment of his extracellular fluid by intravenous infusion of isotonic (normal) saline. Although Option 8 accounts for the peripheral circulatory failure, Option 4 is more appropriate as it includes the underlying mechanism and points to the appropriate treatment.

C. **Option 1**   *Increased total body water.* Inappropriately raised secretion of antidiuretic hormone causes excessive reabsorption of water as fluid passes through the collecting ducts. This dilutes all body fluids as indicated by the low sodium level (osmolality would be correspondingly reduced). The waterlogging of the body cells impairs function and this effect in the brain is manifested by confusion. Restricted water intake would improve the condition.

D. **Option 7**   *Increased blood volume.* Replacement of blood loss is urgent in the elderly, but over-transfusion can increase the blood volume above normal. In the elderly there is an increased risk of heart failure and increasing the blood volume can precipitate this so that the heart cannot adequately clear the venous return. The filling pressure of the two sides of the heart increases, causing pulmonary oedema and breathlessness plus increased systemic venous pressure. Diuretic therapy would reduce blood volume by causing excre-tion of salt and water, thereby lowering extracellular fluid volume.

E. **Option 10**   *Decreased plasma volume.* By damaging capillaries, burns cause increased loss of fluid and proteins from the circulation. In addition large amounts of interstitial fluid are lost through the damaged skin. Both effects lower plasma volume, raising the haematocrit. Low blood volume can lead to peripheral circulatory failure. The standard treatment is to infuse large quantities of normal saline, in proportion to the area of seri-ously burnt skin.

EMQ Question 61

For each blood transfusion problem A–E, select the most appropriate option from the following list.

1. ABO incompatibility.
2. Rhesus incompatibility.
3. Major incompatibility.
4. Minor incompatibility.
5. Multiple repeated transfusions.
6. Massive blood transfusion.
7. Use of stored blood.
8. Use of fresh blood.

A. A patient has been given three units of blood during a surgical operation. Just after the operation the patient is at risk of inadequate tissue oxygenation despite satisfactory arterial blood pressure, haemoglobin and arterial blood oxygen saturation levels.

B. A patient has been given two units of blood on the day before a planned surgical operation. Towards the end of the transfusion the patient was noted to have mild fever, and the next morning slight jaundice was noted in the conjunctivae.

C. A patient admitted with vomiting of blood shows signs of circulatory failure and is given a unit of blood quite rapidly. As the transfusion is nearly completed it is discovered that there has been confusion between two patients with exactly the same first and second names and the patient with the transfusion appears much more unwell than at the start of the transfusion. In fact the group B patient was given group A blood.

D. During emergency surgery for a dissected aortic aneurysm, a condition notorious for severe bleeding during operation, a patient is transfused with 20 units of blood. Despite restoration of a normal blood volume this patient is at risk of hypothermia, tissue hypoxia and coagulation problems.

E. A patient with failure of bone marrow function causing aplastic anaemia is admitted for transfusion as the haemoglobin level has fallen to an unacceptable level. The blood bank report difficulty in finding suitable red cells due to problems with some of the 'minor' blood groups, M and Kell.

EMQ Question 62

For each case of anaemia A–E, select the most appropriate option from the following list.

1. Iron deficiency anaemia.
2. Pernicious anaemia.
3. Microcytic anaemia.
4. Macrocytic anaemia.
5. Normocytic anaemia.
6. Bone marrow disease.
7. Compensatory rise in cardiac output.
8. Decreased blood viscosity.
9. Haemolytic anaemia.
10. Increased bone marrow activity.

A. Normal under the microscope. The mean red cell volume is normal at 90 cubic microns.

B. A patient with long-standing indigestion has noticed increasing lack of energy and tiredness when walking uphill. On questioning he has noticed that the bowel motions are unusually dark from time to time. Due to the indigestion the patient takes a bland diet without much meat or vegetables.

C. A patient with a blood haemoglobin concentration of 60 grams per litre complains of recent palpitations (an abnormal awareness of the heart beat, often rather fast). When at rest, the pulse is 110 per minute and the blood pressure 140/60 mmHg.

D. A woman of 75 has noticed unusual lack of energy recently and feels she is paler than usual. Her haemoglobin level is 110 grams per litre and the red cell count is depressed beyond that expected with the fall in haemoglobin. The circulating level of vitamin B_{12} is very low, but the folate level is normal.

E. A patient with moderate anaemia is found to have a bruit (abnormal murmur) when a stethoscope is used to listen over each of the carotid arteries in the neck. The doctor is inclined to attribute the murmur to a physical effect of the anaemia on the blood rather than to an abnormality of the carotid arteries.

EMQ

Answers for 61

A. **Option 7**   **Use of stored blood.** This blood has the characteristic property of stored blood – a low level of 2:3-DPG. Hence the blood oxygen dissociation curve is shifted to the left, and the blood does not give up adequate oxygen at tissue oxygen tensions.

B. **Option 4**   **Minor incompatibility.** There has been a mild antibody rejection of the donor red cells. A relatively small number of these have been broken down (lysed) to release bilirubin which causes the jaundice. The immune response also releases products, including interleukin-1, which cause the fever.

C. **Option 3**   **Major incompatibility.** This type of mistake carries a high risk of death because the recipient's naturally occurring anti-A antibody (agglutinin) rapidly destroys the transfused group A red cells, releasing huge amounts of deadly toxins.

D. **Option 6**   **Massive blood transfusion.** A massive blood transfusion is defined as one where the volume of blood transfused equals or exceeds the patient's original blood volume. Stored blood carries the problem mentioned in (A) but because large volumes of blood must be given very rapidly there is not time to heat them to body temperature from their initial low temperature, so the patient's core temperature drops (hypothermia). This compounds the shift in the blood oxygen dissociation curve and also slows the coagulation reactions.

E. **Option 5**   **Multiple repeated transfusions.** Such patients require regular blood transfusions on repeated occasions, so their immune system builds up antibodies to minor blood group antigens such as M, N, Kell and Duffy.

Answers for 62

A. **Option 5**   *Normocytic anaemia.* The haemoglobin concentration is about half normal, indicating moderate anaemia. Since the red cells look normal and mean cell volume is also normal this is a normocytic anaemia. It could be due to bone marrow disease, lack of erythropoietin or other chronic disease.

B. **Option 1**   *Iron deficiency anaemia.* This patient has symptoms of anaemia, along with a suggestion of repeated bleeding into the bowel and a diet likely to be low in iron. The most likely explanation is anaemia due to iron deficiency. This is likely to be a microcytic anaemia, but no confirmatory details of the presence of small pale red cells are given in this case.

C. **Option 7**   *Compensatory rise in cardiac output.* This patient has severe anaemia. In order to provide adequate oxygen for the tissues, the low oxygen content per litre must be compensated by increased flow. This patient shows the features – fast pulse, high pulse pressure – of an increased resting cardiac output (hyperdynamic circulation).

D. **Option 2**   *Pernicious anaemia.* This patient has moderately severe anaemia. Because the red cell count is disproportionately low, the cells must be larger than normal – macrocytic. This is explained by the low level of vitamin B_{12} and the normal folate excludes another major macrocytic anaemia. The B_{12} deficiency at this age is usually due to failure of the stomach to produce intrinsic factor – pernicious anaemia. The term pernicious was used because before the discovery of vitamin B_{12} there was no treatment and the condition got worse and worse until the patient died from an extremely low level of haemoglobin.

E. **Option 8**   *Decreased blood viscosity.* A bruit or murmur in the circulation indicates turbulent flow. Turbulent flow is much more likely as the viscosity of blood decreases. Since most of the blood viscosity is due to the haematocrit, moderate anaemia could reduce the viscosity by around half. The increased velocity of flow due to the increased cardiac output mentioned in (C) would also increase the chance of turbulence.

EMQ Question 63

For each lipid-related topic A–E, select the most appropriate option from the following list.
1. Coronary artery disease risk factor.   2. Source of energy.
3. Cell membrane solubility.   4. Cell membrane structure.
5. Metabolic energy per unit mass.   6. Derived from cholesterol.
7. Body lipid stores.   8. Lipase.
9. Carbohydrate hormones.   10. Protein hormones.

A. When explorers were crossing Antarctica trailing all their food in a hand sleigh there was an advantage in taking a high proportion of fat rather than carbohydrate.
B. Oestradiol, testosterone and aldosterone share a property which is not shared by insulin and vasopressin.
C. In life-threatening acute inflammation of the pancreas (pancreatitis) considerable tissue damage is produced by a chemical which is detected in the bloodstream in large amounts.
D. In patients who have had a heart attack due to blockage of the blood supply of the myocardium, drugs may be given to lower the blood cholesterol level.
E. The interior of muscle fibres contains many glycogen granules and lipid droplets.

EMQ Question 64

For each of the descriptions A–E, select the most appropriate option from the following list.
1. Neutrophil polymorphonuclear granulocyte.   2. Platelet.
   3. Lymphocyte.
4. Thrombocytopoenia.   5. Leukaemia.

A. Responsible for ingesting invading bacteria.
B. The blood cell most affected by AIDS.
C. A condition where abnormal white cells invade the bone marrow.
D. The smallest cellular element in the blood.
E. Uniquely capable of becoming sticky.

EMQ Question 65

For each of the descriptions related to body fluids A–E, select the most appropriate option from the following list.
1. Osmolality.   2. Plasma albumin.
3. Glucose.   4. Sodium.
5. Plasma globulin.

A. Responsible for most of the colloid osmotic pressure of the plasma.
B. Responsible for fluid shifts between intracellular and extracellular fluid.
C. Provides about half of osmotically active particles in extracellular fluid.
D. Mainly responsible for opposing the leak of fluid out of capillaries.
E. Determines the freezing point of a solution.

Answers for 63

A.   **Option 5**   *Metabolic energy per unit mass.* Fat liberates just over twice the metabolic energy per unit mass that is liberated by metabolism of carbohydrates. The two substrates are both used by the body to provide energy especially in strenuous exercise. So by dragging relatively large amounts of fat the explorers were minimizing the load on their sleigh and maximizing the energy they obtained from their food.

B.   **Option 6**   *Derived from cholesterol.* Oestradiol, testosterone and aldosterone are all derived in the body from cholesterol. Despite being a risk factor for arterial disease when present in excess in the blood, cholesterol is a precursor of vital hormones and is synthesized in the body. Insulin is a protein hormone and vasopressin a polypeptide hormone.

C.   **Option 8**   *Lipase.* In acute pancreatitis large amounts of lipase escape into the blood and this leads to widespread fat necrosis as part of the life-threatening state when the pancreatic hormones enter the bloodstream.

D.   **Option 1**   *Coronary artery disease risk factor.* Excessive lipids in the blood, including cholesterol, are a risk factor for coronary atheroma. The lipid profile may also be improved by moderate exercise and avoidance of obesity.

E.   **Option 2**   *Source of energy.* During prolonged exercise energy is derived in approximately equal amounts from carbohydrate and fat. The glycogen granules in particular are a major source of energy. They become more prominent with physical training and are depleted after prolonged fasting exercise.

Answers for 64

A.   **Option 1**   *Neutrophil polymorphonuclear granulocyte.* These are the commonest of the white cell types. In an area of serious prolonged infection the 'neutrophils' ingest bacteria, eventually die and accumulate as pus.

B.   **Option 3**   *Lymphocyte.* The lymphocytes are responsible for immunity, so a disease which damages their function leads to immune deficiency.

C.   **Option 5**   *Leukaemia.* Leukaemia is a cancerous multiplication of abnormal white cells which replace normal bone marrow cells, suppressing normal formation of white cells, red cells and other marrow-derived cells.

D.   **Option 2**   *Platelet.* Platelets are about half the diameter of red cells, which in turn are smaller than white cells. Lack of platelets is called thrombocytopoenia.

E.   **Option 2**   *Platelet.* Areas of endothelial damage expose collagen to which platelets are attracted. They adhere to the collagen and become sticky for other platelets so that a platelet plug develops to close the gap and prevent loss of blood.

Answers for 65

A.   **Option 2**   *Plasma albumin.* Colloid osmotic pressure is due to protein molecules which cannot readily cross the capillary wall; albumin constitutes the larger portion of the plasma protein mass, its molecules are smaller than globulin so it exerts much more osmotic pressure.

B.   **Option 1**   *Osmolality.* Water passes across the cell wall by osmotic forces due to the sum of the effects of all dissolved particles – the osmolality.

C.   **Option 4**   *Sodium.* Sodium has a concentration around 135 mmol per litre and provides nearly half of the total osmolality of around 285 mosmol per kg.

D.   **Option 2**   *Plasma albumin.* Because most particles are in equilibrium across the capillary wall they do not contribute to the osmotic force opposing fluid leak. The proteins provide an opposing force and albumin is the commonest protein particle.

E.   **Option 1**   *Osmolality.* Osmolality can be measured by noting the freezing point of the solution being tested.

EMQ Question 66

For each of the intravenous fluids A–E, select the most appropriate option from the following list of infusions.

1. 50 per cent glucose.
2. 1.8 per cent saline.
3. 5 per cent glucose (dextrose).
4. Normal (0.9 per cent) saline (sodium chloride).
5. 8.4 per cent sodium bicarbonate.

A. An isotonic solution which expands mainly the extracellular fluid volume.
B. An isotonic solution which expands both intra- and extracellular fluid volumes.
C. A major nutrient used in intravenous nutrition.
D. A hypertonic fluid with about twice the osmolality of plasma.
E. A fluid occasionally used to treat severe acidosis.

EMQ Question 67

For each of the body fluid disturbances A–E, select the most appropriate option from the following list of abnormalities.

1. Hyper-osmolality.
2. Hypo-osmolality.
3. Hyponatraemia.
4. Hyperkalaemia.
5. Raised haematocrit.

A. Excessive retention of water by the kidneys.
B. Excessive loss of plasma and extracellular fluid as a result of severe burns.
C. Likely to be present if the blood glucose level is 30 (normal 5–8) mmol/litre.
D. Produced by drinking excessive amounts of water.
E. Likely to cause swelling of brain cells.

EMQ

Answers for 66

A. **Option 4** *Normal saline.* Normal saline has the same tonicity (osmolality) as plasma and extracellular fluid. Sodium doesn't enter intracellular fluid appreciably. The chloride and water remain with the sodium in the extracellular space.

B. **Option 3** *5 per cent glucose.* 5 per cent glucose (dextrose) is also isotonic. It has the same number of particles as 0.9 per cent saline. Saline dissociates so the average particle molecular weight is about 30. Dextrose has a molecular weight of 180 and does not dissociate so about six times the mass of dextrose is required for isotonicity.

C. **Option 1** *50 per cent glucose.* A litre of 50 per cent glucose contains 500 grams of glucose, yielding about 2000 kilocalories (about 9 megajoules, MJ), around the resting daily requirement of an adult.

D. **Option 2** *1.8 per cent saline.* This is twice the osmolality of normal saline – around 600 as compared with around 300 mosmoles per kg.

E. **Option 5** *8.4 per cent sodium bicarbonate.* This concentrated bicarbonate solution has a high buffering capacity for hydrogen ions. However correcting acid–base balance is a complex procedure rarely benefiting from such drastic measures.

Answers for 67

A. **Option 2** *Hypo-osmolality.* Excessive retention of water dilutes all the body fluids leading to hypo-osmolality. Water crosses the cell membrane until equilibrium is attained. Inappropriately high levels of antidiuretic hormone could do this.

B. **Option 5** *Raised haematocrit.* As fluid is lost, plasma volume declines, so the red blood cells become an increasing proportion of blood volume.

C. **Option 1** *Hyper-osmolality.* The high glucose raises the osmolality proportionately, so a rise of 25 mmol/litre in the extracellular glucose level would raise the osmolality from 285 to 310 mosmol/kg, an appreciable rise. This would draw fluid from cells, including brain cells, disturbing function.

D. **Option 2** *Hypo-osmolality.* Drinking excessive amounts of water has the same effect as excessive retention by the kidney. However healthy people promptly excrete the excess fluid.

E. **Option 2** *Hypo-osmolality.* Excess water is drawn into brain cells by osmosis. This also disturbs brain function.

MCQs

Questions 68–72

68. Coronary blood flow to the left ventricle increases during
A. Early systole.
B. Myocardial hypoxia.
C. Hypothermia.
D. Stimulation of sympathetic nerves to the heart.
E. Arterial hypertension.

69. Local metabolic activity is the chief factor determining the rate of blood flow to the
A. Heart.
B. Skin.
C. Skeletal muscle.
D. Lung.
E. Kidney.

70. The pressure
A. Drop along large veins is similar to that along large arteries.
B. Drop across the hepatic portal bed is similar to that across the splenic vascular bed.
C. In the hepatic portal vein exceeds that in the inferior vena cava.
D. Drop across the vascular bed in the foot is greater when a subject is in the vertical than when he is in the horizontal position.
E. In foot veins is lower when walking than when standing still.

71. The second heart sound differs from the first heart sound in that it is
A. Related to turbulence set up by valve closure.
B. Longer lasting than the first sound.
C. Higher in frequency.
D. Occasionally split.
E. Heard when the ventricles are relaxing.

72. Pulmonary vascular resistance is
A. Less than one-third that offered by the systemic circuit.
B. Decreased when alveolar oxygen pressure falls.
C. Expressed in units of volume flow per unit time per unit pressure gradient.
D. Decreased during exercise.
E. Regulated reflexly by sympathetic vasoconstrictor nerves.

Answers

68.

A. False   It falls; coronary vessels are compressed by the contracting myocardium.
B. True   A fall in P_{O_2} has a potent vasodilator effect on coronary vessels. Adenosine released from hypoxic myocardium is also a potent vasodilator.
C. False   The fall in metabolic rate and cardiac output in hypothermia reduce cardiac work and lead to a reduction in coronary blood flow.
D. True   Sympathetic stimulation increases the rate and force of contraction; the resulting increase in the rate of production of vasodilator metabolites dilates coronary vessels.
E. True   Myocardial work and metabolism are increased in hypertension.

69.

A. True   There is a close relationship between the work of the heart and coronary flow.
B. False   Skin blood flow is geared mainly to thermoregulation and normally exceeds that needed for skin's modest metabolic requirements.
C. True   Local blood flow is largely determined by the vasoactive metabolites such as rising P_{CO_2}, H^+ concentration and falling P_{O_2}. The changes produced by vasomotornerves are small compared with those produced by metabolites.
D. False   The entire cardiac output must pass through the lungs regardless of the local metabolic needs of the pulmonary tissues. It is greatly in excess of the lungs' metabolic needs.
E. False   As in skin, renal blood flow (about one quarter of total cardiac output) greatly exceeds local metabolic needs. The blood is sent to the kidneys for processing.

70.

A. True   About 10 mmHg or less; both offer little resistance to flow.
B. False   The drop across the splenic vascular bed (about 60 mmHg) is much larger; the hepatic portal bed offers little resistance to flow.
C. True   Otherwise blood would not flow through the portal bed.
D. False   Changing from the horizontal to the vertical position increases arterial and venous pressures equally.
E. True   The muscle pump in the leg decreases venous pressure.

71.

A. False   This applies to both heart sounds.
B. False   It is about 20 per cent shorter.
C. True   About 50 Hz compared with 35 Hz for the first sound.
D. False   Both may be split due to asynchronous valve closure.
E. True   The first sound is due to ventricular systole; the second occurs during ventricular relaxation when the aortic valves snap shut as ventricular pressure falls below aortic.

72.

A. True   The pressure head needed to drive cardiac output through the pulmonary circuit (about 15 mmHg) is much less than that needed in the systemic circuit (about 90 mmHg).
B. False   The reverse is true; low alveolar P_{O_2} may cause pulmonary hypertension.
C. False   These are conductance units, the reciprocal of resistance units.
D. True   Thus there is little rise in pulmonary arterial pressure during exercise despite the increased flow rate. Release of nitric oxide from the pulmonary vascular endothelium may account for the vasodilatation.
E. False   Pulmonary vascular resistance is controlled by local rather than by nervous mechanisms.

Questions 73–78

73. Ventricular filling
A. Depends mainly on atrial contraction.
B. Begins during isometric ventricular relaxation.
C. Gives rise to a third heart sound in some healthy people.
D. Can occur only when atrial pressure is greater than atmospheric pressure.
E. Is most rapid in the first half of diastole.

74. Veins
A. Contain most of the blood volume.
B. Have a sympathetic vasoconstrictor innervation.
C. Receive nutrition from vasa vasorum arising from their lumen.
D. Respond to distension by contraction of their smooth muscle.
E. Undergo smooth muscle hypertrophy when exposed to high pressure through an arterio-venous fistula.

75. In the heart
A. The left atrial wall is about three times thicker than the right atrial wall.
B. Systolic contraction normally begins in the left atrium.
C. Excitation spreads directly from atrial muscle cells to ventricular muscle cells.
D. Atrial and ventricular muscle contracts simultaneously in systole.
E. The contracting ventricles shorten from apex to base.

76. Isometric (static) exercise differs from isotonic (dynamic) exercise in that it causes a greater increase in
A. Venous return.
B. Pressure in the veins draining the exercising muscle.
C. Muscle blood flow.
D. Mean arterial pressure.
E. Cardiac work for the same increase in cardiac output.

77. The net loss of fluid from capillaries in the legs is increased by
A. Arteriolar dilation.
B. Change from the recumbent to the standing position.
C. Lymphatic obstruction.
D. Leg exercise.
E. Plasma albumin depletion.

78. When measuring blood pressure by the auscultatory method
A. The sounds that are heard are generated in the heart.
B. The cuff pressure at which the first sounds are heard indicate systolic pressure.
C. The cuff pressure at which the loudest sounds are heard indicate diastolic pressure.
D. Systolic pressure estimations tend to be lower than those made by the palpatory method.
E. Wider cuffs are required for larger arms.

Answers

73.

A. False   Atrial contraction accounts for only about 20 per cent of filling at rest.
B. False   During this phase the AV valves are closed and ventricular volume is constant.
C. True   This low-pitched sound is sometimes heard in early diastole.
D. False   Filling occurs when atrial pressure exceeds ventricular pressure.
E. True   Due to entry of blood accumulated in the atria during ventricular systole.

74.

A. True   Around three-quarters; veins are referred to as 'capacitance' vessels.
B. True   These modulate venous capacity.
C. False   Their vasa arise from neighbouring arteries.
D. True   This 'myogenic' response helps to limit the degree of distension.
E. True   Another functional adaptation to resist distension.

75.

A. False   Their wall thickness is similar since the workload of the two atria is similar.
B. False   It begins at the sinuatrial node in the right atrium.
C. False   Excitation can only pass from atria to ventricles via specialized conducting tissue in the AV bundle.
D. False   Delay of excitation in the AV bundle makes atrial precede ventricular contraction.
E. True   Due to the spiral arrangement of some muscle fibres; circular fibres reduce ventricular circumference.

76.

A. False   The muscle pump is more effective in dynamic than in static exercise.
B. True   In dynamic exercise, the muscle pump increases venous return and so decreases venous pressure in dependent veins.
C. False   The increase is less since inflow is obstructed by the sustained compression exerted by the contracting muscle.
D. True   There is relatively little fall in total peripheral resistance with static exercise.
E. True   The rise in arterial pressure with static exercise increases cardiac work since cardiac output has to be ejected against a higher aortic pressure.

77.

A. True   This increases capillary hydrostatic pressure.
B. True   In the standing position, capillary pressure increases by the hydrostatic equivalent of the column of blood below the heart.
C. False   Lymphatic obstruction allows tissue fluid to accumulate; the rise in interstitial pressure reduces the capillary transmural hydrostatic pressure gradient.
D. True   Capillary pressure rises during the exercise hyperaemia.
E. True   Hypoproteinaemia decreases the transmural colloid osmotic pressure gradient.

78.

A. False   Korotkoff sounds are produced locally by the turbulence of blood being forced past the narrow segment of a partially occluded artery.
B. True   The sharp taps of Phase 1 are generated as the systolic pressure peaks force blood under the cuff.
C. False   Sudden muffling (Phase 4) or disappearance (Phase 5) of the sounds indicate the diastolic pressure point.
D. False   They are usually higher since palpation may fail to detect the first tiny pulses.
E. True   Otherwise the full cuff pressure may not be transmitted to the artery.

Questions 79–84

79. The absolute refractory period in the ventricles

A. Is the period when the ventricles are completely inexcitable.
B. Corresponds to the period of ventricular depolarization.
C. Corresponds approximately to the period of ventricular contraction.
D. Is shorter than the corresponding period in atrial muscle.
E. Decreases during sympathetic stimulation of the heart.

80. Vascular resistance

A. Increases by 50 per cent when the vascular radius is halved.
B. Is related to the thickness of the wall of the vessel.
C. Is related to the vessel's length.
D. Is affected by blood viscosity.
E. Is greater in the capillary bed than in the arteriolar bed.

81. Sympathetic drive to the heart is increased

A. In exercise.
B. In excitement.
C. In hypotension.
D. When parasympathetic drive is decreased.
E. During a vasovagal attack.

82. In an adult subject standing quietly at rest, venous pressure in the

A. Foot is approximately equal to arterial pressure at heart level.
B. Thorax decreases when the subject inhales.
C. Hand is subatmospheric when the hand is raised above the head.
D. Venous sinuses of the skull are subatmospheric.
E. Superior vena cava is an index of cardiac filling pressure.

83. Hyperaemia in skeletal muscle during exercise is normally associated with

A. Release of sympathetic vasoconstrictor tone in the exercising muscles.
B. Capillary dilation due to relaxation of capillary smooth muscle.
C. A fall in arterial pressure.
D. Reflex vasoconstriction in other vascular beds.
E. An increase in cardiac output.

84. Sinuatrial node cells are

A. Found in both atria.
B. Innervated by the vagus.
C. Unable to generate impulses when completely denervated.
D. Connected to the AV node by fine bundles of Purkinje tissue.
E. Able to generate impulses because their membrane potential is unstable.

Answers

79.

A. True   This is the definition.
B. True   Depolarized cells cannot be excited.
C. True   This prevents tetanic contraction of the heart.
D. False   It is longer, as is the duration of its depolarization.
E. True   Shortening the refractory period permits higher heart rates.

80.

A. False   By more than 90 per cent; resistance is related to the fourth power of the radius.
B. False   Vascular resistance is not related to wall thickness.
C. True   It is directly proportional to length.
D. True   Resistance is related to Viscosity$\times$Length/Radius^4.
E. False   Total arteriolar resistance exceeds total capillary resistance though the reverse is true for single vessels.

81.

A. True   β-adrenergic blocking drugs reduce exercise tachycardia.
B. True   The tachycardia during excitement is also reduced by β-blocking drugs.
C. True   A reflex response to decreased stretch of arterial baroreceptors.
D. False   The two systems can function independently.
E. False   Parasympathetic drive slows the heart during a vasovagal attack; sympathetic drive may stimulate the heart during recovery.

82.

A. True   It is about 90 mmHg, due to the column of blood (about 1 metre) between the heart and the foot.
B. True   The negative intrathoracic pressure during inhalation is transmitted to the veins.
C. False   Limb veins collapse above heart level. Negative pressure cannot be transmitted along a collapsed tube so venous pressure is atmospheric in the raised hand.
D. True   The sinuses are held open by their meningeal attachments and cannot collapse.
E. True   A central venous pressure line is usually placed here.

83.

A. False   Exercise hyperaemia occurs normally in sympathectomized muscles.
B. False   True capillaries have no smooth muscle; they dilate passively with the rise in capillary pressure due to active arteriolar dilation.
C. False   Arterial pressure usually rises.
D. True   Vasoconstriction in kidneys, gut and skin prevent excessive falls in total peripheral resistance.
E. True   This, together with the reflex constriction above, compensate for the fall in muscular vascular resistance and thus prevent arterial pressure falling during exercise.

84.

A. False   The SA node is in the right atrium near its junction with the superior vena cava.
B. True   Vagal activity slows the rate of impulse generation and thus the heart rate.
C. False   The SA node has intrinsic rhythmicity and can generate impulses independently.
D. False   Purkinje tissue is confined to the ventricles; atrial fibres conduct impulses from the SA to the AV node.
E. True   Impulse generation is due to spontaneous diastolic depolarization of the cells.

Questions 85–91

85. The first heart sound corresponds in time with
A. Closure of the aortic and pulmonary valves.
B. The P wave of the electrocardiogram.
C. A rise in atrial pressure.
D. A rise in ventricular pressure.
E. The A wave in central venous pressure.

86. Increased sympathetic drive to the heart increases the
A. Rate of diastolic depolarization in sinuatrial node cells.
B. Coronary blood flow.
C. Rate of conduction in Purkinje tissue.
D. Slope of the Frank–Starling (work versus stretch) curve of the heart.
E. Ejection fraction of the left ventricle.

87. The velocity of blood flow
A. In capillaries is low because they offer high resistance to flow.
B. In veins is greater than in venules.
C. Can fall to zero in the ascending aorta during diastole.
D. Is greater towards the centre of large blood vessels than at the periphery.
E. In the circulation falls as the haematocrit falls.

88. The strength of contraction of left ventricular muscle increases when
A. End-diastolic ventricular filling pressure rises.
B. Serum potassium levels rise.
C. Blood calcium levels fall.
D. Strenuous exercise is undertaken.
E. Peripheral resistance is increased as in hypertension.

89. During isometric ventricular contraction
A. The entry and exit valves of the ventricle are closed.
B. Pressure in the aorta rises.
C. Pressure in the atria falls.
D. Left coronary blood flow falls.
E. The rate of rise in pressure is greater in the right than in the left ventricle.

90. In the electrocardiogram, the
A. QRS complex follows the onset of ventricular contraction.
B. T wave is due to repolarization of the ventricles.
C. PR interval corresponds with atrial depolarization.
D. RT interval is related to ventricular action potential duration.
E. R-R interval normally varies during the respiratory cycle.

91. Cardiac output
A. Is normally expressed as the output of one ventricle in litres/minute.
B. May not increase when heart rate rises.
C. Usually rises when a person lies down.
D. Rises in a hot environment.
E. Does not increase in exercise following denervation of the heart.

Answers

85.

A.	False	It is synchronous with mitral and tricuspid closure.
B.	False	It corresponds with the QRS complex.
C.	True	The mitral and tricuspid valves bulge *back* into the atria.
D.	True	This closes the mitral and tricuspid valves.
E.	False	It corresponds with the C wave; the A wave is due to atrial contraction which precedes the first heart sound.

86.

A.	True	This increases the rate of impulse generation and hence heart rate.
B.	True	The increase in myocardial metabolism generates vasodilator metabolites.
C.	True	Rapid spread of excitation in the ventricles results in more forceful contractions as the ventricular fibres are activated nearly simultaneously.
D.	True	This enhances the force of contraction at any given filling pressure.
E.	True	Due to the increased force of contraction.

87.

A.	False	It is low because the capillary bed has a large total cross-sectional area.
B.	True	The venous bed has a smaller total cross-sectional area than the venular bed.
C.	True	There is a brief period of retrograde flow as the aortic valve closes.
D.	True	Axial flow occurs in large vessels; near the walls, flow velocity is zero.
E.	False	It rises due to the compensatory increase in cardiac output.

88.

A.	True	As seen in the Frank–Starling left ventricular function curve.
B.	False	High K^+ levels decrease cardiac contractility.
C.	False	Calcium channel blockers decrease cardiac contractility.
D.	True	Due to increased sympathetic drive to the ventricles and increased venous return.
E.	True	Initially by increased ventricular filling: later by ventricular hypertrophy.

89.

A.	True	Hence no blood leaves the ventricles.
B.	False	Pressure in the aorta falls as run-off of blood to the tissues continues.
C.	False	It rises as ventricular pressure causes the AV valves to bulge into the atria.
D.	True	The blood vessels are squeezed by the contracting myocardium.
E.	False	The greater force of contraction in the left ventricle gives a greater rate of rise of pressure.

90.

A.	False	The electrical event precedes the mechanical event.
B.	True	This electrical event corresponds with ventricular relaxation.
C.	False	It corresponds to the interval between atrial and ventricular depolarization due to delay of the impulse in the AV bundle.
D.	True	R indicates the beginning, and T the end, of the ventricular action potential.
E.	True	Due to the heart rate changes associated with respiratory sinus arrhythmia.

91.

A.	True	The output from the left and right ventricle is the same.
B.	True	It depends on what happens to stroke volume.
C.	True	Lying down normally increases the filling pressure of the heart.
D.	True	To meet the needs of increased metabolism and increased skin blood flow.
E.	False	The output does increase due to changes in the filling pressure, level of circulating hormones, etc.

Questions 92–97

92. Arterioles
A. Have a smaller wall:lumen ratio than have arteries.
B. Play a major role in regulating arterial blood pressure.
C. Play a major role in regulating local blood flow.
D. Offer more resistance to flow than capillaries.
E. Have a larger total cross-sectional area than do the capillaries.

93. The Purkinje tissue cells in the heart
A. Conduct impulses faster than some neurones.
B. Are larger than ventricular myocardial cells.
C. Lead to contraction of the base before the apex of the heart.
D. Are responsible for the short duration of the QRS complex.
E. Are responsible for the configuration of the QRS complex.

94. In the brachial artery
A. Pulse waves travel at the same velocity as blood.
B. Pulse pressure falls with decreasing elasticity of the wall.
C. Pressure rises markedly when the artery is occluded distally.
D. Pressure falls when the arm is raised above head level.
E. Pulse pressures have a smaller amplitude than aortic pulse pressures.

95. The tendency for blood flow to be turbulent increases when there is a decrease in blood
A. Vessel diameter.
B. Density.
C. Flow velocity.
D. Viscosity.
E. Haemoglobin level.

96. Arterioles offer more resistance to flow than other vessels since they have
A. Thicker muscular walls.
B. Richer sympathetic innervation.
C. Smaller internal diameters.
D. A smaller total cross-sectional area.
E. A greater pressure drop along their length.

97. In the denervated heart, left ventricular stroke work increases when
A. The end-diastolic length of the ventricular fibres increases.
B. Peripheral resistance rises.
C. Blood volume falls.
D. Right ventricular output increases.
E. The veins constrict.

Answers

92.

A. False   In arterioles the ratio is much greater, at about 1:1.
B. True   They provide most of the peripheral resistance.
C. True   Local flow varies directly with the fourth power of their radii.
D. True   The drop in pressure across arterioles is greater than that across capillaries.
E. False   It is smaller, so blood flow velocity is higher in arterioles.

93.

A. True   They conduct at around 4 metres/second. Small diameter nerve fibres conduct impulses at about 1 metre per second.
B. True   This facilitates rapid conduction.
C. False   Purkinje fibres travel to the apex before proceeding to the base of the heart.
D. True   They spread depolarization rapidly over the entire ventricular myocardium.
E. True   Damage to the cells (as in bundle-branch block) changes the pattern of spread of ventricular depolarization, and hence the shape of the QRS complex.

94.

A. False   Pulse waves travel at about ten times the blood velocity.
B. False   It rises; arterial elasticity normally damps the pulse pressure.
C. False   Blood flows off rapidly via collaterals so that little pressure change occurs.
D. True   By the hydrostatic equivalent of the column of blood between it and the heart.
E. False   Brachial arterial pulse pressures are greater due to the superimposition of waves reflected from the end of the arterial tree.

95.

A. False   The tendency is directly proportional to vessel diameter.
B. False   The tendency is directly proportional to fluid density.
C. False   The tendency is directly proportional to velocity.
D. True   The tendency is inversely proportional to viscosity.
E. True   In anaemia, the increase in velocity and decrease in viscosity of blood in the hyperdynamic circulation promote turbulence; bruits may be heard over peripheral arteries.

96.

A. False   Wall thickness is not a factor determining resistance.
B. False   But it suggests that the resistance they offer may be varied by change in nerve activity.
C. False   Capillaries have even smaller internal diameters.
D. False   The aorta has a much smaller *total* cross-sectional area.
E. True   The pressure drop across the arteriolar bed is larger than in other beds indicating that arterioles are responsible for most of the circulation's vascular resistance.

97.

A. True   As stated in the Frank–Starling Law.
B. True   This impedes ventricular outflow, thus increasing end-diastolic fibre length.
C. False   This reduces cardiac filling pressure and hence end-diastolic fibre length.
D. True   This tends to increase left ventricular filling pressure and end-diastolic fibre length.
E. True   This also raises cardiac filling pressure.

Questions 98–103

98. With increasing distance from the heart, arterial

A. Walls contain relatively more smooth muscle than elastic tissue.
B. Flow has a greater tendency to be turbulent.
C. Mean pressure tends to rise slightly.
D. Pulse pressure tends to increase slightly.
E. P_{O_2} falls appreciably.

99. In the estimation of cardiac output by an indicator dilution technique, the

A. Indicator must mix evenly with the entire blood volume.
B. Primary dilution curve may be followed by a secondary rise in indicator concentration.
C. Duration of the dilution curve shortens as cardiac output rises.
D. Mean indicator concentration under the curve increases as cardiac output rises.
E. Injection and monitoring devices may be placed in the pulmonary artery.

100. In the estimation of cardiac output using the Fick principle

A. Pulmonary blood flow is measured.
B. The P_{O_2} of arterial and mixed venous blood are measured.
C. Oxygen uptake is estimated from alveolar P_{O_2} measurements.
D. Pulmonary arterial blood is sampled to measure the oxygen in mixed venous blood.
E. Pulmonary venous blood is sampled to measure the oxygen in arterial blood.

101. Intravenous infusions of adrenaline and noradrenaline have similar effects on

A. Skeletal muscle blood flow.
B. Renal blood flow.
C. Skin blood flow.
D. Diastolic arterial pressure.
E. Heart rate.

102. When the heart suddenly stops beating (cardiac asystole)

A. The physical signs are similar to those of ventricular fibrillation.
B. Consciousness is lost after 1–2 minutes.
C. Cardiac compression should be applied at a rate of 10–15 per minute.
D. Artificial ventilation of the lungs should be given.
E. Electric shocks across the thorax should be applied.

103. Vasovagal fainting or syncope

A. Causes loss of consciousness.
B. Is associated with tachycardia.
C. Is associated with skeletal muscle vasodilation.
D. Is more likely to occur when standing than when lying down.
E. Is more likely to occur in a cold than in a hot environment.

MCQ

Answers

98.

A.	True	The relative amount of smooth muscle increases but that of elastic tissue falls.
B.	False	With the decreasing vessel diameter and flow velocity, the tendency decreases.
B.	False	It falls slightly; blood will only flow down a pressure gradient.
C.	True	Distal arterial pulse pressure is increased by the superimposition of waves reflected back from the end of the arterial tree.
E.	False	Blood cannot release its oxygen until it reaches the exchange vessels.

99.

A.	False	Complete mixing with the blood is required for estimation of blood volume.
B.	True	The secondary peak is due to recirculation of indicator.
C.	True	Due to the more rapid passage of indicator past the sampling site.
D.	False	It falls as the indicator is diluted in a bigger volume.
E.	True	Pulmonary artery blood flow equals cardiac output.

100.

A.	True	Pulmonary blood flow = right ventricular output = cardiac output.
B.	False	The O_2 content of arterial and mixed venous blood are measured.
C.	False	To measure O_2 consumption, the subject breathes from a spirometer filled with oxygen with a CO_2 absorber in the circuit; an open circuit method may also be used.
D.	True	The pulmonary artery is relatively easy to catheterize and the venous blood it contains is thoroughly mixed.
E.	False	Pulmonary veins are difficult to catheterize. Blood from any artery may be used since the O_2 content of peripheral arterial blood is the same as that in the pulmonary vein.

101.

A.	False	Adrenaline increases, and noradrenaline reduces skeletal muscle blood flow.
B.	True	Both decrease renal blood flow.
C.	True	Both cause cutaneous vasoconstriction.
D.	False	Noradrenaline raises diastolic pressure; adrenaline lowers it.
E.	False	Adrenaline increases heart rate; noradrenaline raises mean arterial pressure and causes reflex cardiac slowing.

102.

A.	True	In both cases there is no useful cardiac output.
B.	False	Consciousness is lost within about five seconds.
C.	False	60–80 compressions/minute are needed to maintain flow to the brain.
D.	True	This is needed to maintain oxygenation of the brain.
E.	False	This treatment (applied with a defibrillator) is given for ventricular fibrillation.

103.

A.	True	Due to cerebral ischaemia caused by the abrupt fall in arterial pressure.
B.	False	Increased vagal activity slows the heart and reduces cardiac output.
C.	True	This vasodilation reduces peripheral resistance.
D.	True	Because of gravity, pressure in cerebral arteries is lower when standing than when lying down.
E.	False	The skin vasoconstriction in cold environments raises peripheral resistance.

Questions 104–109

104. Systemic hypertension may be caused by
A. Hypoxia due to chronic respiratory failure.
B. Excessive secretion of aldosterone.
C. Excessive secretion of adrenocorticotrophic hormone (ACTH).
D. Myocardial thickening (hypertrophy) of the left ventricle.
E. The rapid cardiac action of ventricular fibrillation.

105. Peripheral differs from central circulatory failure in that
A. Hypovolaemia is unusual.
B. It leads to underperfusion of the tissues.
C. Cardiac output is usually normal.
D. Central venous pressure is low.
E. Ventricular function is usually normal.

106. In atrial fibrillation
A. The electrocardiogram shows no evidence of atrial activity.
B. Ventricular rate is lower than atrial rate.
C. Respiratory sinus arrhythmia can usually be seen.
D. The ventricular rate is irregular.
E. The QRS complexes have an abnormal configuration.

107. Severe systemic hypertension may result in
A. An increase in the number of myocardial cells in the left ventricle.
B. Increased QRS voltage in certain leads.
C. Increased coronary blood flow.
D. Pulmonary oedema.
E. Impaired vision.

108. Auscultation of the heart can provide evidence of
A. The direction of turbulent flow causing a murmur.
B. Aortic stenosis, if there is a loud pre-systolic murmur in the aortic valve area.
C. Mitral incompetence, if a systolic murmur is heard in the axilla.
D. Ventricular septal defect, if a loud diastolic murmur is heard.
E. Mitral stenosis, if an early diastolic and pre-systolic murmurs are heard.

109. The electrocardiogram shows
A. Irregular P waves in atrial flutter.
B. Regular QRS complexes in atrial fibrillation.
C. Regular QRS complexes in complete heart block.
D. High voltage R waves over the right ventricle in right ventricular hypertrophy.
E. An irregular saw-tooth appearance in ventricular fibrillation.

MCQ

Answers

104.

A.	False	This constricts blood vessels in the lungs causing pulmonary hypertension but dilates systemic vessels.
B.	True	Salt and water retention by the kidneys expands ECF and hence blood volume and cardiac output.
C.	True	The resulting secretion of cortisol also causes salt and water retention.
D.	False	This is a consequence of hypertension, not a cause.
E.	False	This ineffective pumping in ventricular fibrillation causes severe hypotension.

105.

A.	False	Hypovolaemia due to severe haemorrhage is a common cause of peripheral circulatory failure; blood volume may be normal in central circulatory failure.
B.	False	Both types of failure lead to underperfusion of the tissues.
C.	False	It is usually reduced in both types of failure.
D.	True	It is usually raised in central circulatory failure.
E.	True	Reduced ventricular function is the cause of central circulatory failure.

106.

A.	False	Small rapid waves indicate the atrial fibrillation.
B.	True	Atrial rate is higher than ventricular rate as some impulses are filtered out by the atrioventricular node.
C.	False	Sinus arrhythmia indicates normal sinus rhythm.
D.	True	Due to the irregularity of the impulses passing through the AV node.
E.	False	QRS complexes are normal since the pattern of ventricular depolarization is normal.

107.

A.	False	The cells increase in size (*hypertrophy*), not in number (*hyperplasia*).
B.	True	Due to the left ventricular hypertrophy.
C.	True	Due to increased left ventricular work.
D.	True	Due to left ventricular failure.
E.	True	Due to damage to retinal blood vessels.

108.

A.	True	The direction in which the murmur is conducted indicates the direction of flow.
B.	False	The characteristic murmur is a systolic murmur conducted to the neck vessels.
C.	True	This is the direction of flow of the regurgitant blood.
D.	False	The murmur occurs during ventricular contraction and is therefore systolic.
E.	True	Mitral flow is greatest in early diastole but rises again during atrial systole.

109.

A.	False	In atrial flutter, P waves have a high but regular frequency (about 300/minute).
B.	False	Ventricular beats are irregular in rate and strength since impulses pass through the AV node in a random fashion.
C.	True	The beats generated by ventricular pacemakers have slow but regular frequency.
D.	True	The increased muscle bulk generates enhanced voltages during depolarization.
E.	True	Due to chaotic electrical activity in the ventricles.

Questions 110–115

110. The jugular venous
A. Pulse is not visible in normal healthy people.
B. Pulse has greater amplitude in patients with tricuspid incompetence.
C. Pulse can vary widely in amplitude in patients with complete heart block.
D. Pressure is raised in patients with right ventricular failure.
E. Pressure is commonly raised in patients with mediastinal tumours.

111. In heart failure
A. The resting cardiac output may be higher than normal.
B. The arteriovenous oxygen difference during exercise is less than in normal people.
C. There is sodium retention.
D. Oedema occurs in dependent parts of the body.
E. Pulmonary oedema occurs when pulmonary capillary pressure doubles.

112. Respiratory failure (low arterial P_{O_2}; raised arterial P_{CO_2}) leads to
A. Raised pulmonary artery pressure (pulmonary hypertension).
B. Right ventricular failure.
C. Low voltage P waves in the electrocardiogram.
D. Decreased cerebral blood flow.
E. Warm hands and feet.

113. Pain due to poor coronary blood flow (angina) may be relieved by
A. Cutting the sympathetic nerve trunks supplying the heart.
B. Correcting anaemia if present.
C. Providing the patient with a cold environment.
D. β-adrenoceptor stimulating drugs.
E. Drugs causing peripheral vasodilation.

114. Narrowing of the lumen of major arteries supplying the leg is associated with
A. Pain in the calf during exercise which is relieved by rest.
B. Growth of collateral vessels.
C. Reduction in the duration of reactive hyperaemias in the calf.
D. Delayed healing of cuts in leg skin.
E. Reduced arterial pulse amplitude at the ankle.

115. Arterial pulse contours that have
A. Sharp peaks indicate rapid left ventricular ejection.
B. Greatly increased pulse pressures are seen in patients with mitral incompetence.
C. Slowly rising systolic phases are seen in patients with aortic stenosis.
D. Varying beat-to-beat amplitude is seen in patients with atrial fibrillation.
E. Rapid run-offs and low diastolic pressure suggest high peripheral resistance.

Answers

110.
A.   False   It can be seen in healthy people when they lie almost flat.
B.   True   Systolic regurgitation of right ventricular blood can cause giant waves.
C.   True   Periodic giant waves are seen when atrial and ventricular systoles coincide.
D.   True   This is an important sign in right ventricular failure; venous pulsation is present.
E.   True   The jugular veins are distended due to venous obstruction but there is little or no pulsation.

111.
A.   True   In high output failures; however, the ability to raise cardiac output in exercise is impaired in all types of failure.
B.   False   With inadequate output, desaturation of blood in the tissues increases.
C.   True   This increases extracellular fluid and hence blood volume.
D.   True   The back pressure in veins raises capillary hydrostatic pressure and results in oedema in dependent parts where venous pressure is already raised due to gravity.
E.   False   When pulmonary capillary pressure (about 5 mmHg) doubles, it is still less than plasma oncotic pressure (25 mmHg) so fluid does not accumulate in the alveoli.

112.
A.   True   Hypoxia causes generalized pulmonary vasoconstriction.
B.   True   Pulmonary hypertension can lead to right ventricular failure ('cor pulmonale').
C.   False   Atrial hypertrophy in cor pulmonale results in prominent P waves.
D.   False CO_2 dilates cerebral blood vessels.
E.   True CO_2 is a vasodilator and 'cor pulmonale' is a 'high output' failure.

113.
A.   True   Pain sensory fibres from the heart travel with the sympathetic nerves.
B.   True   In anaemia, the capacity of the blood to deliver oxygen is decreased but cardiac work increases due to the rise in cardiac output.
C.   False   Cold vasoconstriction raises arterial pressure and so increases myocardial work.
D.   False   These increase heart rate and force and so increase myocardial work
E.   True   By reducing arterial pressure, vasodilator drugs such as nitrates reduce myocardial work.

114.
A.   True   This is 'intermittent claudication'; pain metabolites accumulate in muscle during exercise in ischaemic limbs and stimulate local pain receptors.
B.   True   When the major arteries are obstructed, collateral vessels open up to help maintain blood flow to the ischaemic tissues.
C.   False   Though the hyperaemias have smaller peak values, their durations are longer.
D.   True   Cuts and ulcers are slow to heal because the supply of nutrients is impaired.
E.   True   Pulses may be absent with severe narrowing.

115.
A.   True   As seen in strenuous exercise.
B.   False   This is typical of aortic incompetence.
C.   True   Due to slow expulsion of blood from the ventricle past the stenosed valve.
D.   True   The variable filling of the ventricle results in variable stroke output.
E.   False   They suggest a low peripheral resistance.

Questions 116–120

116. Murmurs (or bruits) may be detected by auscultation over

A. Vessels in which there is turbulence.
B. Large arteries in healthy adults.
C. Dilations (aneurysms) in arteries.
D. Constrictions (stenoses) in arteries.
E. The heart in healthy young adults in early diastole.

117. Factors ensuring that ventricular muscle has an adequate oxygen supply include the

A. Good functional anastomoses that exist between adjacent coronary arteries.
B. Structural arrangements that prevent vascular compression during systole.
C. High oxygen extraction rate from blood circulating through the myocardium.
D. Sympathetic vasodilator nerve supply to ventricular muscle.
E. Fall in coronary vascular resistance during exercise.

118. When the AV bundle is completely interrupted, as in complete heart block, the

A. Atrial beat becomes irregular.
B. PR interval shows beat-to-beat variability.
C. Ventricular filling shows beat-to-beat variability.
D. QRS complex shows beat-to-beat variability.
E. Ventricular rate falls below 50 beats/minute.

119. Aortic valve incompetence may cause

A. Increase in arterial pulse pressure.
B. Systolic murmurs in the aortic valve area.
C. Hypertrophy of left ventricular muscle.
D. Decreased myocardial blood flow.
E. Left ventricular failure.

120. Ventricular extrasystoles

A. Are usually associated with a normal QRS complex.
B. From the same focus have similar QRS complexes.
C. Usually occur following a compensatory pause.
D. May fail to produce a pulse at the wrist.
E. Indicate serious heart disease.

Answers

116.

A.	True	Turbulent vibrations generate sound waves.
B.	False	Flow is laminar rather than turbulent in normal large arteries.
C.	True	Turbulence is set up as blood flows into the dilated segment.
D.	True	Turbulence is set up as blood squirts through the constricted segment.
E.	True	Rapid ventricular filling in early diastole can cause turbulence in healthy young adults and generate a sound (the third heart sound).

117.

A.	False	Coronary arteries are functional 'end arteries' and have few anastomotic connections; sudden occlusion of an artery usually leads to local muscle death.
B.	False	Coronary vessels are compressed by the contracting myocardium in systole.
C.	True	The extraction rate is about 75 per cent.
D.	False	Reflex vasodilatation is not important in regulating coronary blood flow.
E.	True	The rise in metabolic activity in the exercising heart provides the vasodilator metabolites which adapt coronary flow to supply myocardial oxygen needs.

118.

A.	False	The atria continue to beat regularly at normal sinus rate.
B.	True	In complete block, atria and ventricles beat independently at different rates.
C.	True	Due to loss of the normal sequence of the atrial and ventricular contractions.
D.	False	There is usually a single ventricular pacemaker giving an abnormal but regular QRS complex.
E.	True	The ventricular intrinsic rate of beating is 30–40/minute.

119.

A.	True	Diastolic pressure is abnormally low due to regurgitation of aortic blood into the left ventricle in diastole.
B.	False	Blood regurgitating in diastole causes diastolic turbulence.
C.	True	The greater stroke volume needed to compensate for regurgitating blood increases ventricular workload.
D.	False	Flow increases as ventricular work increases.
E.	True	A persistent increase in ventricular workload can lead to ventricular failure.

120.

A.	False	Extrasystoles are associated with a prolonged abnormal QRS complex; the impulse pathway from the ectopic focus over the myocardium is abnormal and slow.
B.	True	If the focus is the same, the pathway for ventricular excitation will be the same.
C.	False	They are followed by a compensatory pause; the next normal beat may reach the ventricles when they are refractory – a beat is lost.
D.	True	If they occur early in diastole, poor ventricular filling results in weak contractions and small pulses.
E.	False	They occur occasionally in many normal hearts.

Questions 121–126

121. Pulmonary embolism (blood clots impacting in lung blood vessels) usually decreases
A. Pulmonary vascular resistance.
B. Left atrial pressure.
C. Right atrial pressure.
D. Ventilation to perfusion ratios in the affected lung.
E. P_{O_2} in pulmonary venous blood.

122. Hardening of the arterial walls tends to raise
A. Arterial compliance.
B. Systolic arterial pressure.
C. Diastolic arterial pressure.
D. Peripheral resistance.
E. Arterial pulse wave velocity.

123. The 'A' wave of venous pulsation in the neck is
A. Caused by atrial systole.
B. Seen just after the carotid artery pulse.
C. Exaggerated in atrial fibrillation.
D. Exaggerated in tricuspid stenosis.
E. Exaggerated periodically in complete heart block.

124. Left ventricular failure tends to cause an increase in
A. Left atrial pressure.
B. Left ventricular ejection fraction.
C. Pulmonary capillary pressure.
D. Lung compliance.
E. Pulmonary oedema when the patient stands up.

125. In otherwise healthy people, local tissue death follows obstruction of
A. An internal carotid artery.
B. A renal artery.
C. A femoral artery.
D. A retinal artery.
E. The hepatic portal vein.

126. In the measurement of forearm blood flow by venous occlusion plethysmography
A. A continuous record is made of forearm volume.
B. A collecting cuff is applied to the wrist.
C. It is assumed that venous outflow is arrested by the collecting cuff during measurement.
D. The collecting cuff pressure should be greater than diastolic but less than systolic arterial pressure.
E. The forearm must be kept below heart level during the measurements.

Answers

121.

A. False Vascular obstruction tends to increase pulmonary vascular resistance and cause pulmonary hypertension.
B. True   Due to the fall in pulmonary blood flow, atrial pressure tends to fall.
C. False The obstruction tends to dam back blood in the right heart.
D. False It rises since pulmonary capillary perfusion falls.
E. False Blood that traverses pulmonary capillaries is adequately oxygenated; cyanosis in patients with pulmonary embolism is usually peripheral cyanosis due to low cardiac output.

122.

A. False Compliance, the change of arterial volume per unit pressure change, decreases.
B. True   Systolic ejection causes greater pressure rise when arteries are less distensible.
C. False Poor elastic recoil in diastole allows diastolic pressure to fall further.
D. False Stiffness of the wall is not a factor determining vascular resistance.
E. True   Vibrations travel faster in stiff than in lax structures.

123.

A. True   The pressure wave due to atrial contraction passes up freely into the neck.
B. False Atrial systole precedes the ventricular systole that generates the carotid pulse.
C. False It is absent – there is no effective atrial systole in atrial fibrillation.
D. True   Right atrial contraction is more forceful to overcome valvular resistance.
E. True   If the atrial and ventricular systoles coincide, the A and C waves merge to give a giant wave.

124.

A. True   Due to inadequate emptying of the left ventricle in systole.
B. False Stroke volume falls; end-diastolic volume rises.
C. True   The rise may cause pulmonary oedema if pressure exceeds the colloid osmotic pressure of the plasma proteins.
D. False It falls; congestion of pulmonary vessels with blood makes the lungs stiffer.
E. False The decrease in venous return on standing up may relieve pulmonary congestion and hence dyspnoea.

125.

A. False Flow through the circle of Willis normally maintains the viability of the tissue.
B. True   There is no significant collateral circulation.
C. False Normally there is adequate collateral circulation. However, if there is advanced arterial disease, sudden obstruction may cause gangrene.
D. True   The collateral circulation is not good enough to prevent this.
E. False The liver has a dual blood supply; the hepatic artery flow can maintain viability.

126.

A. True   Plethysmography means volume measurement.
B. False It is applied to the upper arm.
C. True   When this is the case, the volume increase equals arterial inflow.
D. False It must be below diastolic so as not to interfere with arterial inflow.
E. False Below heart level, the veins fill with blood and are unable to accommodate more during venous occlusion; the forearm must be above heart level.

EMQs

Questions 127–138

EMQ Question 127

For each of the clinical descriptions (A–E) select the most appropriate options from the following list of circulatory changes.

1. Increased cerebral vascular resistance.	2. Decreased cerebral vascular resistance.
3. Increased coronary resistance.	4. Decreased coronary resistance.
5. Increased splanchnic resistance.	6. Decreased splanchnic resistance.
7. Increased vascular resistance in skin.	8. Decreased vascular resistance in skin.
9. Increased renal vascular resistance.	10. Decreased renal vascular resistance.
11. Increased regional perfusion pressure.	12. Decreased regional perfusion pressure.

A.   A patient with a head injury receives artificial hyperventilation to reduce cerebral oedema.

B.   It has been found that gastric mucosal intracellular acidosis as an indicator of local stagnant hypoxia is useful in assessing splanchnic blood flow in peripheral circulatory failure.

C.   Patients with myocardial infarction show electrocardiological improvement after treatment to convert plasminogen into plasmin within six hours of heart attack.

D.   A patient suffering from chronic respiratory failure with carbon dioxide retention has headaches and is found to have papilloedema.

E.   An elderly patient suffering from diarrhoea and vomiting for several days cannot sit or stand without developing loss of consciousness (syncope).

Answers for 127

A. **Option 1**   *Increased cerebral vascular resistance.* Hyperventilation leads to constriction of cerebral vessels due to washout of carbon dioxide from the body. This leads to decreased cerebral capillary pressure and a reduction in cerebral interstitial fluid volume, thereby reducing the oedema generated by head injury.

B. **Option 5**   *Increased splanchnic resistance.* In circulatory failure, blood pressure is supported by increased peripheral vascular resistance induced by the baroreceptor reflex, particularly in the splanchnic circulation. Splanchnic vasoconstriction occurs early in the condition. The resultant stagnant hypoxia in the alimentary mucosa is thus a sensitive index of the early stages of circulatory failure before more severe effects such as hypotension are obvious.

C. **Option 4**   *Decreased coronary resistance.* Myocardial infarction results from complete or almost complete cessation of perfusion of a region of cardiac muscle due to blocking, often by thrombosis, of a coronary artery or arteries. This reduces flow by a massive increase in resistance and a considerable mass of myocardium is threatened by stagnant hypoxia due to poor flow (ischaemia). Activation of circulating plasminogen to plasmin allows breakdown of blood clot (thrombolysis) and decreases regional coronary resistance to a level which allows recovery of ischaemic areas.

D. **Option 2**   *Decreased cerebral vascular resistance.* Carbon dioxide is an important determinant of cerebral blood flow by its local vasodilator action (in underperfused areas carbon dioxide accumulates and this leads to vasodilation and restoration of normal perfusion). When there is a raised level of carbon dioxide in arterial blood there is generalized cerebral vasodilation and this leads to increased formation of tissue fluid (oedema). The resultant increased intracranial pressure leads to headaches and papilloedema, imitating the effects of an intracranial tumour or abscess.

E. **Option 12**   *Decreased regional perfusion pressure.* With persistent diarrhoea and vomiting, extracellular fluid volume can fall severely. The reduced plasma volume leads to hypotension, especially in the elderly whose compensatory mechanisms are blunted. Sitting and standing trap circulating fluid in the feet causing a severe fall in arterial blood pressure. This decreases cerebral perfusion pressure to a point at which a local decrease in vascular resistance cannot compensate and loss of consciousness (syncope) occurs from cerebral ischaemia (inadequate blood flow).

EMQ Question 128

For each of the clinical scenarios A–E, select the most appropriate option from the cardiovascular parameters listed below.

	Heart rate (per min)	Stroke volume (ml)	Pulse pressure (mmHg)
1.	60	80	40
2.	120	35	20
3.	180	110	110
4.	40	140	50
5.	100	70	70
6.	240	15	15

A. A 30-year-old man has been admitted to hospital for minor elective surgery. He is a long-distance runner of national standard. His cardiac shadow is enlarged on chest X-ray and there is concern about his very slow pulse.

B. A 50-year-old woman has been admitted to hospital for thyroid surgery and is found to have signs of severe uncontrolled hyperthyroidism. Her peripheries are warm and moist and her pulse is rapid and bounding.

C. A 40-year-old woman trains regularly for physical fitness but has been concerned recently about chest discomfort, fearing coronary artery disease. She undertakes cardiological assessment during progressive exercise on a treadmill and the results correspond to the final stage of severity, rarely reached by the patients assessed. At this stage her systolic arterial pressure was 180 mmHg.

D. A 40-year-old woman reports recent episodes of threatened loss of consciousness during exercise and such an episode occurs during treadmill testing in hospital.

E. A 70-year-old man has been admitted to hospital after he collapsed at home and found he could not sit up without feeling he was about to faint. He suffers from epigastric pain treated by a proton pump inhibitor and has recently noticed his bowel motions are loose and very dark. On admission he is pale and sweating with cold peripheries and his systolic arterial pressure is 80 mmHg even with the foot of the bed raised.

Answers for 128

A. **Option 4**   These results are typical of a high level athlete – a normal resting cardiac output of 5.6 litres per minute with a very slow pulse rate compensating for a huge resting stroke volume. Such people have relatively large powerful hearts which contrast dramatically with the large weak hearts of patients with cardiac failure, some of whom may suffer from a pathologically slow heart rate which exacerbates their condition.

B. **Option 5**   Hyperthyroidism leads to a hyperdynamic circulation at rest – rapid strong pulse associated with a high pulse pressure and an increased cardiac output (7 litres per minute in her case). This is required for the increased metabolic rate due to the overactive thyroid. The increased metabolic rate also generates excess heat, hence the sweating.

C. **Option 3**   This woman is typical of patients with chest pain not due to coronary artery disease. In association with regular training she is very fit and can exercise to the maximal level used in the treadmill cardiac stress test. At this stage she shows typical findings of a cardiac output of about 20 litres per minute and arterial blood pressure 180/70 (high systolic due to powerful ejection by the left ventricle and rapidly falling pressure due to very low peripheral resistance). She has achieved the maximal predicted heart rate (220 minus age in years).

D. **Option 6**   Syncope or pre-syncope during exercise can be due to an abnormal ineffective rapid cardiac rhythm (tachycardia). As with the previous case the maximal expected rate is 180 and a rate of 240 does not allow adequate filling for a useful stroke volume. Such a low cardiac output (3.6 litres per minute) would lead to loss of consciousness during mild to moderate exercise.

E. **Option 2**   This patient gives a history suggesting peptic ulcer treated by a drug which raises gastric pH to relieve the pain. The history is strongly suggestive of chronic loss of blood in the faeces (melaena). With an arterial blood pressure of 80/60 he cannot sustain adequate cerebral blood flow in the upright posture. This is because of the reduced venous return experienced by everyone in the upright position. Raising the foot of the bed maximizes venous return. He is suffering from peripheral circulatory failure due to severe blood loss and blood transfusion is urgently indicated.

EMQ Question 129

For each of the physiological characteristics A–E, select the most appropriate option from the types of blood vessels listed below.

1. Veins.
2. Arteries.
3. Arterioles.
4. Venules.
5. Arteria-venous anastomoses.

A. The major source of peripheral resistance.
B. Are important in temperature regulation.
C. Their walls contain relatively more elastic tissue than other blood vessels.
D. Their valves prevent retrograde flow.
E. Have the greatest wall thickness to lumen ratio in blood vessels.

EMQ Question 130

For each of the valvular functions A–E, select the most appropriate option from the valves listed below.

1. Mitral valve
2. Tricuspid valve.
3. Aortic valve.
4. Foramen ovale valve.
5. Pulmonary valve.

A. Preventing regurgitation of right ventricle inflow.
B. Preventing regurgitation of left ventricular outflow.
C. Preventing regurgitation of left ventricular inflow.
D. Preventing regurgitation of right ventricular outflow.
E. Preventing flow from the left to the right atrium after birth.

EMQ Question 131

For each of the physiological responses A–E, select the most appropriate option from the effector mechanisms listed below.

1. Vasodilator metabolites.
2. Autoregulatory responses.
3. Vasodilator nerves.
4. Vasoconstrictor nerves
5. Endothelium derived relaxing factor (EDRF).

A. Minimizing blood flow changes in response to changes in perfusion pressure.
B. Increasing local blood flow by a decrease in their activity.
C. Release of noradrenaline.
D. Baroreceptor reflex responses.
E. Reactive hyperaemia responses.

Answers for 129

A. **Option 3**   *Arterioles.* Arterioles are the main source of peripheral resistance in the circulation since the fall in blood pressure across arteriolar vessels is greater than in any other vascular segment.

B. **Option 5**   *Arterio-venous anastomoses.* The AV anastomoses in the extremities such as the fingers and toes open up when body temperature rises and the resulting increase in blood flow raises skin temperature so that there is greater heat loss from the skin.

C. **Option 2**   *Arteries.* The arteries, especially those near the heart, are highly elastic. This tissue is stretched during systole and the energy so stored is fed back during diastole to maintain the diastolic pressure. Thus the elastic tissue dampens the large pressure gradients generated by the ventricles into the smaller pressure pulses seen in the arterial system.

D. **Option 1**   *Veins.* These valves aid return of blood to the heart. When veins are compressed by surrounding muscles or other organs, the valves do not allow retrograde flow of blood, the blood in the veins is forced forward towards the heart.

E. **Option 3**   *Arterioles.* The walls of arterioles are relatively thick relative to their lumen because of the comparatively high smooth muscle component. This muscle is controlled by vasoactive substances and vasomotor nerves to regulate local blood flow.

Answers for 130

A. **Option 2**   *Tricuspid valve.* This valve closes when right ventricular pressure exceeds right atrial pressure and so prevents regurgitation of blood into the atrium when the right ventricle contracts.

B. **Option 3**   This valve, situated in the mouth of the aorta, closes during diastole when aortic pressure exceeds left ventricular pressure. Incompetence of this valve allows reflux of blood from the aorta back into the ventricle and increases the work of the heart to maintain the same cardiac output.

C. **Option 1**   *Mitral valve.* This valve closes when left ventricular pressure exceeds left atrial pressure and so prevents regurgitation of blood into the atria when the ventricle contracts. When disease results in valve incompetence, a systolic murmur may be heard over the heart.

D. **Option 5**   *Pulmonary valve.* This valve, situated in the mouth of the pulmonary artery, closes during diastole when pulmonary artery pressure exceeds right ventricular pressure.

E. **Option 4**   *Foramen ovale valve.* This valve closes the foramen ovale in the inter-atrial septum when return of blood in the pulmonary veins raises left atrial pressure above right atrial pressure.

Answers for 131

A. **Option 2**   *Autoregulatory responses.* When the perfusion pressure rises, the stretching of the smooth muscle in the walls of blood vessels causes it to contract and so minimize the increase in blood flow that would otherwise occur.

B. **Option 4**   *Vasoconstrictor nerves.* These sympathetic nerves are normally active to exert a steady vasoconstrictor 'tone'. When their activity is decreased, the smooth muscle in the walls of the blood vessels relaxes to cause an increase in local blood flow.

C. **Option 4**   *Vasoconstrictor nerves.* The neurotransmitter for sympathetic vasoconstrictor nerves is noradrenaline

D. **Option 4**   *Vasoconstrictor nerves.* When arterial pressure falls, it is countered by a reflex increase in vasoconstrictor tone that raises peripheral resistance.

E. **Option 1**   *Vasodilator metabolites.* The increase in local blood flow after circulatory arrest (reactive hyperaemia) is due to the accumulation of products of metabolism causing vasodilation during the arrest period.

EMQ Question 132

For each of the reflex systems A–E, select the most appropriate option from the types of receptors listed below.

1. Arterial stretch receptors.
2. Arterial chemoreceptors.
3. Pulmonary stretch receptors.
4. Atrial stretch receptors.
5. Coronary artery chemoreceptors.

A. The reflex regulation of blood pressure.
B. The reflex regulation of ventilation.
C. The reflex regulation of blood volume.
D. System causing reflex hypotension, bradycardia and apnoea.
E. The Hering–Breuer reflex.

EMQ Question 133

For each of the physiological characteristics A–E, select the most appropriate option from the special circulations listed below.

1. Coronary blood flow.
2. Skeletal muscle blood flow.
3. Splanchnic blood flow.
4. Cerebral blood flow.
5. Skin blood flow.

A. Increases during sweating.
B. Greater during diastole than during systole.
C. Passes through a portal circulation.
D. Affected mainly by the P_{CO_2} level in the blood.
E. Increases during fainting.

EMQ Question 134

For each of the cardiac phenomena A–E, select the most appropriate option from the features of the electrocardiogram listed below.

1. The T wave.
2. The P wave.
3. The P–R interval.
4. Depression of the ST segment.
5. A flat record.

A. Cardiac arrest.
B. Repolarization of the ventricles.
C. Inadequate blood flow to ventricular muscle.
D. The delay in impulse conduction in the AV node.
E. Spread of the cardiac impulse over the atria.

EMQ Question 135

For each of the physiological changes A–E, select the most appropriate option from the possible precipitating causes listed below.

1. Fainting.
2. Severe haemorrhage.
3. Severe exercise.
4. Late pregnancy.
5. Hypothermia.
6. Lying down.

A. A fall in the haematocrit.
B. A decrease in heart rate.
C. A decrease in oxygen consumption.
D. A reduction in venous capacity.
E. An increased right atrial pressure.

Answers for 132

A. **Option 1** *Arterial stretch receptors.* Stretch of these receptors by a rise in blood pressure results in a reflex reduction in heart rate and vasoconstrictor tone to limit the rise in pressure.

B. **Option 2** *Arterial chemoreceptors.* A fall in P_{O_2} or pH or a rise in P_{CO_2} stimulates the arterial chemoreceptors to cause a reflex increase in pulmonary ventilation. The main stimulation effect of CO_2 on breathing is via the respiratory centre in the medulla oblongata but the stimulatory effect of hypoxia is via the arterial chemoreceptors only.

C. **Option 4** *Atrial stretch receptors.* Stretch of atrial stretch receptors results in a fall in blood pressure and an increase in urinary output.

D. **Option 5** *Coronary artery chemoreceptors.* C fibres close to the walls of coronary vessels are stimulated by certain circulating substances such as serotonin and veratridine, to cause hypotension, bradycardia and perhaps apnoea (the Bezold–Jarisch reflex).

E. **Option 3** *Pulmonary stretch receptors.* When pulmonary stretch receptors are stretched during inspiration, they send impulses to the brain via the vagus nerves that inhibit the inspiratory centre in the medulla oblongata.

Answers for 133

A. **Option 5** *Skin blood flow.* Skin blood flow increases during sweating due to an active sympathetic cholinergic mechanism.

B. **Option 1** *Coronary blood flow.* Coronary blood flow is decreased during systole because of compression of the vessels by the contracting ventricular myocardium.

C. **Option 3** *Splanchnic blood flow.* Splanchnic blood flow passes through two capillary beds in one circuit of the circulation, firstly through the capillaries in the alimentary tract and then through a portal capillary bed in the liver.

D. **Option 4** *Cerebral blood flow.* Cerebral blood flow is little affected by cardiovascular reflexes. However it is very sensitive to changes in the P_{CO_2} of the perfusing blood.

E. **Option 2** *Skeletal muscle blood flow.* Vasodilatation in skeletal muscle during fainting causes a large fall in peripheral resistance and is one of the factors leading to the fall in arterial pressure that results in the faint.

Answers for 134

A. **Option 5** *A flat record.* During asystole no ECG complexes can be detected.

B. **Option 1** *The T wave.* The T wave marks the end of the ventricular depolarization that gives rise to systole.

C. **Option 4** *Depression of the ST segment.* Depression of the ST segment is a sign of ischaemia during cardiac treadmill testing.

D. **Option 3** *The P–R interval.* This delay allows the atria to contract before the ventricles contract.

E. **Option 2** *The P wave.* Abnormalities in the P waves indicate atrial dysfunction.

Answers for 135

A. **Option 4** *Late pregnancy.* The relative increase in plasma volume in late pregnancy results in a low haematocrit.

B. **Option 1** *Fainting.* The vagal element of the vaso-vagal faint can cause severe bradycardia.

C. **Option 5** *Hypothermia.* The decrease in the metabolic rate in hypothermia reduces oxygen consumption.

D. **Option 2** *Severe haemorrhage.* The intense reflex venoconstriction in severe haemorrhage may make it difficult to insert catheters for introducing intravenous fluids.

E. **Option 6** *Lying down.* Due to the increase in venous return to the heart.

EMQ Question 136

For each of the features of the capillary circulation A–E, select the most appropriate option from the possible locations and precipitating causes listed below.

1. In the brain.
2. In Vitamin C deficiency.
3. In exercising muscle.
4. After haemorrhage.
5. In the spleen.

A. High permeability.
B. Low permeability.
C. High fragility.
D. Net outflow of fluid.
E. Net inflow of fluid.

EMQ Question 137

For each of the functional characteristics of heart muscle A–E, select the most appropriate option from the types of heart muscle listed below.

1. The sinoatrial node.
2. The Purkinje system.
3. The AV node.
4. Atrial muscle.
5. Ventricular muscle.

A. The fastest conduction rate in the heart.
B. The slowest conduction rate in the heart.
C. The fastest pacemaker in the heart.
D. Associated with the P wave of the electrocardiogram.
E. The longest action potentials.

EMQ Question 138

For each of the circulatory features A–E, select the most appropriate option from the special circulations listed below.

1. Hypothalamic circulation.
2. Coronary circulation.
3. Pulmonary circulation.
4. Fetal circulation.
5. Cerebral circulation.

A. A low-pressure circulation.
B. A portal capillary system.
C. Functional end arteries.
D. A ductus arteriosus.
E. An elaborate anastomotic system.

Answers for 136

A.   **Option 5**   *In the spleen.* Splenic capillaries, because of the large slits between adjacent endothelial cells, are freely permeable to most solutes.

B.   **Option 1**   *In the brain.* Because of the 'blood–brain barrier', cerebral capillaries are much less permeable than capillaries elsewhere in the body so that tissue fluid in the brain differs in composition from that of plasma.

C.   **Option 2**   *In Vitamin C deficiency.* Capillary (petechial) haemorrhages are a feature of scurvy caused by Vitamin C deficiency.

D.   **Option 3**   *In exercising muscle.* Because the arteriolar vasodilation raises capillary pressure.

E.   **Option 4**   *After haemorrhage.* Because arteriolar constriction decreased capillary pressure.

Answers for 137

A.   **Option 2**   *The Purkinje system.* The modified heart muscle fibres in the Purkinje system can conduct the impulse at about 8 metres/second.

B.   **Option 3**   *The AV node.* The slow conduction of the impulse through the AV node allows the atrial muscle to contract before ventricular contraction begins.

C.   **Option 1**   *The sinoatrial node.* The sinoatrial node normally generates impulse faster than any other cardiac pacemaker and so in responsible for the normal heart rate.

D.   **Option 4**   *Atrial muscle.* The P wave results from the spread of excitation from the sinoatrial node over the atria.

E.   **Option 5**   *The longest action potentials.* Ventricular muscle action potentials are much longer than those in atrial muscle.

Answers for 138

A.   **Option 3**   *Pulmonary circulation.* Pressure in the pulmonary circuit is much lower than that in the systemic circuit since it offers much less resistance to flow.

B.   **Option 1**   *Hypothalamic circulation.* The capillary bed in the hypothalamus is connected by blood vessels to a second capillary bed in the anterior pituitary gland. This allows hormones secreted in the hypothalamus to be carried to the pituitary where they lead to the release of certain pituitary gland hormones.

C.   **Option 2**   *Coronary circulation.* Coronary arteries, though they are connected by anastomotic vessels act as functional end arteries so that when one is blocked the ventricular muscle served by that artery dies.

D.   **Option 4**   *Fetal circulation.* During fetal life, blood returning from the placenta to the right atrium bypasses the pulmonary circuit by (i) passing through the foramen ovale; and (ii) being diverted from the proximal part of the pulmonary artery via the ductus arteriosus to the aorta.

D.   **Option 5**   *Cerebral circulation.* The circle of Willis is a vascular arrangement at the base of the brain into which all the main arteries to the brain connect so that if one artery should block, the brain can still be supplied by the other arteries in this anastomotic arrangement.

MCQs

Questions 139–144

139. In a person breathing normally at rest with an environmental temperature of 25°C, the partial pressure of

A. CO_2 in alveolar air is about twice that in room air.
B. Water vapour in alveolar air is less than half the alveolar P_{CO_2} level.
C. Water vapour in alveolar air is greater than that in room air even at 100 per cent humidity.
D. O_2 in expired air is greater than in alveolar air.
E. CO_2 in mixed venous blood is greater than in alveolar air.

140. As blood passes through systemic capillaries

A. pH rises.
B. HCO_3^- ions pass from red cells to plasma.
C. Cl^- ion concentration in red cells falls.
D. Its oxygen dissociation curve shifts to the right.
E. Its ability to deliver oxygen to the tissues is enhanced.

141. The respiratory centre

A. Is in the hypothalamus.
B. Sends impulses to inspiratory muscles during quiet breathing.
C. Sends impulses to expiratory muscles during quiet breathing.
D. Is involved in the swallowing reflex.
E. Is involved in the vomiting reflex.

142. The carotid bodies

A. Are stretch receptors in the walls of the internal carotid arteries.
B. Have a blood flow per unit volume similar to that in the brain.
C. Are influenced more by blood P_{O_2} than by its oxygen content.
D. Generate more afferent impulses when blood H^+ ion concentration rises.
E. And the aortic bodies are mainly responsible for the increased ventilation in hypoxia.

143. Pulmonary surfactant increases

A. The surface tension of the fluid lining alveolar walls.
B. Lung compliance.
C. In effectiveness as the lungs are inflated.
D. In amount when pulmonary blood flow is interrupted.
E. In amount in fetal lungs during the last month of pregnancy.

144. As people age, there is usually a decrease in their

A. Ratio of lung residual volume to vital capacity.
B. Percentage of vital capacity expelled in one second.
C. Lung volume level at which small airways start to close during expiration.
D. Lung elasticity.
E. Resting arterial blood P_{O_2}.

Answers

139.

A.   False   Room air P_{CO_2} (0.2 mmHg; 0.03 kPa) is negligible compared with alveolar air P_{CO_2} (40 mmHg; 5.3 kPa).

B.   False   Alveolar H_2O vapour pressure at 37°C is 47 mmHg (6.3 kPa).

C.   True   Alveolar air is saturated with water vapour at 37˚C. At 25˚C saturated vapour pressure is 24 mmHg (3.2 kPa), about half that at 37˚C.

D.   True   Expired air is alveolar air plus dead space air.

E.   True   This is necessary for CO_2 excretion by diffusion.

140.

A.   False   It falls, due largely to CO_2 uptake.

B.   True   Incoming CO_2 is converted to HCO_3^- (carbonic anhydrase in RBCs catalyses the reaction $CO_2 + H_2O = H^+ + HCO_3^-$; HCO_3^- migrates out as its concentration rises.

C.   False   It rises as Cl^- moves in to replace departing HCO_3^- in the 'chloride shift'.

D.   True   Due largely to the rise in blood P_{CO_2}.

E.   True   Due to the shift of the oxygen dissociation curve.

141.

A.   False   It is in the medulla oblongata.

B.   True   Causing expansion of the thorax cage.

C.   False   Expiration at rest is passive.

D.   True   It is inhibited during swallowing so preventing aspiration of food.

E.   True   Expiratory, including abdominal muscle contraction with the oesophagus relaxed and the glottis closed helps expel gastric contents in vomiting.

142.

A.   False   The stretch receptors in internal carotid arteries are carotid sinus baroreceptors; the carotid bodies are separate structures nearby.

B.   False   They have the greatest flow rate/unit volume yet described in the body.

C.   True   They are not excited in anaemia where P_{CO_2} is normal but O_2 content is low.

D.   True   Acidosis stimulates ventilation.

E.   True   When carotid and aortic bodies are denervated, hypoxia depresses respiration.

143.

A.   False   It decreases surface tension.

B.   True   It permits the lungs to be more easily inflated.

C.   False   The decreasing effect as lungs inflate helps prevent overinflation.

D.   False   It decreases; this may lead to local collapse of the lung.

E.   True   Premature babies may have breathing problems due to surfactant deficiency.

144.

A.   False   Residual volume increases and vital capacity decreases.

B.   True   This gradually falls with normal ageing.

C.   False   The 'closing volume' increases with age.

D.   True   This increases residual and closing volumes.

E.   True   There is, however, little change in oxygen saturation.

Questions 145–151

145. During inspiration
A. Intrapleural pressure is lowest at mid inspiration.
B. Intrapulmonary pressure is lowest around mid-inspiration.
C. Intraoesophageal pressure is lowest at mid-inspiration.
D. The rate of air flow is greatest at end-inspiration.
E. The lung volume/intrapleural pressure relationship is the same as in expiration.

146. Carbon dioxide
A. Is carried as carboxyhaemoglobin on the haemoglobin molecule.
B. Uptake by the blood increases its oxygen-binding power.
C. Uptake by the blood leads to similar increases in H^+ and HCO_3^- ion concentrations.
D. Stimulates ventilation when breathed at a concentration of 20 per cent.
E. Content is greater than oxygen content in arterial blood.

147. In normal lungs
A. The rate of alveolar ventilation at rest exceeds the rate of alveolar capillary perfusion.
B. The ventilation/perfusion (V/P) ratio exceeds 1.0 during maximal exercise.
C. The V/P ratio is higher at the apex than at the base of the lungs when a person is standing.
D. Oxygen transfer can be explained by passive diffusion.
E. Dead space increases during inspiration.

148. Alveolar ventilation is increased by breathing
A. 21 per cent O_2 and 79 per cent N_2.
B. 17 per cent O_2 and 83 per cent N_2.
C. 2 per cent CO_2 and 98 per cent O_2.
D. 10 per cent CO_2 and 90 per cent O_2.
E. A gas mixture which raises arterial P_{CO_2} by 10 per cent.

149. Bronchial smooth muscle contracts in response to
A. Bronchial mucosal irritation.
B. Local beta adrenoceptor stimulation.
C. A fall in bronchial P_{CO_2}.
D. Inhalation of cold air.
E. Circulating noradrenaline.

150. In early inspiration there is a fall in
A. Intrapulmonary pressure.
B. Intrathoracic pressure.
C. Intra-abdominal pressure.
D. Dead space P_{O_2}.
E. Pressure in the superior vena cava.

151. Compliance of the lungs is greater
A. When they are expanded above their normal tidal volume range.
B. In adults than in infants.
C. Than the compliance of the lungs and thorax together.
D. When they are filled with normal saline than when they are filled with air.
E. In standing than in recumbent subjects.

Answers

145.

A. False   It is lowest at the end of inspiration.

B. True   After mid-inspiration, intrapulmonary pressure rises as air is drawn into the lungs.

C. False   Its pattern is similar to that of intrapleural pressure.

D. False   It is greatest at mid-inspiration; it depends on the mouth:alveoli pressure gradient.

E. False   Volume changes lag behind pressure changes to give a hysteresis loop.

146.

A. False   It is carried as carbaminohaemoglobin; carboxyhaemoglobin is the combination of haemoglobin with carbon monoxide.

B. False   It decreases as the oxygen dissociation curve is shifted to the right.

C. False HCO_3^- ions increase more; H^+ ions are largely buffered by haemoglobin.

D. False   Breathing 20 per cent CO_2 causes respiratory depression; stimulation of respiration by CO_2 is maximal when breathed at concentrations of around 5 per cent.

E. True CO_2 content in arterial blood is about 500 ml/l; O_2 content is about 200 ml/l.

147.

A. False   Alveolar ventilation at rest is about 4 l/min; perfusion is about 5 l/min.

B. True   In maximal exercise, alveolar ventilation may rise to about 80 l/min whereas alveolar perfusion (cardiac output) rises to about 25 l/min.

C. True   Perfusion decreases from base to apex; ventilation does also but to a lesser extent.

D. True   There is no evidence of O_2 secretion in the lungs.

E. True   The trachea and bronchi expand as the lungs expand.

148.

A. False   This is the normal composition of air.

B. False   The O_2 level must fall to around 15 per cent before breathing is stimulated.

C. True   The stimulating effect of high P_{CO_2} is little affected by high P_{O_2} levels.

D. False   This level of carbon dioxide depresses breathing.

E. True   This is enough to double the volume breathed per minute.

149.

A. True   Via a reflex with a parasympathetic efferent pathway.

B. False   This leads to relaxation.

C. True   This tends to limit local overventilation.

D. True   This is minimized normally by the warming of air in the upper airways.

E. False   This causes relaxation via beta receptors.

150.

A. True   This creates a pressure gradient between mouth and lungs.

B. True   Due to an increase in the dimensions of the thoracic cage.

C. False   It rises due to descent of the diaphragm.

D. False   It rises as inspired air replaces alveolar air.

E. True   It falls as intrathoracic pressure falls.

151.

A. False   Compliance is maximal in the tidal volume range.

B. True   Compliance is extremely small in infants.

C. True   It is nearly twice as great.

D. True   There are no surface tension forces to overcome in fluid-filled lungs.

E. True   Lungs are less stiff when their blood content falls.

Questions 152–158

152. At a high altitude where atmospheric pressure is halved, there is an increase in

A. Pulmonary ventilation.
B. Alveolar H_2O vapour pressure.
C. Arterial P_{O_2}.
D. Arterial pH.
E. Cerebral blood flow.

153. During inspiration

A. Venous return to the heart is increased.
B. More energy is expended than during expiration.
C. Lung expansion is assisted by surface tension forces in the alveoli.
D. Lung expansion begins when intrapleural pressure falls below atmospheric.
E. Lung expansion ends when intrapulmonary pressure falls to atmospheric.

154. The residual volume is

A. The gas remaining in the lungs at the end of a full expiration.
B. Greater on average in men than in women.
C. 3–4 litres on average in young adults.
D. Measured directly using a spirometer.
E. Smaller in old than in young people.

155. A rise in arterial P_{CO_2} leads to an increase in

A. Ventilation due to stimulation of peripheral chemoreceptors.
B. Ventilation due to stimulation of central chemoreceptors.
C. Arterial pressure.
D. Cerebral blood flow.
E. The plasma bicarbonate level.

156. Ventilation is increased during

A. Periods when cerebrospinal fluid pH is reduced.
B. Chronic renal failure.
C. Periods when plasma bicarbonate level is raised.
D. Deep sleep.
E. Exercise because of the ensuing fall in arterial P_{O_2}

157. Voluntarily hyperventilation increases the

A. Negative charge on the plasma proteins.
B. Level of ionized calcium in blood.
C. Alveolar P_{O_2} three-fold when ventilation is increased three-fold.
D. Arterial blood oxygen saturation by 10–15 per cent when ventilation is increased by 10–15 per cent.
E. The renal excretion of bicarbonate.

158. If the carotid and aortic chemoreceptors are denervated

A. Increasing alveolar P_{CO_2} by 25 per cent fails to stimulate ventilation.
B. Halving the alveolar P_{O_2} fails to stimulate ventilation.
C. The resting ventilation rate is depressed by more than 40 per cent.
D. Ventilation does not increase during exercise.
E. The ability to adapt to life at high altitude is impaired.

MCQ

Answers

152.
A. True   Due to stimulation of chemoreceptors by oxygen lack.
B. False This remains at the saturated pressure at body temperature.
C. False The fall in arterial P_{O_2} stimulates the carotid bodies to increase ventilation.
D. True   Hyperventilation causes respiratory alkalosis.
E. False The fall in P_{CO_2} causes cerebral vasoconstriction.

153.
A. True   By decreasing intrathoracic venous pressure.
B. True   Expiration is assisted by the elastic recoil of the lungs and thoracic cage.
C. False Surface tension is a force to be overcome in inspiration.
D. False Expansion begins when intrapulmonary pressure falls below atmospheric.
E. True   There is no pressure gradient at this point to drive air.

154.
A. True   This is its definition.
B. True   Men, on average, have bigger thoracic cages than women.
C. False It is around 1–1.5 litres
D. False Residual air cannot be exhaled; it is measured indirectly by a dilution technique.
E. False It increases with age since the elastic recoil of the lungs decreases with age.

155.
A. True   Via the carotid and aortic bodies.
B. True   The central effect predominates.
C. True   Reflex vasoconstriction and cardiac stimulation predominate over the direct vasodilator effects of CO_2.
D. True   The cerebral vessels are little affected by sympathetic reflexes so the direct vasodilator effect of CO_2 predominates.
E. True   To compensate for the respiratory acidosis.

156.
A. True CO_2 acts centrally by reducing the pH of CSF.
B. True   Because of the ensuing metabolic acidosis.
C. False The metabolic alkalosis depresses ventilation.
D. False Ventilation falls during deep sleep.
E. False Arterial P_{O_2} is well maintained in exercise.

157.
A. True   It makes it more negative by raising blood pH.
B. False It decreases as protein binding of calcium increases.
C. False Alveolar P_{O_2} cannot exceed the P_{O_2} of the air being breathed (160 mmHg, 21 kPa).
D. False The blood is normally almost fully saturated (95–98 per cent).
E. True   To compensate for the respiratory alkalosis.

158.
A. False Raised P_{CO_2} can still stimulate breathing by acting on central chemoreceptors.
B. True   In fact, hypoxia depresses ventilation by its action on the respiratory centre.
C. False Normal ventilation is driven mainly by the effect of CO_2 on central chemoreceptors.
D. False Central and other peripheral effects increase respiratory drive in exercise.
E. True   The individual is unable to increase ventilation in response to hypoxia.

Questions 159–165

159. Pulmonary
A. Arterial mean pressure is about one-sixth systemic mean arterial pressure.
B. Blood flow/minute is similar to systemic blood flow/minute.
C. Vascular resistance is about 50 per cent that of systemic vascular resistance.
D. Vascular capacity is similar to systemic vascular capacity.
E. Arterial pressure increases by about 50 per cent when cardiac output rises by 50 per cent.

160. Carbon dioxide is carried in the blood in
A. Combination with the haemoglobin molecule.
B. Combination with plasma proteins.
C. Physical solution in plasma.
D. Greater quantity in red blood cells than in plasma.
E. Greater quantity as HCO_3^- ions than as other forms.

161. A shift of the oxygen dissociation curve of blood to the right
A. Occurs in the pulmonary capillaries.
B. Occurs if blood temperature rises.
C. Favours oxygen delivery to the tissues.
D. Favours oxygen uptake from the lungs by alveolar capillary blood.
E. Increases the P_{50} (the P_{O_2} value giving 50 per cent blood oxygen saturation).

162. The work of breathing increases when
A. Lung compliance increases.
B. The subject exercises.
C. The rate of breathing increases even though the minute volume stays constant.
D. The subject lies down.
E. Functional residual capacity increases.

163. The compliance of the lungs and chest wall is
A. Expressed as volume change per unit change in pressure.
B. Minimal during quiet breathing.
C. Increased by the surface tension of the fluid lining the alveoli.
D. Increased by surfactant.
E. Changed by parallel displacement of the line relating lung volume to distending pressure.

164. Respiratory dead space
A. Saturates inspired air with water vapour before it reaches the alveoli.
B. Removes all particles from inspired air before it reaches the alveoli.
C. Decreases when blood catecholamine levels rise.
D. Decreases during a deep inspiration.
E. Decreases during a cough.

165. Vital capacity is
A. The volume of air expired from full inspiration to full expiration.
B. Reduced as one grows older.
C. Greater in men than in women of the same age and height.
D. Related more to total body mass than to lean body mass.
E. The sum of the inspiratory and expiratory reserve volumes.

Answers

159.
A. True   About 15 compared with 90 mmHg in the systemic circuit.
B. True   Otherwise blood would accumulate in one or other bed.
C. False From (A) and (B) above, it is only about 17 per cent of systemic resistance.
D. False Its capacity is about one-third of systemic capacity.
E. False Pulmonary vascular resistance falls when cardiac output rises, due possibly to endothelial release of nitric oxide.

160.
A. True   Attached to amino groups as carbaminohaemoglobin (Hb-NH.COOH).
B. True   Attached to amino groups as carbaminoprotein (Pr-NHCOOH).
C. True   It is the CO_2 in solution that exerts the P_{CO_2} and is diffusible.
D. False Plasma carries the greater quantity, mainly as bicarbonate.
E. True   Bicarbonate accounts for 80–90 per cent of the total CO_2 in blood.

161.
A. False It occurs in the systemic capillaries.
B. True   This occurs when tissue metabolic activity increases.
C. True   More oxygen is released at any given P_{O_2}.
D. False Less oxygen is taken up at any given P_{O_2}.
E. True   For example, a rise in temperature raises the P_{50}.

162.
A. False Compliant lungs are easier to inflate.
B. True   Since the rate and depth of ventilation are increased.
C. True   The work of breathing is minimal around the normal rate of breathing.
D. True   The increase in pulmonary blood volume increases lung stiffness and abdominal pressure on the diaphragm rises.
E. True   Lung compliance falls at higher lung volumes.

163.
A. True   The normal value is about 0.1 litre/cm H_2O (1 litre/kPa).
B. False It is maximal over this range of chest movement.
C. False The surface tension of alveolar fluid decreases compliance.
D. True   This decreases the surface tension.
E. False The slope of this line indicates compliance and is unchanged by a parallel shift.

164.
A. True   This prevents drying of the alveolar surface.
B. False Particles less than about two microns can reach the alveoli.
C. False Catecholamines relax airway muscle and constrict mucosal vessels.
D. False Expansion of the lungs expands airways as well as alveoli.
E. True   This allows air to be expelled at high airway velocity.

165.
A. True   This is how it is usually measured.
B. True   It falls on average by about a litre between age 20 and age 70.
C. True   By half to one litre.
D. False It is related closely to lean body mass.
E. False The tidal volume must be added.

Questions 166–171

166. In pulmonary capillary blood

A. Carbonic anhydrase in erythrocytes catalyses the formation of H^+ and HCO_3^-.
B. Hydrogen ions dissociate from haemoglobin.
C. The rise in P_{O_2} is of greater magnitude than the fall in P_{CO_2}.
D. The oxygen content is linearly related to alveolar P_{O_2}.
E. The pH is lower than in blood in the pulmonary artery.

167. Oxygen debt is

A. The amount of O_2 consumed after cessation of exercise.
B. Incurred because the pulmonary capillary walls limit O_2 uptake during exercise.
C. Possible since skeletal muscle can function temporarily without oxygen.
D. Associated with a rise in blood lactate.
E. Associated with metabolic acidosis.

168. The CO_2 dissociation curve for whole blood shows that

A. Its shape is sigmoid.
B. Blood saturates with CO_2 when P_{CO_2} exceeds normal alveolar levels.
C. Blood contains some CO_2 even when the P_{CO_2} is zero.
D. Oxygenation of the blood drives CO_2 out of the blood.
E. Adding CO_2 to the blood drives O_2 out of the blood.

169. The oxygen content of mixed venous blood is

A. Measured using blood sampled from the right atrium.
B. Increased during generalized muscular exercise.
C. Increased in a warm environment.
D. Increased in cyanide poisoning.
E. Decreased in circulatory failure.

170. Bronchial asthma is likely to be relieved by

A. Stimulation of cholinergic receptors.
B. Stimulation of beta adrenoceptors.
C. Histamine aerosols.
D. Drugs which stabilize mast cell membranes.
E. Glucocorticoids.

171. Air in the pleural cavity (pneumothorax)

A. Allows intrapleural pressure to rise to atmospheric pressure.
B. Causes the underlying lung to collapse by compressing it.
C. Increases the functional residual capacity.
D. Leads to a slight outward movement of the chest wall.
E. Reduces vital capacity.

Answers

166.
A. False   It catalyses the conversion of H_2CO_3 to CO_2 and H_2O.
B. True   Oxygenation of haemoglobin favours this dissociation.
C. True P_{O_2} rises by at least 40 mmHg whereas P_{CO_2} falls by only 6 mmHg.
D. False   It follows the sigmoid oxygen dissociation curve.
E. False   It is higher due to the diffusion of CO_2 out of the blood to the alveoli.

167.
A. False   It is the amount of O_2 in excess of resting needs consumed after exercise stops.
B. False O_2 uptake across pulmonary capillary walls is not usually diffusion limited.
C. True   The O_2 debt incurred during anaerobic metabolism is repaid later.
D. True   This is generated during anaerobic metabolism.
E. True   Due to the lactic acid, blood HCO_3^- falls as the lactic acid is buffered.

168.
A. False   The curves start and finish differently. The CO_2 curve has a steep initial slope which gradually decreases, but there is no plateau. It is the O_2 curve which is sigmoid in shape.
B. False   Content continues to rise as P_{CO_2} rises above normal alveolar levels.
C. False CO_2 content is zero when P_{CO_2} is zero.
D. True   Oxyhaemoglobin is a stronger acid than reduced haemoglobin; the liberated H^+·ions drive the reaction $H^+ + HCO_3^- \rightarrow H_2CO_3 \rightarrow CO_2 + H_2O$.
E. False   This is shown by the oxygen dissociation curve, not the carbon dioxide dissociation curve.

169.
A. False   For adequate mixing, pulmonary artery blood is needed.
B. False   It falls due to increased oxygen extraction by the active muscles.
C. True   Due to large volumes of well oxygenated blood returning from skin.
D. True   Cyanide blocks uptake of oxygen by tissue enzyme systems.
E. True   Oxygen extraction is increased in stagnant hypoxia.

170.
A. False   This causes bronchoconstriction.
B. True   This causes relaxation of bronchial muscle.
C. False   Histamine is a bronchoconstrictor.
D. True   The chromoglycate drugs are thought to work like this and reduce release of bronchoconstrictor agents from mast cells.
E. True   These suppress bronchoconstrictor and inflammatory mechanisms.

171.
A. True   Air flows in since the pressure in the cavity is normally subatmospheric.
B. False   Except in tension pneumothorax, pleural pressure does not exceed intrapulmonary pressure (atmospheric); collapse is due to elastic recoil of the lungs.
C. False   It decreases as the lung collapses.
D. True   The elastic recoil of the lung is no longer applied to the chest wall.
E. True   The lungs cannot be fully inflated.

Questions 172–177

172. A patient with chronic respiratory failure
A. Shows an enhanced respiratory sensitivity to inhaled carbon dioxide.
B. Shows little or no respiratory response to hypoxia.
C. Is likely to have a low blood bicarbonate level.
D. Responds well when given 100 per cent oxygen to breathe.
E. Must have been breathing oxygen-enriched air if alveolar P_{CO_2} is 150 mmHg (20 kPa).

173. Loss of pulmonary elastic tissue in 'emphysema' reduces
A. Physiological dead space.
B. Anatomical dead space.
C. Residual volume.
D. Vital capacity.
E. The percentage of the vital capacity expired in one second.

174. Complete obstruction of a major bronchus usually results in
A. Collapse of the alveoli supplied by the bronchus.
B. A rise in local intrapleural pressure.
C. An increase in physiological dead space.
D. An increase in blood flow to the lung tissue supplied by the bronchus.
E. Cyanosis.

175. A shift of the oxygen dissociation curve of blood to the left
A. Decreases the O_2 content of blood at a given P_{O_2}.
B. Impairs O_2 delivery to the tissues at the normal tissue P_{O_2}.
C. Occurs in blood perfusing cold extremities.
D. Occurs in blood stored for several weeks.
E. Is characteristic of fetal blood when compared with adult blood.

176. Obstructive airways disease (COPD) is similar to restrictive lung disease (RLD) in that it reduces
A. Vital capacity (VC).
B. The forced expiratory volume in one second (FEV_1).
C. The ratio FEV_1/VC.
D. Residual volume.
E. Peak expiratory flow rate to the same degree.

177. A diver breathing air at a depth of 30 metres under water
A. Is exposed to a pressure of about four times that at the surface.
B. Has a raised pressure of nitrogen in the alveoli.
C. Has a four-fold increase in the oxygen content of blood.
D. Has a four-fold increase in alveolar water vapour pressure.
E. Expends less energy than normal on the work of breathing.

Answers

172.

A. False   There is increased tolerance of high P_{CO_2} levels.
B. False   Sensitivity to low P_{O_2} remains and is important in maintaining ventilation.
C. False HCO_3^- levels rise to compensate for the raised P_{CO_2} in respiratory acidosis.
D. False   This could arrest ventilation by removing hypoxic drive; 24–28 per cent O_2 would do.
E. True   When breathing air, $P_{O_2} + P_{CO_2}$ equal about 140 mmHg (19 kPa).

173.

A. False   It increases as the walls between alveoli break down to form large sacs.
B. True   Destruction of elastic fibres holding airways open allows them to narrow.
C. False   It is increased as airways close more readily than usual during expiration.
D. True   It decreases as the residual volume increases.
E. True   Thus it is a typical obstructive airways disease.

174.

A. True   This 'atelectasis' is due to absorption of trapped air.
B. False   Local collapse of the lung lowers local intrapleural pressure.
C. False   Since the affected lung is collapsed it does not count as dead space.
D. False   Local hypoxia in the unventilated segment causes local vasoconstriction.
E. False   Vasoconstriction in the collapsed segment prevents deoxygenated blood passing through to the systemic circulation.

175.

A. False   It increases content, especially at tissue P_{O_2}.
B. True   The blood does not release its oxygen adequately.
C. True   Cold shifts the curve to the left and may reduce O_2 delivery to cold tissues.
D. True   Such blood when transfused may not release its O_2 content adequately.
E. True   Fetal blood can thus take up O_2 at the low P_{O_2} levels seen in the placenta but fetal tissue P_{O_2} has to be low to permit its release.

176.

A. True   In COPD by air trapping and in RLD by reducing total lung volume.
B. True   In COPD by slowing flow and in RLD by restricting volume.
C. False   Only COPD which slows flow reduces it.
D. False   It rises in COPD and falls in RLD.
E. False   COPD typically causes marked reduction, RLD typically has little effect.

177.

A. True   10 metres of water = approximately one atmosphere.
B. True   Total alveolar pressure = four atmospheres.
C. False   Haemoglobin is already saturated with O_2 at sea level and cannot take up more; the amount of dissolved oxygen increases raising total O_2 content by less than 10 per cent.
D. False   This depends on temperature alone.
E. False   More energy is needed to move air made more viscous by compression.

Questions 178–183

178. Cyanosis
A. May be caused by high levels of carboxyhaemoglobin in the blood.
B. May be caused by high levels of methaemoglobin in the blood.
C. Is seen in fingers of hands immersed in iced water.
D. Occurs more easily in anaemic than in polycythaemic patients.
E. Is severe in cyanide poisoning.

179. A patient with carbon dioxide retention is likely to have
A. Metabolic acidosis.
B. Alkaline urine.
C. Cool extremities.
D. Raised cerebral blood flow.
E. Raised plasma bicarbonate.

180. Surgical removal of one lung reduces the
A. FEV_1 by about 10 per cent.
B. Percentage saturation of arterial blood with oxygen.
C. Exercise tolerance.
D. Residual volume.
E. Ventilation/perfusion ratio by about 50 per cent.

181. Coughing
A. Is reflexly initiated by irritation of the alveoli.
B. Is associated with relaxation of airways smooth muscle.
C. Depends on contraction of the diaphragm for expulsion of air.
D. Differs from sneezing in that the glottis is initially closed.
E. Is depressed during anaesthesia.

182. The severity of an obstructive airways disease is indicated by the degree of change in the
A. Total ventilation/perfusion ratio.
B. Peak expiratory flow rate.
C. Respiratory quotient.
D. Tidal volume.
E. Work of breathing.

183. A 50 per cent fall in the ventilation/perfusion ratio in one lung would
A. Lower systemic arterial oxygen content.
B. Have effects similar to those of a direct right to left atrial shunt.
C. Increase the physiological dead space.
D. Lower systemic arterial carbon dioxide content.
E. Be compensated (with respect to oxygen uptake) by a high ratio in the other lung.

Answers

178.

A.   False   Carboxyhaemoglobin is pink and gives the skin a pinkish colour.
B.   True   This blue pigment is a rare cause of central cyanosis.
C.   False   The fingers are red; cold inhibits oxygen dissociation and reduces metabolism.
D.   False   Cyanosis occurs when arterial blood contains more than 5 g/dl reduced haemoglobin; low haemoglobin values in anaemia make it difficult to reach this level.
E.   False   Cyanide poisons the enzymes involved in O_2 uptake by the tissues; in cyanide poisoning the blood remains fully oxygenated and the skin is pink.

179.

A.   False CO_2 retention causes respiratory acidosis.
B.   False   In respiratory acidosis there is increased secretion of H^+ ions in urine.
C.   False   Carbon dioxide dilates peripheral blood vessels.
D.   True   The vasodilator effect of high P_{CO_2} on cerebral vessels may lead to cerebral oedema and headaches.
E.   True   The kidney manufactures bicarbonate to compensate the respiratory acidosis.

180.

A.   False   It reduces it by at least half.
B.   False   A single lung can maintain normal oxygenation at rest.
C.   True   Maximum ventilation and maximum oxygen uptake are reduced.
D.   True   It leads to a restrictive lung disease pattern.
E.   False   The ratio is little affected.

181.

A.   False   It is initiated by irritation of the trachea and bronchi.
B.   False   Contraction narrows airways and increases velocity of flow.
C.   False   It depends on expiratory muscles, particularly abdominal muscles.
D.   True   Thus it is more explosive than sneezing.
E.   True   This may lead to retention of mucous secretions.

182.

A.   False   It may well be normal.
B.   True   It is a sensitive indicator.
C.   False   RQ is related to the mixture of substrates being metabolized.
D.   False   This also may be normal.
E.   True   This is related to the increased airway resistance.

183.

A.   True   It constitutes a physiological shunt.
B.   True   This would be an anatomical shunt.
C.   False   Physiological dead space is relatively overventilated.
D.   False   It would tend to raise it.
E.   False   Increased ventilation cannot increase oxygen saturation; compensation for carbon dioxide retention can occur.

Questions 184–187

184. In the forced expiratory volume (FEV$_1$) measurement, an adult patient

A. With normal lungs should expire 95 per cent of vital capacity (VC) in 1 second.
B. With restrictive disease may expire a greater than predicted per cent of VC in the first second.
C. Who is female would be expected to expire a greater per cent of VC in 1 second than a male of the same age.
D. With obstructive disease may take more than 5 second to complete the expiration.
E. With normal lungs should achieve a peak flow rate of at least 200 litres/minute.

185. The hypoxia in chronic respiratory failure

A. May cause central cyanosis.
B. May cause peripheral cyanosis.
C. Leads to increased formation of erythropoietin.
D. Raises pulmonary vascular resistance.
E. May lead to right heart failure.

186. 'Blue Bloaters' (patients with chronic obstructive pulmonary disease showing marked cyanosis and oedema) differ from 'Pink Puffers' (patients with chronic obstructive pulmonary disease showing dyspnoea but not cyanosis) by having a lower

A. Forced expiratory volume in one second.
B. Peak expiratory flow rate.
C. Arterial blood pH.
D. Sensitivity to carbon dioxide.
E. Pulmonary arterial pressure.

187. The total amount of O$_2$ carried by the circulation to the tissues/min. (oxygen delivery or total available oxygen)

A. Normally equals the rate of O$_2$ consumption by the body/min.
B. Is normally more than 95 per cent combined with haemoglobin.
C. Must fall by about half if haemoglobin concentration is halved.
D. Is more closely related to P$_{O2}$ than to percentage saturation of the blood with O$_2$.
E. Must double if body oxygen consumption doubles.

Answers

184.

A. False   The normal is about 85 per cent at age 20, falling to about 70 per cent at age 60–70.
B. True   The airways are not obstructed and vital capacity volume is reduced.
C. True   Females have, on average, smaller vital capacities than males.
D. True   This is typical of moderately severe obstructive airways disease.
E. True   200 litres/min is a low figure; most subjects, other than small elderly females, should do better.

185.

A. True   Reduced V/P ratios allow deoxygenated blood to be shunted to the left side of the heart.
B. False   The peripheral circulation in chronic respiratory failure is usually adequate.
C. True   This in turn leads to the secondary polycythaemia typical of the condition.
D. True   Hypoxia constricts pulmonary vessels and may cause pulmonary hypertension.
E. True   Persistent pulmonary hypertension can lead to right heart failure.

186.

A. False   This is not a differentiating feature.
B. False   This tends to parallel the FEV_1.
C. True   They have a respiratory acidosis due to CO_2 retention.
D. True   They do not respond adequately to their high P_{CO_2}.
E. False   Pulmonary hypertension in 'Blue Bloaters' leads to heart failure and oedema.

187.

A. False   At rest, O_2 consumption (about 250 ml/min) is about 25 per cent of the total available.
B. True   All but 3 of the 200 ml/l is combined with haemoglobin, the rest is dissolved.
C. False   In anaemic hypoxia, cardiac output rises to compensate for the reduced oxygen content per litre of blood.
D. False   If P_{O_2} falls by 25 per cent from normal, there is relatively little change in the blood oxygen content.
E. False   The extraction ratio rises as oxygen consumption rises, e.g. during exercise.

EMQs

Questions 188–194

EMQ Question 188

For each description of respiratory pressures A–E, select the most appropriate option from the following list.

1. Intrapleural pressure.
2. Intra-abdominal pressure.
3. Intra-alveolar pressure.
4. Intra-oesophageal pressure.
5. Atmospheric pressure.

A. Intra-alveolar pressure at end-inspiration and end-expiration.
B. Shows transient rises and falls during the respiratory cycle peaking at mid-expiration and mid-inspiration respectively.
C. Approximates to intrapleural pressure.
D. Rises markedly during the vomiting reflex.
E. Determines the pressure gradient for inspiration and expiration.

EMQ Question 189

For each person described below A–E, select the most appropriate set of arterial blood gas results (pH and bicarbonate are included) from the following list.

	pH	P_{O_2}	P_{CO_2}	Bicarbonate
1.	Normal	Normal	Normal	Normal
2.	Normal	Reduced	Normal	Normal
3.	Reduced	Reduced	Increased	Normal
4.	Reduced	Reduced	Increased	Increased
5.	Reduced	Increased	Increased	Increased
6.	Reduced	Increased	Reduced	Reduced
7.	Increased	Increased	Reduced	Normal
8.	Increased	Reduced	Reduced	Reduced

A. A healthy 25-year-old has climbed from sea level to a height of 1000 metres (about 3000 feet), feels fine and is enjoying the view.
B. A 40-year-old known diabetic on insulin has been admitted to hospital, semi-conscious with ketoacidosis and is breathing deeply.
C. A healthy 30-year-old is on a high-altitude adventure holiday with initially several days at moderate altitude where ventilation is definitely increased. Later, while climbing at 4500 metres (about 15 000 feet) severe headache, retching and inability to continue climbing develop.
D. A 55-year-old patient with long-standing cough and sputum has been admitted with signs of serious chest infection and a general bluish colour. Initial treatment has included treatment with oxygen through a facemask.
E. A 30-year-old is admitted to hospital with signs of serious renal damage. The patient is drowsy and is breathing deeply.

Answers for 188

A. **Option 5**   *Atmospheric pressure.* Intra-alveolar pressure returns to atmospheric pressure at the end of each inspiratory and expiratory phase.

B. **Option 3**   *Intra-alveolar pressure.* This dips transiently during inspiration and rises to a similar extent during expiration.

C. **Option 4**   *Intra-oesophageal pressure.* Since the oesophagus and the intrapleural spaces are normally closed cavities within the chest, intra-oesophageal pressure normally approximates to intrapleural pressure.

D. **Option 2**   *Intra-abdominal pressure.* During vomiting this rises markedly to compress the gut while the way out through the lower oesophageal (cardiac) sphincter is open due to relaxation of oesophageal smooth muscle.

E. **Option 3**   *Intra-alveolar pressure.* The difference between this and atmospheric pressure constitutes the pressure gradient which determines the flow of air into or out of the lungs.

Answers for 189

A. **Option 2** P_{O_2} *reduced, others normal.* At 1000 metres, atmospheric pressure and hence ambient oxygen pressure fall by about 10 per cent. This reduces alveolar and hence arterial P_{O_2} by slightly more, since alveolar water vapour pressure and P_{CO_2} do not change. However, due to the plateau of the oxygen dissociation curve, arterial saturation falls only slightly. Bodily function is unaffected, with no change in ventilation, so carbon dioxide, pH and bicarbonate do not change.

B. **Option 6**   *All reduced, apart from Po_2, which is increased.* The ketoacidosis is due to abnormal accumulation of highly acidic metabolites. Hence the pH is reduced. Bicarbonate ions have buffered most of the surplus hydrogen ions to minimize the fall in pH, hence bicarbonate is reduced. The acidosis stimulates ventilation. This reduces P_{CO_2} and also limits pH fall; the increased ventilation also increases P_{O_2}, though as in (A) the effect on saturation is minute.

C. **Option 8**   *pH increased, others reduced.* In this case, serious 'hypoxic hypoxia' leads to increased ventilation reflexly via the carotid and aortic bodies. Increased ventilation improves P_{O_2}, but it remains well below normal, causing general tissue hypoxia. The increased ventilation acts mainly by lowering P_{CO_2}, allowing oxygen to replace some of the carbon dioxide in the alveoli. However, lowered P_{CO_2} causes a respiratory alkalosis so pH rises. To compensate for the respiratory alkalosis, the renal tubules reduce secretion of hydrogen ions and lower blood bicarbonate level. However, all these compensations merely reduce the abnormalities. The combination of tissue hypoxia, decreased cerebral blood flow (due to the low P_{CO_2}), and alkalosis seriously disturb bodily function. Some people tolerate this quite well, but others, like this person, feel wretched and are at risk of serious and even fatal complications.

D. **Option 5**   *pH reduced, others increased.* The 55-year-old has inadequate ventilation related to chronic respiratory disease. The inadequate ventilation is shown by the bluish colour (cyanosis) due to excessive desaturated haemoglobin. This is another variety of 'hypoxic hypoxia'. The inadequate ventilation also raises the P_{CO_2}, causing a respiratory acidosis. As with (C), but in the opposite direction, the renal tubules raise the blood bicarbonate level. The increased P_{O_2} can only be explained by the administration of oxygen. Before this the oxygen level would have been reduced. Such patients require careful monitoring of their blood gases and control of the administered oxygen.

E. **Option 6**   *All reduced, apart from P_{O_2}, which is increased.* Here the renal damage impairs hydrogen ion excretion in the urine and addition of bicarbonate to the blood. Just like (B) this patient has a metabolic acidosis. The respiratory compensation and its effects are explained in the same way.

EMQ

EMQ Question 190

For each person A–E, select the most appropriate set of results for respiratory function tests from the following list, where VC = vital capacity; $FEV_{1.0}$ = forced expiratory volume in one second; RV = residual volume all litres; PEFR = peak expiratory flow rate in litres per second.

	VC	$FEV_{1.0}$RV	$FEV_{1.0}$/VC	Per cent	PEFR
1.	5.0	4.0	1.5	80	600
2.	3.0	2.1	1.2	70	350
3.	4.5	5.0	1.2	90	200
4.	4.0	2.0	2.5	50	120
5.	3.0	2.4	0.8	80	620
6.	4.0	3.4	1.2	85	450

A. A woman of 19 years who had occasional asthma as a child but is now free of symptoms.
B. A man of 32 who is having respiratory function testing as part of a routine health check.
C. A woman of 77 who is acting as a normal control in a research project.
D. When this patient comes to discuss the results of respiratory testing, the doctor apologizes that there seems to have been a mistake as the results do not make sense.
F. A man of 45 with a long history of chronic obstructive pulmonary disease (COPD).

EMQ Question 191

For each item A–E related to control of ventilation, select the most appropriate option from the list below.

1. Voluntary hyperventilation.
2. Reflex hyperventilation.
3. Hypoventilation.
4. Ventilation controlled from the medulla oblongata.
5. Ventilation controlled from above the medulla oblongata.
6. Ventilation associated with dyspnoea.

A. An athlete's ventilation may increase from a normal value of 6 litres per minute to over 100 litres per minute while running a race.
B. A student breathes a mixture of 5 per cent carbon dioxide and finds that, without apparent effort, the breathing is much deeper than normal.
C. Another student is asked to breathe rapidly and deeply for three minutes. Towards the end of the time there is a strong wish to reduce the breathing and there is a feeling of lightness and discomfort in the head.
D. In normal people breathing continues steadily during sleep.
E. In people with COPD the lungs are over-inflated and it may be harder to breathe in than breathe out.

Answers for 190

A. **Option 6** This is a normal vital capacity for a young female where volumes are smaller than in males. $FEV1_{1.0}$ is 85 per cent of VC which is normal in young people; RV is also in keeping. PEFR is also normal for a female. Option 2 would be the next best option but note the comments in (C).

B. **Option 1** These are all normal values for an average male of this age.

C. **Option 2** These are normal values for a woman of this age. VC is smaller in females and falls with age. $FEV_{1.0}/FVC$ also falls with age and this is normal at her age. RV tends to rise with age, although the value is quite small it is a higher proportion of total lung capacity (VC + RV) here than in Option 1. This is a normal PEFR for a woman of this age.

D. **Option 3** This is a nonsense result. $FEV_{1.0}$ cannot be greater than VC; they may have been reversed, which would correspond with the percentage of 90. However, these results would not then correspond with the low PEFR.

E. **Option 4** These results are typical of fairly severe COPD. $FEV_{1.0}$ is only half the vital capacity, RV is considerably increased and PEFR is much reduced. The changes would be those expected in someone whose predicted normal results correspond to Option 1. If this man had developed restrictive disease, then Option 5 would be appropriate parallel reductions in all volumes including RV, but a well preserved and even increased PEFR as the airways are not affected by restrictive disease.

Answers to 191

A. **Option 4** *Ventilation controlled from above the medulla oblongata.* The commonest situation for this huge minute volume is strenuous exercise in a normal person. This is not a reflex from a fall in arterial oxygen levels, which remain normal, but is controlled from higher levels where circulatory and respiratory activities are coordinated with muscular activity. This activity is sometimes identified with 'the exercise centre' though this is more a function of the brain than a localized area.

B. **Option 2** *Reflex hyperventilation.* The increased ventilation is reflexly produced via chemoreceptors in the region of the medulla oblongata. These respond to the huge rise in hydrogen ions produced centrally from the rise in carbon dioxide level.

C. **Option 1** *Voluntary hyperventilation.* The hyperventilation lowers the carbon dioxide level. This causes a respiratory alkalosis and constricts cerebral arterioles. There has been a suggestion that people who are most distressed by this activity are the most likely to suffer from severe symptoms at high altitudes where such changes are the result of reflex hyperventilation.

D. **Option 4** *Ventilation controlled from the medulla oblongata.* The spontaneous rhythmicity in the inspiratory and expiratory centres here generate the basic breathing pattern upon which other more complicated activities, including voluntary control as in respiratory function testing, are built.

E. **Option 6** *Ventilation associated with dyspnoea.* With severe over-inflation lung compliance falls; this increases the work of breathing in and may be less severe when breathing out (patients vary in this). The extra effort is interpreted as something wrong with the breathing (dyspnoea means bad breathing). In Option 1 the problem is not with the breathing but with the effects it produces. In Option 2 the increased breathing is not experienced as particularly unpleasant. In Option 5 the increased breathing of exercise is recognized as normal.

EMQ Question 192

For each item A–E related to oxygen transport, select the most appropriate option from the list below:

1. Sigmoid.
2. Plateau.
3. Oxygen in solution.
4. Percentage saturation.
5. Oxygen content, ml oxygen per litre of blood.
6. Shift of the curve to the right.
7. Shift of the curve to the left.

A. When the y axis of the oxygen dissociation curve of blood is labelled thus, the curve for severe anaemia is very similar to that for normal blood.
B. The form in which oxygen passes from blood to tissues.
C. This leads to proportionately greater release of oxygen to the tissues.
D. A property of the oxygen dissociation curve which is related to the varying affinities of haemoglobin for oxygen particularly at very low oxygen pressures and at the pressures around the normal range for alveolar oxygen pressures.
E. The reason the 'plateau' phase of the oxygen dissociation curve is not completely horizontal.

EMQ Question 193

For each item A–E related to carbon dioxide transport, select the most appropriate option from the list below.

1. Dissolved carbon dioxide.
2. Carbon dioxide combined with haemoglobin.
3. Carbon dioxide in red cells.
4. Carbon dioxide in plasma.
5. Carbaminohaemoglobin.
6. Carboxyhaemoglobin.
7. Ability of desaturated haemoglobin to buffer hydrogen ions.

A. This has a particularly unfavourable effect on the ability of blood to carry adequate oxygen.
B. The action of carbonic anhydrase is particularly important here.
C. The relationship of this to partial pressure is quantitatively different than is the case with oxygen.
D. This favours carriage of carbon dioxide by the law of mass action.
E. This form of transport is influenced more by the saturation of the haemoglobin with oxygen than the partial pressure of carbon dioxide in the blood.

Answers for 192

A. **Option 4**   *Percentage saturation.* Regardless of the haemoglobin content, the oxygen content of blood at a given oxygen pressure will always be very similar, expressed as a percentage of the capacity. The very slight differences are due to the fact that in severe anaemia the amount of dissolved oxygen relative to oxygen combined with haemoglobin is slightly greater since there is a higher proportion of plasma.

B. **Option 3**   *Oxygen in solution.* Only dissolved gases can pass through the tissue fluids.

C. **Option 6**   *Shift of the curve to the right.* When the oxygen dissociation curve of blood shifts to the right on the x axis, the oxygen content of blood at a given oxygen pressure shifts downwards on the y axis. Thus the blood retains less oxygen and more is released to the tissues.

D. **Option 1**   *Sigmoid.* Sigmoid means S-shaped. The first bend of the S is produced by the increasing affinity of haemoglobin for oxygen; at low pressures the curve becomes increasingly steep and then straightens to a steep fairly linear rise. The second bend is produced as full saturation is approached and the steep rise curves to join the plateau.

E. **Option 3**   *Dissolved oxygen.* As the partial pressure of oxygen increases above the normal alveolar value, the content rises very gradually as the dissolved oxygen increases in proportion to the pressure. In hyperbaric oxygen conditions this dissolved amount can be significant. For example if 3 ml are dissolved per litre when P_{O2} is 100 mmHg (13.5 kPa), then at two atmospheres of oxygen, with a P_{O2} around 1500 mmHg (200 kPa), the dissolved oxygen amounts to 45 ml/litre. This can be helpful when haemoglobin has been disabled by combination with carbon monoxide.

Answers for 193

A. **Option 6**   *Carboxyhaemoglobin.* This is formed when people breathe even low concentrations of carbon monoxide. The great affinity of carbon monoxide for haemoglobin displaces most of the oxygen so that most haemoglobin is rendered useless and the patient suffers from potentially fatal anaemic hypoxia.

B. **Option 3**   *Carbon dioxide in red cells.* Carbonic anhydrase is located in red cells rather than plasma. It provides the necessary acceleration of the formation of carbonic acid and hence bicarbonate during the short time available for the uptake of carbon dioxide at tissue level. Without it the dissolved carbon dioxide would build up a pressure which would seriously slow diffusion from the tissues.

C. **Option 1**   *Dissolved carbon dioxide.* At any given partial pressure carbon dioxide is many times more soluble than oxygen.

D. **Option 7**   *Ability of desaturated haemoglobin to buffer hydrogen ions.* As mentioned in (B), generation of bicarbonate is necessary for adequate carriage of carbon dioxide. Desaturated haemoglobin has a greater ability to buffer hydrogen ions than has oxyhaemoglobin. The law of mass action predicts that the removal of hydrogen ions by buffering favours further conversion of carbon dioxide to bicarbonate. In addition, diffusion of bicarbonate ions from red cells to plasma lowers the concentration of the other product of the reaction.

E. **Option 5**   *Carbaminohaemoglobin.* Oxyhaemoglobin cannot carry as much CO_2 in the carbamino compound as can reduced haemoglobin.

EMQ Question 194

For each item A–E related to oxygen delivery and uptake by tissues, select the most appropriate option from the list below.

1. Total available oxygen.
2. Cardiac output.
3. Blood haemoglobin concentration.
4. Arterial blood oxygen saturation.
5. Venous blood oxygen saturation.
6. Pulmonary arterial blood oxygen saturation.

A. Abnormality here is the fundamental cause of hypoxic hypoxia at high altitudes.
B. The normal value for this in the resting average adult is around one litre per minute.
C. Abnormality here is the fundamental cause of anaemic hypoxia.
D. Abnormality here is the fundamental cause of hypoxic hypoxia in respiratory disease.
E. This is reduced in stagnant hypoxia, in anaemic hypoxia and also in hypoxic hypoxia.

Answers to 194

A. **Option 4**   *Arterial blood oxygen saturation.* At high altitudes the alveolar oxygen pressure falls to levels at which blood passing through the lungs is inadequately saturated with oxygen. Therefore arterial blood oxygen saturation is seriously reduced and this is the fundamental cause of impaired delivery of oxygen at high altitudes.

B. **Option 1**   *Total available oxygen.* This equals the oxygen in five litres of normally saturated blood with a normal haemoglobin content.

C. **Option 3**   *Blood haemoglobin concentration.* Here the reduction in total available oxygen is reduced in proportion to the reduction in the blood haemoglobin concentration.

D. **Option 4**   *Arterial blood oxygen saturation.* As with (A) the hypoxic hypoxia is due to inadequate saturation of blood in the lungs. However this time the cause is impaired lung function rather than reduced inspired oxygen.

E. **Option 1**   *Total available oxygen.* This depends on cardiac output, blood oxygen capacity and arterial blood saturation percentage. Impaired cardiac output causes *stagnant hypoxia,* impaired blood oxygen capacity causes *anaemic hypoxia* and reduced arterial blood saturation causes *hypoxic hypoxia.*

MCQs

Questions 195–199

195. Bile

A. Contains enzymes required for the digestion of fat.
B. Contains unconjugated bilirubin.
C. Salts make cholesterol more water-soluble.
D. Pigments contain iron.
E. Becomes more alkaline during storage in the gallbladder.

196. Saliva

A. From different salivary glands has a similar composition.
B. Contains enzymes essential for the digestion of carbohydrates.
C. Has less than half the ionic calcium level of plasma.
D. Has more than twice the iodide level of plasma.
E. Has a pH between 5 and 6.

197. Swallowing is a reflex which

A. Has its reflex centres in the cervical segments of the spinal cord.
B. Includes inhibition of respiration.
C. Is initiated by a voluntary act.
D. Is dependent on intrinsic nerve networks in the oesophagus.
E. Is more effective when the person is standing rather than when lying down.

198. Appetite for food is lost when

A. Certain hypothalamic areas are stimulated.
B. Certain hypothalamic areas are destroyed.
C. The stomach is distended.
D. The stomach is surgically removed.
E. Blood glucose falls.

199. Secretion of saliva increases when

A. Touch receptors in the mouth are stimulated.
B. The mouth is flushed with acid fluids with a pH of about 4.
C. A subject thinks of unappetizing food.
D. Vomiting is imminent.
E. Their sympathetic nerve supply is stimulated.

Answers

195.

A. False   Bile contains no digestive enzymes; its bile salts assist in the emulsification and absorption of fat.
B. False   The bilirubin is conjugated by the hepatocytes before excretion.
C. True   By forming cholesterol micelles.
D. False   Iron is removed from haem in the formation of bilirubin.
E. False   It becomes more acid, which improves the solubility of bile solids.

196.

A. False   Serous glands such as the parotids produce a watery juice; mucous glands such as the sublinguals produce a thick viscid juice.
B. False   The functions of salivary amylase (ptyalin) can be affected by enzymes from other digestive glands.
C. False   It is saturated with calcium ions; calcium salts are laid down as plaque on the teeth.
D. True   Saliva is an important route of iodide excretion; its concentration in saliva is 20–100 times that in plasma.
E. False   Saliva has a neutral pH; acidity in the mouth tends to dissolve tooth enamel.

197.

A. False   The reflex centres lie in the medulla oblongata.
B. True   This plus closure of the glottis prevents food being aspirated into the airways.
C. True   The voluntary act is propulsion of a bolus of food onto the posterior pharyngeal wall.
D. True   These are essential for the peristaltic phase.
E. True   Gravity can assist the reflex; tablets are more difficult to swallow when lying down.

198.

A. True   For example, when the 'satiety' centres are stimulated.
B. True   For example, when the 'hunger' centres are damaged.
C. True   Appetite is relieved after a meal before the food products of digestion are absorbed into the blood.
D. False   The drive to eat does not depend on an intact stomach.
E. False   It increases as hypothalamic '*glucostats*' detect the low glucose and excite the 'hunger' centres to generate the emotional drive to eat.

199.

A. True   Food, foreign bodies and the dentist are effective stimuli.
B. True   E.g. lemon juice; saliva is a useful buffer to protect teeth from acid.
C. False   Thinking of appetizing food results in salivary secretion by a conditioned reflex; conversely, thinking of unappetizing food inhibits secretion.
D. True   Saliva helps to buffer the acid vomitus when it reaches the mouth.
E. True   Sympathetic stimulation produces a scanty viscid juice; parasympathetic stimulation produces a copious watery juice.

MCQ

Questions 200–205

200. Defaecation is a reflex action
A. That is coordinated by reflex centres in the sacral cord.
B. Whose afferent limb carries impulses from stretch receptors in the colon.
C. Whose efferent limb travels mainly in sympathetic autonomic nerves.
D. Which is more likely to be initiated just after a meal than just before it.
E. Which can be voluntarily inhibited or facilitated.

201. Thirst sensation occurs when
A. Osmoreceptors in the sensory cortex are activated.
B. Blood osmolality is raised but blood volume is normal.
C. Blood volume is reduced but blood osmolality is normal.
D. The mouth is dry.
E. A patient has severe diabetic keto-acidosis.

202. In the stomach
A. pH rarely falls below 4.0.
B. Pepsinogen is converted to pepsin by hydrochloric acid.
C. Ferrous iron is reduced to ferric iron by hydrochloric acid.
D. Acid secretion is inhibited by pentagastrin.
E. There is a rise in the bacterial count after histamine H_1 receptor blockade.

203. Intestinal secretions contain
A. Potassium in a concentration similar to that in extracellular fluid.
B. Enzymes that are released when the vagus nerve is stimulated.
C. Enzymes that hydrolyze disaccharides.
D. Enzymes that hydrolyze monosaccharides.
E. Enzymes that activate pancreatic proteolyic enzymes.

204. Pancreatic secretion
A. In response to vagal stimulation is copious, rich in bicarbonate but poor in enzymes.
B. In response to acid in the duodenum is scanty but rich in enzymes.
C. In response to secretin secretion is low in bicarbonate.
D. Contains enzymes that digest neutral fat to glycerol and fatty acids.
E. Contains enzymes that convert disaccharides to monosaccharides.

205. The liver is the principal site for
A. Synthesis of plasma albumin.
B. Synthesis of plasma globulins.
C. Synthesis of vitamin B_{12}.
D. Storage of vitamin C.
E. Storage of iron.

Answers

200.

A. True   Reflex defaecation can occur after complete spinal cord transection.
B. False   The stretch receptors triggering the reflex are in the rectal wall.
C. False   Parasympathetic nerves are the main motor nerves for defaecation.
D. True   The wish to defaecate that follows a meal is attributed to a 'gastrocolic reflex'.
E. True   Forced expiration against a closed glottis facilitates the reflex by raising intra-abdominal pressure and pushing faeces into the rectum; contraction of the voluntary muscle of the external sphincter can inhibit it.

201.

A. False   The emotional drive to drink depends on 'thirst centres' in the hypothalamus.
B. True   Presumably due to stimulation of hypothalamic osmoreceptors.
C. True   Presumably due to stimulation of vascular volume receptors.
D. True   Afferents from the upper alimentary tract can influence 'thirst centre' activity.
E. True   Probably due to osmoreceptor stimulation by the hyperglycaemic blood and a reduction in the activity of vascular volume receptors.

202.

A. False   Values around pH 2–3 are normal.
B. True   Pepsin is the active proteolyic form of pepsinogen.
C. False   HCl reduces trivalent ferric iron to the divalent ferrous form in which it can be absorbed in the small intestine.
D. False   Pentagastrin is a powerful pharmacological stimulant of mucosal cells to produce HCl.
E. False   But it rises markedly after H_2 blockade which blocks gastric acid secretion.

203.

A. False   The concentration is higher, due partly to potassium released from cast off cells.
B. False   Intestinal secretion is not under vagal control; its enzymes are thought to be constituents of the mucosal cells and released when these are cast off into the lumen.
C. True   The mucosal cell brush border contains these enzymes, e.g. maltase and lactase.
D. False   Monosaccharides are end-products of digestion and absorbed as such.
E. True   For example, enterokinase which converts trypsinogen to trypsin.

204.

A. False   It is scanty and rich in enzymes; it is secreted reflexly in the 'cephalic' phase of pancreatic secretion when food is thought about or chewed.
B. False   It is copious, bicarbonate rich and poor in enzymes; it buffers the acid secretions entering the duodenum from the stomach.
C. False   This is the hormone released when acid enters the duodenum that stimulates the pancreas to produce the juice described in (B) above.
D. True   Pancreatic lipase.
E. False   Pancreatic amylase breaks down carbohydrates to dextrins and polysaccharides.

205.

A. True   Plasma albumin concentration falls in liver failure.
B. False   Immunoglobulins are produced by ribosomes in lymphocytes.
C. False   Vitamin B_{12} is ingested in food, absorbed complexed with *intrinsic factor* in the terminal ileum and stored in the liver.
D. False   Vitamin C is not stored; any in excess of requirements is excreted in urine.
E. True   Iron released from haem from broken down RBCs is stored in the liver for future haemopoiesis.

Questions 206–211

206. In the colon
A. A greater volume of water is absorbed than in the small intestine.
B. Mucus is secreted to lubricate the faecal contents.
C. Faecal transit time is normally about 7 days.
D. Faecal transit time is inversely related to its fibre content.
E. Bacteria normally account for about three quarters of the faecal weight.

207. Gastric juice
A. Is secreted when the vagus nerves are stimulated.
B. Is secreted in vagotomized animals when food is chewed but not swallowed.
C. Inactivates the digestive enzymes secreted with saliva.
D. Does not digest the gastric mucosa because it is protected by a pepsin inactivator.
E. Irritates the oesophageal mucosa if regurgitated from the stomach.

208. An increase in body fat increases the
A. Percentage of water in the body.
B. Survival time during fasting.
C. Survival time in cold water.
D. Specific gravity of the body.
E. Probability of increased morbidity and premature mortality.

209. The respiratory quotient
A. Is the ratio of the volume of O_2 consumed to the volume of CO_2 produced.
B. Depends essentially on the type of substrate being metabolized.
C. Is 1.0 when glucose is the substrate metabolized.
D. Is between 0.9 and 1.00 in the second week of fasting.
E. For the brain is around 1.0.

210. Oxygen consumption tends to increase when the
A. Concentration of oxygen in inspired air rises.
B. Metabolic rate falls.
C. Body temperature rises.
D. Environmental temperature falls.
E. After a meal is ingested.

211. Saliva is necessary for
A. Digestion of food.
B. Swallowing of food.
C. Normal speech.
D. Antisepsis in the mouth.
E. Taste sensation.

Answers

206.

A.   False   The colon absorbs 1–2 litres/day; 8–10 litres is absorbed per day in the small intestine.

B.   True   Mucous cells are the predominant cells on the colonic mucosal surface.

C.   False   The average transit time from caecum to pelvic colon is about 12 hours but passage from the pelvic colon to the anus may take days.

D.   True   Fibre (cellulose, lignin etc.) in the colonic contents stimulates peristaltic movements by adding 'bulk' to the food residues.

E.   False   But bacteria such as Escherichia coli make up about a third of faecal weight.

207.

A.   True   Vagal stimulation increases acid and pepsinogen secretion; this action is mediated by acetylcholine and gastrin-releasing peptide released from the vagal nerve endings.

B.   False   After vagotomy, food must enter the stomach to stimulate gastric secretions.

C.   True   Salivary enzymes are not effective at the low pH of gastric juice.

D.   False   But mucosal cells are protected by a coat of mucus impregnated with bicarbonate.

E.   True   This is normally prevented by the cardiac sphincter.

208.

A.   False   The reverse is true, since fat tissue contains little water

B.   True   Fat is the main energy store of the body.

C.   True   It favours survival by increasing skin insulation.

D.   False   Fat has a lower specific gravity than the lean body mass.

E.   True   Actuarial tables show this to be true.

209.

A.   False   It is the inverse of this ratio.

B.   True   The respiratory quotients for carbohydrate, fat and protein metabolism are different.

C.   True $C_6H_{12}O_6 + 6O_2 = 6CO_2 + 6H_2O$; each molecule of O_2 consumed results in the production of one molecule of CO_2.

D.   False   It approaches 0.7, the value when fat is the main substrate being metabolized.

E.   True   Carbohydrate is the main substrate for brain metabolism.

210.

A.   False   The concentration of oxygen in the air breathed is not a determinant of oxygen consumption.

B.   False   It rises; metabolic rate is the prime determinant of oxygen consumption.

C.   True   This increases metabolic rate by increasing the rate of cellular metabolism.

D.   True   More thermogenesis is required to maintain body temperature.

E.   True   Due to the specific dynamic action of the food, particularly protein.

211.

A.   False   Other digestive tract enzymes can take over if salivary enzymes are absent.

B.   False   But swallowing solids is difficult without saliva's moisturizing and lubricant effects.

C.   True   Nervous orators with dry mouths continually sip water.

D.   True   In the absence of saliva, the mouth becomes infected and ulceration occurs.

E.   True   Substances must go into solution before they can stimulate taste receptors.

Questions 212–217

212. The stomach
A. Is responsible for absorbing about 10 per cent of the ingested food.
B. Contains mucosal cells containing high concentrations of carbonic anhydrase.
C. Peristaltic contractions start from the pyloric region.
D. Motility increases when fat enters the duodenum.
E. Relaxes when food is ingested so that there is little rise in intra-gastric pressure.

213. Brown fat is
A. Relatively more abundant in adults than in infants.
B. Richer in mitochondria than ordinary fat.
C. More vascular than ordinary fat.
D. Stimulated to generate more heat when its parasympathetic nerve supply is stimulated.
E. Is more important than shivering in neonatal thermoregulation.

214. Nitrogen balance
A. Is the relationship between the body's nitrogen intake and nitrogen loss.
B. Is positive in childhood.
C. Becomes more positive when dietary protein is increased.
D. Becomes negative when a patient is immobilized in bed.
E. Becomes less negative in the final stages of fatal starvation.

215. The normally innervated stomach
A. Is stimulated to secrete gastric juice when food is chewed, even if it is not swallowed.
B. Cannot secrete HCl when its H_1 histamine receptors are blocked.
C. And the denervated stomach can secrete gastric juice after a meal is ingested.
D. Empties more quickly than the denervated stomach.
E. Is stimulated to secrete gastric juice by the hormone secretin

216. The passage of gastric contents to the duodenum may cause
A. Copious secretion of pancreatic juice rich in bicarbonate.
B. Decreased gastric motility.
C. Contraction of the gallbladder.
D. Contraction of the sphincter of Oddi.
E. Release of pancreozymin.

217. Bile salts
A. Are the only constituents of bile necessary for digestion.
B. Have a characteristic molecule, part water-soluble and part fat-soluble.
C. Are reabsorbed mainly in the upper small intestine.
D. Are derived from cholesterol.
E. Inhibit bile secretion by the liver.

Answers

212.

A.   False   Little food is absorbed in the stomach other than alcohol.

B.   True   This is needed to generate the H^+ ions required for HCl secretion; carbonic anhydrase inhibitors reduce acid secretion.

C.   False   They begin at the other end, the fundus.

D.   False   Fat in the duodenum inhibits gastric motility.

E.   True   This 'receptive relaxation' allows the stomach to store large volumes of food without discomfort.

213.

A.   False   The reverse is true.

B.   True   It has a higher metabolic rate than ordinary fat.

C.   True   Its higher metabolic rate merits a higher rate of blood flow.

D.   False   Metabolic activity in brown fat is stimulated by sympathetic nerve stimulation.

E.   True   Infants do not shiver well.

214.

A.   True   It is positive when more nitrogen is taken in than is lost.

B.   True   Nitrogen intake is greater than nitrogen loss during active tissue growth.

C.   False   The additional nitrogen intake is balanced by additional nitrogen loss as the extra protein is metabolized and its nitrogen excreted in the urine.

D.   True   Muscles waste and the protein released is metabolized.

E.   False   It becomes more negative when little but protein remains to be metabolized.

215.

A.   True   This depends on a vagal reflex.

B.   False   Blockade of histamine H_2 receptors blocks gastric acid secretion.

C.   True   The denervated stomach is still affected by gastrin released from the gastric mucosa when food enters the stomach.

D.   True   Gastric motility is more effective when it is coordinated by vagal nerve activity.

E.   False   Secretin, which stimulates pancreatic secretion, decreases gastric secretion.

216.

A.   True   This is caused by the hormone secretin released from the duodenal mucosa.

B.   True   This postpones further gastric emptying.

C.   True   Due to the action of cholecystokinin released from the mucosal cells.

D.   False   The sphincter of Oddi must relax to allow bile to enter the gut.

E.   True   Pancreozymin stimulates the pancreas to secrete a scanty, enzyme rich juice.

217.

A.   True   They emulsify fat creating a greater surface area for lipase to act on.

B.   True   This property allows them form to micelles for fat transport.

C.   False   They are absorbed in the terminal ileum.

D.   True   They are synthesized from cholesterol in the liver.

E.   False   They are 'choleretics', substances which stimulate bile secretion.

Questions 218–222

218. Absorption of
A. Fat is impaired if either bile or pancreatic juice is not available.
B. Undigested protein molecules can occur in the newborn.
C. Laevo-amino acids occurs more rapidly than absorption of the dextro-forms.
D. Iron is at a rate proportional to body needs.
E. Sodium is at a rate proportional to body needs.

219. The specific dynamic action of food
A. Is the increase in metabolic rate that results from ingestion of food.
B. Persists for about an hour after a meal is ingested.
C. Is due to the additional energy expended in digesting and absorbing the food.
D. Results in about 30 per cent of the energy value of ingested protein being unavailable for other purposes.
E. Results in about 20 per cent of the energy value of ingested fat and carbohydrate being unavailable for other purposes.

220. Secretion of gastric juice
A. Increases when food stimulates mucosal cells in the pyloric region.
B. Is associated with a decrease in the pH of venous blood draining the stomach.
C. In response to food is reduced after vagotomy.
D. Is essential for protein digestion.
E. Is essential for absorption of vitamin B_{12}.

221. In the small intestine
A. The enzyme concentration in intestinal juice is lower in the ileum than in the jejunum.
B. Vitamin B_{12} is absorbed mainly in the jejunum.
C. Water absorption is dependent on the active absorption of sodium and glucose.
D. Absorption of calcium occurs mainly in the terminal ileum.
E. Glucose absorption is dependent on sodium absorption.

222. The cells of the liver
A. Help to maintain the normal blood glucose level.
B. Deaminate amino acids to form NH_4^+ which is excreted as ammonium salts in the urine.
C. Synthesize Vitamin D_3 (cholecalciferol).
D. Manufacture most of the immune globulins.
E. Inactivate steroid hormones manufactured in the gonads.

Answers

218.

A. True   If either is absent, undigested fat appears in the faeces.
B. True   Maternal antibodies (globulins) in colostrum are so absorbed.
C. True   Transport mechanisms are isomer-specific.
D. True   An active carrier-mediated transport mechanism is involved which reduces the danger of iron toxicity with excessive intake.
E. False   Most ingested sodium is absorbed; if absorption is above the body requirements, the excess is excreted by the kidneys.

219.

A. True   This is its definition.
B. False   It persists for about six hours.
C. False   It is due mainly to the additional energy expended on processing absorbed material for detoxification, metabolism and storage.
D. True   Mainly because of the energy required to deaminate amino acids.
E. False   The figures are around 4 per cent for fat and 6 per cent for carbohydrate.

220.

A. True   Cells in the pylorus release gastrin when food enters the stomach.
B. False   Venous blood pH rises as bicarbonate enters the circulation in the 'alkaline tide'.
C. True   Vagal activity plays an important role in gastric juice secretion.
D. False   Pancreatic trypsin and chymotrypsin can digest proteins.
E. True   Without gastric 'intrinsic factor', Vitamin B_{12} is not absorbed from the gut.

221.

A. True   Being proteins, enzymes are digested by proteolytic enzymes as they pass down the gut.
B. False   It is absorbed mainly in the terminal ileum.
C. True   Water is absorbed passively down the osmotic gradient set up by active sodium and glucose absorption.
D. False   It occurs mainly in the duodenum.
E. True   Sodium is required at the luminal surface for glucose to be absorbed by an active carrier-mediated process.

222.

A. True   When blood glucose falls, liver glycogen is broken down to form glucose; when glucose levels rise above normal, glucose is taken up by the liver and stored as liver glycogen.
B. False   The NH_4^+ is converted into urea and excreted in the urine; NH_4^+ is toxic.
C. False   Cholecalciferol in produced in skin by the action of sunlight; the liver converts it to 25-hydroxycholecalciferol and the kidney completes its activation by further hydroxylation.
D. False   They manufacture most of the plasma proteins but lymphocytes manufacture immune globulins.
E. True   The failure to inactivate oestrogens in men with liver failure can lead to breast enlargement.

Questions 223–228

223. Absorption of dietary fat
A. Can only occur after the neutral fat has been split into glycerol and fatty acids.
B. Involves fat uptake by both the lymphatic and blood capillaries.
C. Is impaired following gastrectomy.
D. Is required for normal bone development.
E. Is required for normal blood clotting.

224. One gram of
A. Carbohydrate, metabolized in the body, yields the same energy as when oxidized in a bomb calorimeter.
B. Fat, metabolized in the body, yields 10 per cent more energy than 1g of carbohydrate.
C. Protein, metabolized in the body, yields the same energy as when oxidized in a bomb calorimeter.
D. Carbohydrate, metabolized in the body, yields about the same energy as 1g of protein.
E. Protein per kg body weight is an adequate daily protein intake for a sedentary adult.

225. Cholesterol
A. Can be absorbed from the gut by intestinal lymphatics following its incorporation into chylomicrons.
B. Can be synthesized in the liver.
C. In the diet comes mainly from vegetable sources.
D. Is eliminated from the body mainly by metabolic degradation.
E. Is a precursor of adrenal cortical hormones.

226. Free (non-esterified) fatty acids in plasma
A. Account for less than 10 per cent of the total fatty acids in plasma.
B. Are complexed with the plasma proteins.
C. Decrease when the level of blood adrenaline rises.
D. Can be metabolized to release energy in cardiac and skeletal muscle.
E. Can be metabolized to release energy in the brain.

227. The risk of developing gallstones increases
A. When cholesterol micelles are formed in the gall bladder.
B. As the bile salt:cholesterol ratio increases.
C. As the lecithin:cholesterol ratio increases.
D. When supplementary bile salts are taken by mouth.
E. In patients with haemolytic anaemia.

228. Modifying gastric function
A. By cutting vagal fibres to the pylorus increases the emptying rate.
B. By enlarging the pyloric orifice increases the emptying rate.
C. By making a side-to-side anastomosis between the stomach and jejunum may cause peptic ulceration in the jejeunum.
D. To allow rapid gastric emptying may lead to low blood glucose levels after a meal.
E. To allow rapid gastric emptying may lead to a fall in blood volume and blood pressure after a large meal.

Answers

223.

A.   False   Unsplit neutral fat can be absorbed if emulsified into sufficiently small particles.

B.   True   The smaller fatty acids pass directly into blood; the larger ones are esterified, packaged into chylomicrons and taken into lymphatics.

C.   True   The loss of gastric storage capacity results in rapid transit of food through the small intestine and insufficient time for complete digestion and absorption of fat.

D.   True   Vitamin D is required for normal bone development; it is a fat-soluble vitamin and absorbed along with the fat.

E.   True   Vitamin K which is needed for the synthesis of certain clotting factors in the liver is also a fat-soluble vitamin.

224.

A.   True   In both cases the carbohydrate is oxidized to carbon dioxide and water.

B.   False   Fat yields approximately 125 per cent more energy.

C.   False   It yields about 40 per cent less when metabolized in the body, urea derived from protein is excreted in the urine and its free energy is not released to the body.

D.   True   The free energy released by carbohydrate and protein in the body is similar.

E.   True   This is probably a high figure; protein requirements increase with increasing levels of energy expenditure.

225.

A.   True   Most of it is incorporated into very low density lipoproteins(VLDL) and circulates as such.

B.   True   Its synthesis is determined mainly by saturated fat intake.

C.   False   The main sources are egg yolk and animal fat.

D.   False   It is eliminated mainly by excretion in the bile.

E.   True   It is a precursor of a number of steroid hormones.

226.

A.   True   Most are esterified to glycerol and cholesterol.

B.   True   This is necessary for solubility.

C.   False   They rise due to release from adipose tissue.

D.   True   They are an important source of energy for contraction.

E.   False   Glucose is the only normal substrate for energy production here.

227.

A.   False   This is a vital solubilizing mechanism.

B.   False   This favours formation of micelles.

C.   False   Lecithin also contributes to the formation of micelles.

D.   False   This can decrease the risk temporarily.

E.   True   Excess bilirubin can give rise to pigment stones.

228.

A.   False   Emptying is slowed as vagal coordination of gastric motility is lost.

B.   True   This may compensate for the slowing effects of vagotomy.

C.   True   Acid-pepsin can cause a jejunal stomal ulcer.

D.   True   Rapid glucose absorption leads to excessive insulin secretion and a consequent fall in blood glucose.

E.   True   This is a further feature of the 'dumping syndrome'. The sudden arrival of osmotically active particles in the intestine draws extracellular fluid into the gut.

Questions 229–234

229. Impaired intestinal absorption of
A. Iron occurs frequently following removal of most of the stomach.
B. Iodide leads to a reduction in size of the thyroid gland.
C. Water occurs in infants who cannot digest disaccharides.
D. Calcium may occur following removal of the terminal ileum.
E. Bile salts may occur following removal of the terminal ileum.

230. Peptic ulcer pain is typically relieved by
A. Raising the pH of the fluid bathing the ulcer.
B. Oral administration of sodium bicarbonate.
C. Oral administration of a non-absorbable antacid.
D. A drug which interferes with the action of acetylcholinesterase.
E. A drug which blocks the gastric proton pump.

231. Fat stores in the adult
A. Make up less than 5 per cent of average body weight.
B. Make up a smaller percentage of body weight in women than in men.
C. Release fatty acids when there is increased sympathetic nerve activity.
D. Release fatty acids when insulin is injected.
E. Enlarge by increasing the number of adipocytes they contain.

232. Metabolic rate can be estimated from measurements of
A. Total heat production.
B. The calorific value of the food consumed in the previous 24 hours.
C. Oxygen consumption provided the type of food being metabolized is known.
D. Oxygen consumption and the respiratory quotient.
E. Carbon dioxide production and the respiratory quotient.

233. Intestinal obstruction causes
A. Constipation.
B. Crampy pain due to intermittent vigorous peristalsis.
C. Distension due to fluid and gas proximal to the obstruction.
D. Hypotension.
E. Vomiting which is more severe with low than with high bowel obstruction.

234. The cause of jaundice is likely to be
A. Liver disease, if albumin is low and bilirubin mainly unconjugated.
B. Bile duct obstruction, if the urine is paler than normal.
C. Haemolysis, if the prothrombin level is below normal.
D. Haemolysis, if the urine is darker than normal.
E. A post-hepatic cause, if the bilirubin level in the blood is high.

Answers

229.

A. **True**   Due to loss of gastric acid which reduces ferric to the ferrous iron, the form in which it is absorbed. Another problem affecting iron absorption is rapid intestinal transit.

B. **False**   The size increases to cause 'goitre' due to increased TSH stimulation.

C. **True**   The unabsorbed disaccharides such as lactose cause osmotic diarrhoea.

D. **False**   Calcium is absorbed mainly in the duodenum.

E. **True**   The terminal ileum is the main site of bile salt absorption.

230.

A. **True**   Acid is the cause of pain in these ulcers.

B. **True**   But this is absorbed and may cause alkalosis.

C. **True**   This also reduces acidity, but for a short time only.

D. **False**   This would increase vagal acid production.

E. **True**   This can give long lasting relief.

231.

A. **False**   The normal value is around 15–20 per cent.

B. **False**   Fat, as a percentage of body weight, is 5–10 per cent higher in women than in men.

C. **True**   This is mediated via beta adrenergic receptor stimulation.

D. **False**   Insulin favours deposition of fat in the fat stores.

E. **False**   In obesity, adipocytes increase in size rather than number.

232.

A. **True**   Total energy expenditure must eventually appear as heat.

B. **False**   Energy production is related to the metabolism of food, not its intake.

C. **True**   Since oxygen is consumed only in metabolism, total oxygen consumption is an index of metabolic rate; the energy produced per unit of oxygen consumed varies somewhat with different substrates.

D. **True**   Respiratory quotient indicates the mix of substrates used.

E. **True**   Metabolic rate is proportional to carbon dioxide formation.

233.

A. **True**   This is complete when the bowel below the block is empty.

B. **True**   Intermittent colic is typical of early obstruction.

C. **True**   This may be severe when the obstruction is in the lower gut.

D. **True**   Due to hypovolaemia as secretions accumulate in the lumen of the intestines above the obstruction.

E. **False**   Vomiting is worse with high obstruction since the copious upper alimentary secretions cannot be absorbed from the intestines below the obstruction where most absorption normally takes place.

234.

A. **True**   Both indicate impairment of liver function.

B. **False**   Urine is dark in jaundice due to bile duct obstructions since conjugated bilirubin can pass the glomerular filter.

C. **False**   A low prothrombin suggests impaired liver function.

D. **False**   Haemolysis raises the level of unconjugated bilirubin which is protein-bound and not excreted in the urine (acholuric jaundice).

E. **False**   It is high with all causes of jaundice.

Questions 235–241

235. Complications that may arise after total gastrectomy include
A. Inadequate food intake.
B. Depletion of vitamin B_{12} stores in the liver.
C. Malabsorption of fat due to rapid intestinal transit.
D. Impaired defaecation due to loss of the gastrocolic reflex.
E. Inability to digest protein.

236. Severe diarrhoea causes a decrease in
A. Body potassium.
B. Body sodium.
C. Extracellular fluid volume.
D. Total peripheral resistance.
E. Blood pH.

237. Diminished liver function may result in an increase in the
A. Albumin to globulin ratio in the blood.
B. Size of male breasts.
C. Level of unconjugated bilirubin in the blood.
D. Tendency to bleed.
E. Variability of the blood glucose level.

238. Peptic ulceration tends to heal after
A. Division of the vagal nerve supply to the stomach.
B. Surgical removal of the pyloric antrum.
C. Glucocorticoid drug treatment.
D. Elimination of the bacterium *Helicobacter pylori* from the stomach.
E. Treatment with histamine H_2 blocking drugs.

239. Urobilinogen is
A. A mixture of colourless compounds also known as stercobilinogen.
B. Formed in the reticuloendothelial system from bilirubin.
C. Converted into the dark pigment, urobilin, on exposure to air.
D. Absorbed from the intestine.
E. Excreted mainly in the urine.

240. Surgical removal of 90 per cent of the small intestine may cause a decrease in
A. The fat content of the stools.
B. Bone mineralization (osteomalacia).
C. Extracellular fluid volume.
D. Blood haemoglobin level.
E. Body weight.

241. Lack of pancreatic juice in the duodenum may lead to
A. The presence of undigested meat fibres in the stools.
B. An increase in the fat content of the faeces.
C. Faeces with a high specific gravity.
D. A tendency for the faeces to putrefy.
E. A high prothrombin level in blood.

Answers

235.

A. True   Due to loss of the 'reservoir' function of the stomach.
B. True   Due to loss of gastric 'intrinsic factor', required for absorption of the vitamin.
C. True   The mechanism regulating food delivery to the small intestine is lost.
D. False   This 'reflex' is not essential for defaecation.
E. False   Pancreatic enzymes can make up for the loss of pepsin.

236.

A. True   Due to loss of secretions rich in potassium.
B. True   Sodium is the main cation lost in diarrhoea.
C. True   Body sodium is the 'skeleton' of extracellular fluid volume.
D. False   This is raised to maintain arterial blood pressure as plasma volume falls.
E. True   Loss of intestinal bicarbonate causes metabolic acidosis.

237.

A. False   Albumin, which is manufactured in the liver tends to fall relative to globulin in plasma.
B. True   Due to loss of the liver's ability to conjugate oestrogens and progestogens.
C. True   The liver normally conjugates bilirubin with glucuronic acid.
D. True   Due to reduced synthesis of clotting factors such as prothrombin by the liver.
E. True   Due to the liver's reduced ability to store and mobilize glycogen.

238.

A. True   This reduces gastric acidity.
B. True   Gastrin which stimulates acid secretion is produced in the pyloric antrum.
C. False   Glucocorticoids by inhibiting tissue repair may make the ulceration worse.
D. True   This bacterium appears to play an important part in the pathogenesis of peptic ulcers.
E. True   These reduce acidity and are widely used in the treatment of peptic ulceration.

239.

A. True   It is present in both urine and faeces.
B. False   It is formed in the intestine.
C. True   Urine rich in urobilinogen (due to haemolysis) darkens on exposure to light.
D. True   And carried back to the liver in the enterohepatic circulation.
E. False   It is excreted mainly in the bile.

240.

A. False   Fat absorption is incomplete and this causes steatorrhoea.
B. True   There is poor absorption of fat-soluble vitamin D.
C. False   Adequate salt and water absorption still occur.
D. True   Vitamin B_{12} and iron absorption are impaired and this may cause anaemia.
E. True   Due to the malabsorption of food.

241.

A. True   Due to lack of the proteinases trypsin and chymotrypsin.
B. True   Due to impaired fat digestion and absorption caused by lack of pancreatic lipase.
C. False   A high fat content lowers specific gravity; stools may float.
D. True   Due to the high level of nutrients in the faeces, bacteria flourish.
E. False   It is reduced; malabsorption of fat reduces absorption of fat-soluble vitamin K that is needed for prothrombin production.

Questions 242–247

242. In liver failure there is likely to be

A. Salt and water retention.
B. Oedema in dependent extremities such as the feet and ankles.
C. Raised blood urea.
D. Impaired absorption of fat.
E. Intoxication after eating a high protein meal.

243. Gastric

A. Acid secretion in response to a lowered blood sugar is mediated by the hormone gastrin.
B. Emptying is facilitated by sympathetic nerve activity.
C. Acid secretion increases when histamine H_2, muscarinic M_1 or gastrin receptors are activated.
D. Acid secretion is inhibited by the presence of food in the duodenum.
E. Contraction waves pass over the stomach at a rate of about ten per minute.

244. In portal hypertension

A. The total vascular resistance of the hepatic sinusoids is increased.
B. Portal blood flow through the liver is increased.
C. The volume of fluid in the peritoneal cavity increases.
D. A porto-caval shunt (anastomosis between portal vein and inferior vena cava) can decrease the tendency to bleed into the alimentary tract.
E. A porto-caval shunt increases the risk of coma after bleeding into the alimentary tract.

245. Constipation is a recognized consequence of

A. Sensory denervation of the rectum.
B. Psychological stress.
C. Abnormality of the autonomic nerve supply to the colon.
D. A diet that leaves little unabsorbed residue in the gut.
E. Over-activity of the thyroid gland as in thyrotoxicosis.

246. Absorption of glucose by intestinal mucosal cells

A. Relies on a carrier mechanism in the cell membrane.
B. Is blocked by the same agents that block renal reabsorption of glucose.
C. Is enhanced by blockade of active sodium transport in the cells.
D. Involves the same carriers that are used for the absorption of galactose.
E. Takes place mainly in the ileum.

247. Vomiting

A. Is caused by violent rhythmic contractions of gut smooth muscle.
B. Is coordinated by a vomiting centre in the mid brain.
C. Of green fluid suggests that duodenal contents have regurgitated into the stomach.
D. May be accompanied by a fall in arterial blood pressure.
E. Is more marked in low intestinal obstruction than in high intestinal obstruction.

MCQ

Answers

242.
A. True   Due in part to the liver's failure to conjugate salt-retaining hormones such as aldosterone.
B. True   Due to the above plus depletion of plasma albumin.
C. False   It falls due to impaired urea synthesis from NH_4^+ released in deamination.
D. True   Due to impaired formation and excretion of bile salts.
E. True   Due to inadequate detoxification of toxins derived from proteins in the diet.

243.
A. False   It is mediated through a vagal reflex and is absent in vagotomized stomachs.
B. False   This delays gastric emptying.
C. True   Histamine from mast-like cells activates H_2 receptors, acetylcholine from parasympathetic nerve endings activates M_1 receptors and gastrin activates gastrin receptors.
D. True   The neural/hormonal mechanisms responsible for the inhibition are not certain.
E. False   The normal rate is around 3/minute.

244.
A. True   This is the cause of the hypertension.
B. False   It is decreased as blood is diverted to alternative routes back to the great veins.
C. True   Raised hydrostatic pressure increases filtration from visceral capillaries; fluid accumulates in the peritoneal cavity to cause ascites.
D. True   By diverting blood away from oesophageal varices.
E. True   The failure of the liver to detoxicate toxic end-products of protein metabolism in liver failure can lead to hepatic encephalopathy; bypassing the liver with a portocaval shunt may aggravate the condition, especially after an intestinal bleed.

245.
A. True   This breaks the reflex arc on which defaecation depends.
B. True   Stress may modify the reflex to cause either constipation or diarrhoea.
C. True   In children this may cause megacolon.
D. True   Frequency of defaecation is related to the bulk of food residues.
E. False   This leads to increased frequency of defaecation.

246.
A. True   This facilitates transport from the lumen.
B. True   Phloridzin has this action; the carrier mechanisms at the two sites are similar.
C. False   It is impaired, suggesting that sodium absorption facilitates glucose absorption.
D. True   But different carriers are involved in fructose absorption.
E. False   It takes place mainly in the duodenum and jejunum.

247.
A. False   Forced expiratory efforts by skeletal muscles in the presence of a closed glottis and pylorus are responsible for compressing the stomach.
B. False   It is coordinated by a vomiting centre in the medulla oblongata.
C. True   Bile pigments enter the gut in the duodenum.
D. True   This is one of several types of associated autonomic disturbance.
E. False   It is more marked in high obstruction because the copious digestive secretion cannot be absorbed by the gut below the obstruction.

Questions 248–249

248. Obesity

A. Is unlikely to occur on a high protein diet even if the calorific value of the food exceeds daily energy expenditure.
B. Is associated with increased demands on pancreatic islet beta cells.
C. Can be assessed by multiple measurements of skin fold thickness.
D. Can be assessed by weighing the body in air and in water.
E. Is not diagnosed until body weight is 40 per cent above normal.

249. Muscle tone in the lower oesophagus is

A. Greater than tone in the middle oesophagus.
B. A major factor in preventing heartburn.
C. Increased in pregnancy.
D. Increased by gastrin.
E. Increased by anticholinergic drugs

MCQ

Answers

248.

A. False   If food energy intake exceeds energy expenditure, obesity develops regardless of the predominant food in the diet.

B. True   Mild maturity-onset diabetes mellitus may be relieved by decreasing body weight.

C. True   Subcutaneous fat is a good indicator of the severity of obesity.

D. True   Body specific gravity which is inversely related to body fat content can be calculated from these values.

E. False   The conventional threshold is 10 per cent.

249.

A. True   The high-pressure zone indicates the 'cardiac sphincter'.

B. True   It prevents reflux of acid into the oesophagus.

C. False   It is decreased and heartburn is common in pregnancy.

D. True   This prevents reflux during gastric contractions.

E. False   These reduce tone, suggesting that cholinergic nerves have a role in maintaining normal tone.

EMQs

Questions 250–260

EMQ Question 250

For each of the absorptive functions A–E, select the most appropriate absorption site from the following list of alimentary tract sites.

    1. Stomach.
    2. Upper small intestine.
    3. Lower small intestine.
    4. Colon.
    5. Rectum.

A.   The site where most of the intestinal water is absorbed.
B.   The site where most of the intestinal sodium is absorbed.
C.   The main site of iron absorption.
D.   The main site of Vitamin B_{12} absorption.
E.   The main site of bile salt absorption.

EMQ Question 251

For each of the digestive functions A–E, select the most appropriate digestive secretion from the following list of secretions.

    1. Salivary secretion.
    2. Gastric secretion.
    3. Pancreatic secretion.
    4. Bile.
    5. Intestinal secretion.

A.   Splitting disaccharides.
B.   Splitting triglycerides.
C.   Absorption of vitamin B_{12}.
D.   Emulsification of fat.
E.   Digestion of nucleic acids.

EMQ Question 252

For each of the examples of intestinal motility A–E, select the most appropriate stimulus from the following list of stimuli:

    1. Release of CCK-PZ.
    2. Distension of the viscus wall.
    3. Release of secretin.
    4. Release of gastrin.
    5. Sympathetic nerve activity.

A.   Gastro-colic reflex.
B.   Receptive relaxation.
C.   Peristalsis.
D.   Contraction of the cardiac (oesophogeal-gastric) sphincter.
E.   Contraction of the gallbladder.

Answers for 250

A. **Option 2**   *Upper small intestine.* About four fifths of intestinal water is absorbed by the osmotic gradient created by glucose and sodium absorption in the small intestine, the remaining fifth is absorbed in the colon.

B. **Option 2**   *Upper small intestine.* Most sodium is absorbed by active transport in the upper small intestine but some is also absorbed in the lower small intestine and in the colon.

C. **Option 2**   *Upper small intestine.* Iron is absorbed in the ferrous state using an intra-cellular iron carrier mainly in the upper small intestine but some is also absorbed in the lower small intestine.

D. **Option 3**   *Lower small intestine.* Vitamin B_{12} is absorbed complexed with intrinsic factor in the terminal ileum.

E. **Option 3**   *Lower small intestine.* Like Vitamin B_{12}, bile salts are reabsorbed in the lower small intestine to be returned to the liver as part of the enterohepatic circulation.

Answers for 251

A. **Option 5**   *Intestinal secretion.* Intestinal juice contains the enzymes maltase, lactase and sucrase that split maltose, lactose and sucrose respectively.

B. **Option 3**   *Pancreatic secretion.* Pancreatic lipase splits neutral fat into glycerol and fatty acids.

C. **Option 2**   *Gastric secretion.* Gastric juice contains the intrinsic factor needed for the absorption of Vitamin B_{12}.

D. **Option 4**   *Bile.* Bile salts help to emulsify fat so that the fat droplets offer a large sur-face area to the action of lipases.

E. **Option 3**   *Pancreatic secretion.* Nucleic acids are split by pancreatic nucleases in the small intestine.

Answers for 252

A. **Option 2**   *Distension of the viscus wall.* For this reflex, the distension of the stomach wall following ingestion of a meal is thought to stimulate colonic motility that results in defaecation.

B. **Option 2**   *Distension of the viscus wall.* When food is ingested, the smooth muscle in the stomach wall relaxes so that the added bulk can be accommodated without much increase in intragastric pressure.

C. **Option 2**   *Distension of the viscus wall.* When a bolus of food distends a hollow viscus it sets up a wave of contraction preceded by a wave of relaxation that carries the bolus along the viscus. Though peristalsis can be modified by autonomic nerves, the mechanism is based on local nerve networks in the wall of the viscus.

D. **Option 4**   *Release of gastrin.* Gastrin secreted in response to a meal increases tone in the cardiac sphincter and so prevents regurgitation of gastric contents into the oesopha-gus during stomach contractions.

E. **Option 5**   *Release of CCK-PZ.* CCK-PZ released from the bowel wall when fat enters the duodenum causes the gall bladder to contract to empty its contents into the second part of the duodenum. It also inhibits gastric emptying.

EMQ Question 253

For each of the structures and substances found in the alimentary tract A–E, select the most appropriate function from the list below.

1. Fat transport.
2. Secrete alkaline mucus.
3. Activates enzymes in pancreatic secretion.
4. Secrete serotonin.
5. Ingest bacteria.

A. Enterochromaffin cells.
B. Brunner's glands.
C. Micelles.
D. Kupffer cells.
E. Enterokinase.

EMQ Question 254

For each of the digestive functions A–E, select the most appropriate digestive enzymes from the following list of enzymes.

1. Rennin.
2. Endopeptidases.
3. Sucrase.
4. Alpha-amylase.
5. Deoxyribonuclease.

A. Acts on protein to produce polypeptides and amino acids.
B. Acts on DNA to produce nucleotides.
C. Acts on a disaccharide to produce fructose and glucose.
D. Acts on starch to produce dextrins and maltose.
E. Acts on milk to produce a clot.

EMQ Question 255

For each of the absorptive functions A–E, select the most appropriate co-factor(s) required for absorption from the list below.

1. A sodium dependent carrier system.
2. Apoferritin.
3. Vitamin D.
4. Intrinsic factor.
5. Bile salts.

A. Fat absorption.
B. Iron absorption.
C. Glucose absorption.
D. Calcium absorption.
E. Vitamin B_{12} absorption.

Answers for 253

A. **Option 4.**   *Secrete serotonin.* Certain duodenal cells called enterochromaffin cells contain serotonin and the polypeptide 'motilin' that are thought to influence smooth muscle motility in the gut.

B. **Option 2**   *Secrete alkaline mucus.* Brunner's glands in the duodenum secrete a thick alkaline mucus that protects the duodenal mucosa against acid when gastric juice enters the duodenum.

C. **Option 1**   *Fat transport.* Micelles are complexes of lipids and bile salts. The complexes are water-soluble and this aids their take up by the enterocytes lining the intestinal mucosa.

D. **Option 5**   *Ingest bacteria.* Kupffer cells are macrophages in the capillary sinusoids of the liver; when they are deficient due to liver disease there is increased risk of organisms passing from the gut to the systemic circulation via the portal circulation.

E. **Option 3**   *Activates enzymes in pancreatic secretion.* Trypsinogen is a proenzyme secreted by the pancreas that is activated in the lumen of the small intestine by the enzyme enterokinase secreted by the intestinal mucosa.

Answers for 254

A. **Option 2**   *Endopeptidases.* Secreted by the pancreas in an inactive form, the endopeptidases that include trypsin, chymotrypsin and elastase split the peptide bonds in polypeptides.

B. **Option 5**   *Deoxyribonuclease.* RNA is split by ribonuclease.

C. **Option 3**   *Sucrase.* Two other disaccharidases present in intestinal secretions, lactase and maltase, split lactose and maltose into galactose and glucose and glucose and glucose respectively.

D. **Option 4**   *Alpha-amylase.* Alpha amylase is produced by the salivary glands as well as by the pancreas.

E. **Option 1**   *Rennin.* Found in the gastric juice of infants, rennin aids in milk digestion by causing it to clot and slow its passage out of the stomach.

Answers for 255

A. **Option 5**   *Bile salts.* Bile salts aid fat absorption by helping to emulsify the fat into very small globules which present a large surface area that can be attacked by pancreatic lipase. They then form part of the micelles that fit neatly between the microvilli of the enterocytes.

B. **Option 2**   *Apoferritin.* Apoferritin is an intracellular carrier that carries the iron molecules from the mucosal surface of the enterocytes to the inner surface where it is delivered to the carrier molecule, transferrin, in the plasma.

C. **Option 1**   *A sodium dependent carrier system.* The co-transporter molecule for glucose is called SGLT (sodium dependent glucose transporter).

D. **Option 3**   *Vitamin D.* In Vitamin D deficiency, calcium is not taken up by the intestinal mucosa. This results in weakening of the bones as in rickets and osteomalacia.

E. **Option 4**   *Intrinsic factor.* Vitamin B_{12} has to be complexed with intrinsic factor in gastric juice before it can be absorbed from the gut.

EMQ Question 256

For each of the deficiencies of digestive secretions A–E, select the most appropriate consequence from the list below.

1. Pale stools.
2. Local infections.
3. Steatorrhoea.
4. Milk intolerance.
5. Anaemia.

A. Saliva deficiency.
B. Biliary obstruction.
C. Lactase deficiency.
D. Pancreatic juice deficiency.
E. Gastric juice deficiency.

EMQ Question 257

For each of the factors affecting intestinal activity A–E, select the most appropriate response from the list below.

1. Inhibition of gastric secretion.
2. Stimulation of gastric secretion.
3. Increase in gastric motility.
4. Decrease in gastric motility.
5. Gall bladder contraction.

A. CCK-PZ.
B. Fat in the duodenum.
C. Pentagastrin.
D. Blockade of H_2 receptors.
E. Adrenaline injection.

EMQ Question 258

For each of the structures in the alimentary tract A–E, select the most appropriate option from the list below.

1. Controls entry of bile into the intestine.
2. Fat absorption.
3. Glucose absorption.
4. Secretion of gastric acid.
5. Lymphoid aggregations in the intestines involved with immunity.

Intestinal structures

A. Lacteals.
B. Brush border.
C. Oxyntic cells.
D. Sphincter of Oddi.
E. Peyer's patches.

Answers to 256

A. **Option 2**   *Local infections.* The flow of saliva helps to control the multiplication of bacteria in the mouth.

B. **Option 1**   *Pale stools.* Bile entering the alimentary tract is responsible for the normal brown colour of the stools.

C. **Option 4**   *Milk intolerance.* Lactase deficiency is seen in a proportion of the population. There is an inability to digest and absorb milk sugar. This results in an osmotic diarrhoea that can be a problem especially in babies where milk forms a large part of the dietary intake.

D. **Option 3**   *Steatorrhoea.* Steatorrhoea, the presence of unsplit fat in the faeces, is seen in the absence of pancreatic juice since dietary fat cannot be hydrolysed and consequently cannot be absorbed.

E. **Option 5**   *Anaemia.* A macrocytic anaemia develops because there is no intrinsic factor to facilitate the absorption of Vitamin B_{12}.

Answers for 257

A. **Option 5**   *Gallbladder contraction.* CCK, produced by the mucosal cells in the duodenal wall when fat or other nutrients enter that part of the gut, travels in the blood to the gall bladder so that the bile contents are sent to the duodenum to help in the digestion and absorption of fat.

B. **Option 4**   *Decrease in gastric motility.* Fat in the duodenum slows the transit of gastric contents into the small gut and so slows and delays the digestion of the gastric contents.

C. **Option 2**   *Stimulation of gastric secretion.* Pentagastrin is a pharmacological product containing five of the amino acids in gastrin that can act like gastrin to stimulate gastric secretion. It is used to test the functional efficiency of the gastric mucosa to secrete gastric juice.

D. **Option 1**   *Inhibition of gastric secretion.* Histamine is the neurotransmitter at vagal nerve endings in the stomach and acts on H_2 receptors. Thus H_2 receptor blockers can reduce acid secretion by the gastric mucosa.

E. **Option 4**   *Decrease in gastric motility.* Adrenaline and similar adrenergic agents cause intestinal smooth muscle to relax.

Answers for 258

A. **Option 2**   *Fat absorption.* Most of the absorbed fat is taken up directly by lacteals, so called for their white colour following a fatty meal due to the fat globules in the lymph.

B. **Option 3**   *Glucose absorption.* The brush border that is characteristic of the luminal surface of enterocytes is made up of tiny microvilli protruding into the lumen of the gut and offering a huge surface area for absorption of the products of digestion.

C. **Option 4**   *Secretion of gastric acid.* These cells, sometimes also called parietal cells, are found in the mucosa of the body and fundus of the stomach and are responsible for HCl secretion.

D. **Option 1**   *Controls entry of bile into the intestine.* The sphincter of Oddi lies in the second part of the duodenum where the bile duct and the pancreatic ducts meet and controls the flow of bile and pancreatic secretions into the duodenum.

E. **Option 5**   *Lymphoid aggregations in the intestines involved with immunity.* These patches are composed of lymphoid tissue and are responsible for immune reactions and responses in the gut.

EMQ Question 259

For each of the surgical interventions (-ectomy means removal) carried out on the alimentary tract A–E, select the most appropriate possible consequence from the list below.

    1. No digestive consequences.   2. Bulky liquid stools.
    3. Dumping syndrome.   4. Steatorrhoea.
    5. Indigestion after fatty meals.

A.   Gastrectomy.
B.   Pancreatectomy.
C.   Colectomy.
D.   Cholecystectomy.
E.   Appendicectomy.

EMQ Question 260

For each of polypeptides secreted by the enteric nervous system in the alimentary tract A–E, select the most appropriate effect on the gut from the list below.

    1. Release of gastrin.   2. Relaxation of sphincters.
    3. Increase in small intestinal motility.   4. Inhibition of gut motility.
    5. Inhibition of gastric emptying.

A.   VIP.
B.   CCK-PZ.
C.   Somatostatin.
D.   Substance P.
E.   GRP.

Answers for 259

A. **Option 3** *Dumping syndrome.* When the stomach is removed, ingested food passes very rapidly to the small intestine and can lead to the unpleasant consequences of fluid loss to the intestinal lumen and excessive insulin secretion. The syndrome is called the 'dumping syndrome'.

B. **Option 4** *Steatorrhoea.* This may be seen following pancreatectomy because lack of lipase allows undigested fat to appear in the faeces.

C. **Option 2** *Bulky liquid stools.* Removal of the colon limits the ability of the alimentary tract to reabsorb water and this results in the passage of watery stools.

D. **Option 5** *Indigestion after fatty meals.* The loss of the gall bladder's ability to send bile to the duodenum after a fatty meal results in poor digestion and absorption of the meal and hence abdominal discomfort.

E. **Option 1** *No digestive consequences.* The appendix has no known function other than as a lymphoid organ and its immune function can be taken over by other lymphoid tissue in the intestines.

Answers for 260

A. **Option 2** *Relaxation of sphincters.* Vasoactive intestinal polypeptide (VIP) also causes vasodilatation by relaxing vascular smooth muscle.

B. **Option 5** *Inhibition of gastric emptying.* Besides its main action of stimulating the gall bladder to contract, cholecystokinin (CCK) decreases the rate of emptying of the stomach.

C. **Option 4** *Inhibition of gut motility.* Somatostatin, the growth hormone-inhibiting hormone, originally isolated in the hypothalamus, is secreted by D cells in the intestinal mucosa. It inhibits the release of several gut hormones including motilin and so inhibits gut motility.

D. **Option 3** *Increase in small intestinal motility.* Substance P, a polypeptide found in intestinal mucosal endocrine cells, acts locally to increase gut motility.

E. **Option 1** *Release of gastrin.* Gastrin-releasing polypeptide (GRP) is released by the postganglionic vagal fibres that innervate the G cells in the lateral walls of the glands in the pyloric antrum. Activity in these nerves causes release of the gastrin granules in the G cells.

MCQs

Questions 261–266

261. A reflex action
A. Is initiated at a sensory receptor organ.
B. May result in endocrine secretion.
C. Involves transmission across at least two central nervous synapses in series.
D. May be excitatory or inhibitory.
E. Is independent of higher centres in the brain.

262. In skeletal muscle neuromuscular junctions
A. The motor end plate is the motor nerve terminal.
B. Spontaneous (miniature) potentials may be recorded in the motor nerve terminal.
C. Motor nerve terminals have vesicles containing acetylcholine.
D. There is a high concentration of acetylcholinesterase.
E. Transmission is facilitated by botulinum toxin.

263. Cerebrospinal fluid
A. Is formed in the arachnoid granulations.
B. Provides the brain with most of its nutrition.
C. Protects the brain from injury when the head is moved.
D. Has a lower pressure than that in the cerebral venous sinuses.
E. Flow around the adult brain is around half a litre per day.

264. A skeletal muscle fibre
A. Membrane is negatively charged on the inside with respect to the outside at rest.
B. Contains intracellular stores of calcium ions.
C. Is normally innervated by more than one motor neurone.
D. Becomes more excitable as its resting membrane potential falls.
E. Becomes less excitable as the extracellular ionized calcium levels fall.

265. In sensory receptors
A. Stimulus energy is converted into a local depolarization.
B. The generator potential is graded and self-propagating.
C. A generator potential can be produced by only one form of energy.
D. The frequency of action potentials generated doubles when the strength of the stimulus doubles.
E. Serving touch sensation, constant suprathreshold stimulation causes action potentials to be generated at a constant rate.

266. A somatic lower motor neurone
A. Innervates fewer fibres in an eye muscle than does one innervating a leg muscle.
B. Conducts impulses at a speed similar to that in an autonomic postganglionic neurone.
C. Is unmyelinated.
D. Conducts impulses which cause relaxation in some skeletal muscles.
E. Synapse with skeletal muscle but not with other neurones.

Answers

261.

A. True   Stimulation of the receptor generates impulses in the afferent limb.
B. True   Stimulation of osmoreceptors reflexly modifies ADH output from the posterior pituitary gland.
C. False   The knee jerk reflex arc contains only one central nervous synapse.
D. True   In the knee jerk extensors of the knee contract, while flexors relax (reciprocal inhibition).
E. False   Higher centres can facilitate or inhibit many reflex actions such as micturition.

262.

A. False   It is the modified muscle membrane adjacent to the nerve terminal.
B. False   They may be recorded at the motor end plate.
C. True   This neurotransmitter, released by exocytosis, excites the end plate membrane.
D. True   This makes acetylcholine's action transient.
E. False   Botulinum toxin blocks transmission by an action on the motor nerve terminals.

263.

A. False   It is formed in choroid plexuses by active and passive processes.
B. False   Most of the brain's nutrition comes from the blood.
C. True   This is its main function and it does so through cushioning and buoyancy.
D. False   Its higher pressure allows drainage by filtration to the dural venous sinuses via the arachnoid villi.
E. True   This is about four times its volume.

264.

A. True   This 'resting membrane potential' is about -90 mV.
B. True   These are released on excitation.
C. False   A single neurone supplies a group of muscle fibres.
D. True   It becomes more excitable as its membrane potential approaches the firing threshold (about -70 mV).
E. False   Decreasing extracellular Ca^{2+} increases excitability and may lead to spontaneous contractions (tetany), possibly by increasing sodium permeability.

265.

A. True   This is the generator potential.
B. False   It is graded but not propagated.
C. False   But sensitivity is greatest to one form of energy – the 'adequate stimulus'.
D. False   Frequency is related to the logarithm of the strength of the stimulus.
E. False   Frequency falls with time due to adaptation.

266.

A. True   The more precise the movement required, the fewer the fibres supplied by one motor neurone.
B. False   Somatic motor neurones conduct at 60–120 m/sec; autonomic at about 1 m/sec.
C. False   Fast-conducting fibres are large and myelinated.
D. False   Impulses carried by somatic motor neurones are excitatory to skeletal muscle.
E. False   Some carry impulses to inhibitory (Renshaw) cells in the anterior horn.

Questions 267–272

267 Impulses serving pain sensation in the left foot are relayed

A. Across synapses in the left posterior root ganglion.
B. By fibres in the left spinothalamic tract.
C. By the same spinal cord tract which serves heat and cold sensation.
D. To the thalamus on the right side.
E. To the cerebral cortex before entering consciousness.

268. An excitatory post-synaptic potential

A. Is the depolarization of a post-synaptic nerve cell membrane that occurs when a pre-synaptic neurone is stimulated.
B. Involves reversal of polarity across the post-synaptic nerve cell membrane.
C. May be recorded from a posterior root ganglion cell.
D. Is propagated at the same rate as an action potential.
E. Is caused by the electrical field induced by activity in the pre-synaptic nerve terminals.

269. The ascending reticular formation

A. When stimulated tends to increase alertness.
B. Transmits impulses to higher centres via a multisynaptic pathway.
C. Is activated by collateral branches of sensory neurones.
D. Neurones project to most parts of the cerebral cortex.
E. Increases its activity during deep sleep.

270. The cerebellum

A. Modifies the discharge of spinal motor neurones.
B. Is essential for finely coordinated movements.
C. Has an afferent input from the motor cortex.
D. Has an afferent input from muscle proprioceptors.
E. Has an afferent input from the vestibular system.

271. During deep sleep there is a fall in

A. Hand skin temperature.
B. Arterial P_{CO_2}.
C. Blood growth hormone/cortisol ratio.
D. Metabolic rate.
E. Urine formation.

272. Sympathetic

A. Ganglionic transmission is mediated by acetylcholine.
B. Neuromuscular transmission at the heart is mediated by adrenaline.
C. Neuromuscular transmission in hand skin arterioles is mediated by acetylcholine.
D. Neuroglandular transmission at sweat glands is mediated by noradrenaline.
E. Neuromuscular transmission at the iris is mediated by noradrenaline.

Answers

267.

A.	False	The ganglion contains sensory cell bodies but no synapses; primary pain fibres carrying these impulses synapse with secondary neurones in the left posterior horn.
B.	False	They cross to the right spinothalamic tract.
C.	True	Pain and temperature fibres travel together.
D.	True	Sensations other than smell are relayed in the thalamus.
E.	False	They enter consciousness at a subcortical level.

268.

A.	True	An inhibitory potential is a hyperpolarization.
B.	False	It is a transient (about 5 msec), small (about 5 mV) depolarization towards the threshold for firing.
C.	False	It may be recorded from a motor neurone.
D.	False	It is not propagated.
E.	False	It is caused by transmitters changing permeability in post-synaptic membranes.

269.

A.	True	Associated with increased electrical activity in cortical regions.
B.	True	Diffuse cortical activity following sensory stimulation occurs later than local postcentral gyrus activity.
C.	True	Sensory fibres ascending to the thalamus send collaterals to reticular nuclei.
D.	True	The diffuse cortical activity following sensory stimulation is abolished by damage to the reticular formation.
E.	False	Decreased activity leads to a higher arousal threshold during sleep.

270.

A.	True	Hence it influences skeletal muscle activity.
B.	True	Damage to it leads to movements being clumsy (ataxia).
C.	True	This provides information of the desired movement.
D.	True	This provides information of the actual movement.
E.	True	It has an important role in maintaining balance.

271.

A.	False	Skin temperature rises due to vasodilation.
B.	False	The level rises due to hypoventilation.
C.	False	Growth hormone level is higher, cortisol lower in sleep.
D.	True	Due to slowing of metabolism and a fall in catecholamine level.
E.	True	The antidiuretic hormone level is higher in sleep.

272.

A.	True	This applies to parasympathetic ganglia also.
B.	False	The transmitter is noradrenaline.
C.	False	The transmitter is noradrenaline here also.
D.	False	These sympathetic fibres are cholinergic.
E.	True	Sympathetic adrenergic fibres innervate radial muscle in the iris; cholinergic parasympathetic fibres innervate the circular muscle.

Questions 273–278

273. The blood–brain barrier
A. Slows equilibration of solutes between blood and brain tissue fluids.
B. Is a more effective barrier for fat-soluble substances than water-soluble substances.
C. Is a more effective barrier in infants than in adults.
D. Is a more effective barrier for CO_2 than for O_2.
D. Permits hydrogen ions to pass freely.

274. Nerve impulses
A. Can travel in one direction only in a nerve fibre.
B. Can travel in one direction only across a synapse.
C. Travel at the speed of an electric current.
D. Correspond in duration to that of the nerve refractory period.
E. Can be transmitted at higher frequencies in autonomic than in somatic nerves.

275. In skeletal muscle
A. Contraction occurs when its pacemaker cells depolarize sufficiently to reach the threshold for firing.
B. Calcium is taken up by the sarcotubular system when it contracts.
C. Actin and myosin filaments shorten when it contracts.
D. The sarcomeres shorten during contraction.
E. Contraction strength is related to initial length of the muscle fibres.

276. The electroencephalogram normally shows voltage waves
A. Whose amplitude is related to intelligence.
B. Of smaller amplitude during deep sleep than during alert wakefulness.
C. Of lower frequency during deep sleep than during alert wakefulness.
D. Of greater amplitude than those of the electrocardiogram.
E. Which are bilaterally symmetrical.

277. Saltatory conduction
A. Occurs only in myelinated fibres.
B. Does not depend on depolarization of the nerve membrane.
C. Has a slower velocity in cold than in warm conditions.
D. Is faster than non-saltatory conduction in nerve fibres with diameters around 10 μm.
E. Transmits impulses with a velocity proportional to fibre diameter.

278. Parasympathetic nerves
A. Have opposite effects to sympathetic nerves on intestinal smooth muscle.
B. Have opposite effects to sympathetic nerves on iris smooth muscle.
C. Cause vasodilatation in skeletal muscle during prolonged exercise.
D. Cause sweat secretion in skin when body temperature rises.
E. Have longer postganglionic than preganglionic fibres.

Answers

273.

A. True   Capillary permeability is lower in the brain than in other tissues.
B. False   Fat-soluble substances cross readily due to the lipid in cell membranes.
C. False   The reverse is true; bilirubin, which cannot pass in the adult, does so in infants.
D. False   Both CO_2 and O_2 cross the blood–brain barrier easily.
E. False   This protects brain tissues against sudden changes in the pH of blood.

274.

A. False   In axons, impulses travel in both directions from a point of electrical stimulation.
B. True   The transmitter vesicles are in the pre-synaptic terminal.
C. False   Impulse propagation is a different process and much slower than electrical current.
D. True   Nerves cannot be re-excited while their membrane polarity is reversed.
E. False   The shorter refractory periods in somatic nerves allow higher frequencies.

275.

A. False   Skeletal muscle has no pacemaker cells and shows no spontaneous activity.
B. False   Calcium is released from intracellular stores when it contracts.
C. False   The filaments do not shorten but slide together over one another.
D. True   There is greater overlap of the actin and myosin fibrils.
E. True   Moderate stretch increases contraction strength as in the heart.

276.

A. False   EEG is no index of intelligence.
B. False   High amplitude waves occur in deep sleep; the reverse is true of wakefulness.
C. True   The high amplitude waves in sleep are of low frequency; the reverse is true of the low amplitude waves in wakefulness.
D. False   EEG voltages are much smaller than ECG voltages.
E. True   Asymmetry is a sign of disease.

277.

A. True   Excitation leaps from node to node across the myelinated segments.
B. False   The membrane does depolarize at the nodes.
C. True   Cooling slows sodium conductance at the nodes.
D. True   Theoretically, saltatory conduction becomes the slower in nerve fibres with diameters less than 1 μm.
E. True   And to the distance between nodes.

278.

A. True   Parasympathetic nerves stimulate, and sympathetic nerves inhibit, intestinal smooth muscle contractions.
B. False   Both contract iris smooth muscle; however parasympathetics constrict the pupil by contracting circular muscle, sympathetics dilate it by contracting radial muscle.
C. False   Skeletal muscle has no parasympathetic nerve supply; local metabolites are responsible for the vasodilatation.
D. False   Skin has no parasympathetic innervation; sympathetic cholinergic nerves are responsible for the increase in sweating when body temperature rises.
E. False   The reverse is the case.

Questions 279–284

279. α (alpha) adrenoceptors

A. Are located on myofilaments in smooth muscle cells.
B. Are distinguishable from β (beta) receptors using electron microscopy.
C. Can be stimulated by both adrenaline and noradrenaline.
D. Are involved in the vasoconstrictor responses in skin to adrenaline.
E. Are involved in the heart rate responses to noradrenaline.

280. Neurones serving conscious muscle proprioception

A. Conduct impulses at a similar rate to somatic motor neurones.
B. Have their cell bodies in the ipsilateral posterior horn of the spinal cord.
C. Use a different pathway from the primary neurones serving unconscious proprioception.
D. Synapse with secondary neurones whose axons project up the ipsilateral posterior (dorsal) columns of the spinal cord.
E. Synapse with neurones which cross the midline of the body in the brainstem.

281. The α (alpha) rhythm of the electroencephalogram

A. Disappears when the eyes are closed.
B. Is an electrical potential with an amplitude around one millivolt.
C. Has a frequency of 8–12 Hz.
D. Has a lower frequency than the δ (delta) rhythm.
E. Indicates that the subject is awake.

282. Nerve fibres continue to conduct impulses when

A. Extracellular sodium is replaced by potassium.
B. Extracellular sodium is replaced by a non-diffusible cation.
C. Temperature is lowered from 37 to 30°C.
D. Temperature is lowered to below 0°C provided freezing does not occur.
E. The sodium-potassium pump is inactivated.

283. The primary sensory ending of a muscle spindle is stimulated by

A. Shortening of an antagonist muscle.
B. Relaxation of the muscle concerned when under load.
C. Shortening of the extrafusal fibres.
D. Stimulation of the gamma efferent fibres.
E. Striking the appropriate tendon with a tendon hammer.

284. In the spinal cord

A. Pain impulse traffic may be modulated in the posterior horn.
B. Autonomic motor neurones arise in the lateral horn.
C. Gamma-aminobutyric acid may act as an excitatory neurotransmitter.
D. Reflex centres are normally inhibited by descending impulses from supra-spinal centres.
E. Post-synaptic excitation may be mediated by amino acid derivatives acting as neuro-transmitters.

MCQ

Answers

279.

A. False   They are located in the cell membranes.
B. False   They cannot be visualized; chemical evidence suggests their structure is similar.
C. True   Also by drugs such as ephedrine which has a similar structure.
D. True   Alpha receptors predominate in skin arterioles.
E. False   Cardiac adrenoceptors are predominantly beta receptors.

280.

A. True   Both are fast fibres and reflexes involving them have a short reflex delay.
B. False   They are in the posterior root ganglion.
C. True   Unconscious proprioception impulses travel in the spino-cerebellar tracts.
D. False   The primary neurone axons pass up the ipsilateral posterior columns before synapsing with secondary neurones at the top of the spinal cord.
E. True   The secondary neurones cross in the medulla oblongata.

281.

A. False   It is best seen when the subject's eyes are closed.
B. False   It is much smaller, at around 50 microvolts.
C. True   It is described in terms of frequency and amplitude.
D. False   The upper limit of the delta rhythm is 3.5 Hz.
E. True   It disappears with the onset of sleep.

282.

A. False   This would depolarize the fibres completely.
B. False   Influx of cations is essential for depolarization.
C. True   However, conduction is slowed.
D. False   Nerve fibres stop conducting before tissue freezing occurs.
E. True   They continue to conduct until the electrochemical gradients created by the pump decline.

283.

A. True   This stretches the agonist and its spindles.
B. True   This also stretches the spindles.
C. False   This reduces the stretch of the spindle.
D. True   Muscle contraction at each end of the spindle stretches the nuclear bag.
E. True   The knee jerk is initiated by striking the patellar tendon which stretches spindles in the quadriceps muscle.

284.

A. True   In the substantia gelatinosa; endorphins may inhibit pain impulse transmission.
B. True   These are the preganglionic autonomic motor neurones.
C. False   It is an inhibitory transmitter thought to be responsible for IPSPs at post-synaptic membranes.
D. False   Loss of supraspinal facilitation is responsible for the areflexia in spinal shock.
E. True   Glutamate and aspartate are thought to be responsible for much of excitatory transmission in the CNS.

Questions 285–289

285. In the cerebral cortex
A. Neuronal connections are innate and immutable.
B. Language and non-language skills are represented in different hemispheres.
C. The areas concerned with emotional behaviour are concentrated in the frontal lobes.
D. The cortical area devoted to sensation in the hand is larger than that for the trunk.
E. Stimulation of the motor cortex causes contractions of individual muscles on the opposite side of the body.

286. When a nerve cell membrane is depolarized by 5 mV
A. Its permeability to sodium increases.
B. Sodium ions move into the cell to cause further depolarization.
C. Potassium ions move outwards down their electrochemical gradient.
D. Chloride ions move inwards down their electrochemical gradient.
E. An action potential is generated.

287. Generalized sympathetic activity is characterized by
A. Contraction of the radial muscle in the iris.
B. Increased urinary excretion of catecholamines.
C. Lipolysis in adipose tissue.
D. Decreased conduction rate in the atrio-ventricular bundle.
E. Relaxation of sphincteric smooth muscle in the alimentary tract.

288 Stimulation of the vagus nerves causes
A. A reduction in the strength of ventricular contraction.
B. Secretion and vasodilatation in the salivary glands.
C. Mucous secretion from bronchial mucosal cells.
D. The spleen to contract.
E. The gallbladder to contract.

289. An action potential in a nerve fibre
A. Occurs when its membrane potential is hyperpolarized to a critical level.
B. Is associated with a transient increase in membrane permeability to sodium.
C. Is associated with a transient decrease in membrane permeability to potassium.
D. Induces local electrical currents in adjacent segments of the fibre.
E. Has an amplitude which varies directly with the strength of stimulus.

Answers

285.

A. False   The connections of brain neurones can be changed fairly rapidly to reflect new patterns of activity and sensory experience; this is referred to as neuronal plasticity.

B. True   The left hemisphere is dominant for speech in most people and the right is dominant for skills requiring appreciation of time and space relationships.

C. False   They are found mainly in the limbic cortex.

D. True   The cortical area given to a particular skin area is related to the richness of its sensory innervation, not its anatomic size.

E. False   Stimulation causes integrated movements not individual muscle contractions.

286.

A. True   Depolarization opens sodium channels in the membrane.

B. True   Positively charged sodium ions move down their electrochemical gradient making the inside of the fibre more positive.

C. True   The fall in membrane potential increases the outward electrochemical gradient for the positively charged potassium ions; their exit tends to stabilize the membrane potential.

D. True   The fall in membrane potential increases the inward electrochemical gradient for chloride; this again tends to restore the resting membrane potential.

E. False   Not unless it reaches the threshold for firing.

287.

A. True   This dilates the pupil.

B. True   Derived from activity in the adrenal medulla and sympathetic nerve endings.

C. True   This provides fatty acids for energy production.

D. False   It increases and the PR interval shortens; higher heart rates are made possible.

E. False   Sympathetic activity inhibits most smooth muscle in gut but contracts the sphincters.

288.

A. False   Ventricles have little vagal innervation.

B. False   The vagus does not supply parasympathetic nerves to the salivary glands.

C. True   It also contracts bronchial smooth muscle.

D. False   It is sympathetic activity that causes the spleen to contract.

E. True   This together with relaxation of the sphincter of Oddi drives bile into the duodenum.

289.

A. False   It occurs when the membrane potential is reduced to its threshold for firing.

B. True   This leads to rapid depolarization towards the sodium equilibrium potential.

C. False   Permeability to K^+ increases and the resulting K^+ efflux contributes to membrane repolarization.

D. True   This depolarizes the adjacent axon and leads to propagation of the impulse.

E. False   Because of the 'all or none' law, impulse configuration is independent of stimulus strength.

Questions 290–294

290. Non-myelinated axons differ from myelinated axons in that they are
A. Not sheathed in Schwann cells.
B. Not capable of regeneration after section.
C. Found only in the autonomic nervous system.
D. Less excitable.
E. Refractory for a longer period after excitation.

291. Resting nerve cell membranes are more permeable to
A. Organic anions than to Cl^- anions.
B. K^+ ions than to Cl^- ions.
C. Na^+ ions than to K^+ ions.
D. Oxygen molecules than to glucose molecules.
E. Water molecules than to H^+ ions.

292. Acetylcholine
A. Acts on the same type of receptor on postganglionic fibres in sympathetic and parasympathetic ganglia.
B. Acts on the same type of receptor on target organs at cholinergic sympathetic and parasympathetic nerve terminals.
C. Acts on the same type of receptor at autonomic ganglia and at somatic neuromuscular junctions.
D. Acts as an excitatory transmitter in the basal ganglia.
E. In blood is hydrolyzed by the same cholinesterase as is found at neuromuscular junctions.

293. Visceral smooth muscle differs from skeletal muscle in that
A. It contracts when stretched.
B. It is not paralyzed when its motor nerve supply is cut.
C. Its cells have unstable resting membrane potentials.
D. It contains no actin or myosin.
E. Excitation depends more on influx of extracellular calcium than release of calcium from endoplasmic reticulum.

294. An inhibitory post-synaptic potential
A. May be recorded in a post-ganglionic sympathetic neurone.
B. May be recorded in an anterior horn motor neurone.
C. Does not exceed one millivolt in amplitude.
D. Moves membrane potential towards the equilibrium potential for potassium.
E. May summate in space and time with other excitatory and inhibitory potentials in the same neurone.

Answers

290.

A.   False   Both types have Schwann cell sheaths.

B.   False   Following section, the central end of the axon buds and grows down the Schwann cell sheath until it reaches its target organ.

C.   False   Some sensory fibres serving pain and temperature are unmyelinated C fibres.

D.   True   Myelinated fibres have a lower threshold for stimulation.

E.   True   2 ms compared with 0.5 ms in well myelinated nerves; myelinated fibres can transmit impulses at higher frequencies than unmyelinated nerves.

291.

A.   False   Organic anions cannot cross the membrane readily.

B.   False   The permeability to Cl^- is about twice that to K^+.

C.   False K^+ permeability is about 100 times that of Na^+.

D.   True O_2, being a small, nonpolar, lipophilic molecule dissolves in the membrane lipid and crosses more easily than the larger glucose molecule.

E.   True   The bilipid layer is more permeable to water than to the charged hydrogen ion.

292.

A.   True   These are 'nicotinic' receptors and the action is blocked at both sites by drugs such as hexamethonium.

B.   True   These are 'muscarinic' receptors and the action is blocked at both sites by atropine.

C.   False   The receptors are different; curare blocks transmission at somatic neuromuscular junctions but not at ganglia.

D.   True   Anticholinergic drugs are sometimes useful in the treatment of muscle rigidity in Parkinsonism.

E.   False   The 'pseudocholinesterase' found in blood differs from the 'true cholinesterase' found near neuromuscular junctions.

293.

A.   True   The intrinsic 'myogenic' response in smooth muscle opposes stretch; skeletal muscle requires a nerve reflex arc for this type of response.

B.   True   It continues to contract due to local pacemakers.

C.   True   They show spontaneous depolarization between contractions.

D.   False   In smooth muscle, actin and myosin filaments occur but are less obvious on microscopy.

E.   True   Smooth muscle has a less well-developed sarcoplasmic reticulum.

294.

A.   False   No such potentials have been recorded here.

B.   True   The hyperpolarization of the anterior horn cell reduces the likelihood of the cell firing action potentials by moving the membrane potential further from the firing threshold.

C.   False   Its amplitude is about 5 mV and its duration about 5 msec.

D.   True   It may be produced by increased permeability to potassium or to chloride ions.

E.   True   In this way the post-synaptic cell integrates the various signals it receives.

Questions 295–300

295. A volley of impulses travelling in a pre-synaptic neurone causes
A. An identical volley in the post-synaptic neurone.
B. An increase in the permeability of the pre-synaptic nerve terminals to calcium.
C. Vesicles in the nerve endings to fuse with the cell membrane and release their contents.
D. The generation of at least one action potential in the post-synaptic neurone.
E. Neurotransmitter to travel down the nerve axon.

296. Pain receptors are
A. Similar in structure to Pacinian corpuscles.
B. Stimulated by a rise in the local K^+ concentration.
C. Quick to adapt to a constant stimulus.
D. More easily stimulated in injured tissue.
E. Stimulated in the wall of the gut by agents which damage the tissues.

297. A property shared by
A. Skeletal and cardiac muscle is their striated microscopical appearance.
B. Skeletal and multiunit smooth muscle is that they are paralysed when their motor nerves are cut.
C. Cardiac and visceral smooth muscle is their spontaneous activity when denervated.
D. Skeletal and cardiac ventricular muscle is their stable resting membrane potential.
E. All varieties of muscle is that contraction strength is related to their initial length.

298. The equilibrium potential (E) for
A. An ion species is the membrane potential observed when its concentrations on each side of the membrane are in equilibrium.
B. Na^+ is about -50 mV in squid axon.
C. An ion species depends on the ratio of the concentrations of the ion outside (I_o) and inside (I_i) the cell.
D. An ion species is the potential the membrane potential would approach if it became freely permeable to that ion.
E. An ion species would be zero if the concentrations of the ion on each side of the membrane were equal.

299. Histological and physiological study of skeletal muscle shows that the
A. Distance between two Z lines remains constant during contraction.
B. Width of the anisotropic A band is constant during contraction.
C. Tension developed is maximal when actin and myosin molecules just fail to overlap.
D. Stimulus needed to cause contraction is minimal when applied at the Z line.
E. The T system of transverse tubules opens into the terminal cisterns of the sarcoplasmic reticulum.

300. Rapid eye movement (REM) sleep differs from non-REM sleep in that
A. The EEG shows waves of higher frequency.
B. Muscle tone is higher.
C. Heart rate and respiration are more regular.
D. Secretion of growth hormone is increased.
E. Dreaming is more common.

Answers

295.

A. False   The synapse may amplify or attenuate the signal.

B. True   The uptake of Ca^{2+} by the nerve ending facilitates release of transmitter.

C. True   The neurotransmitter contained in the vesicles is released by exocytosis.

D. False   The impulses may be inhibitory; even if they are excitatory, the post-synaptic neurone may be strongly inhibited by inputs from other pre-ganglionic neurones.

E. True   Neurotransmitter is thought to be synthesized and packaged in the Golgi apparatus in the neurone cell body before travelling down the axon to the nerve terminals.

296.

A. False   They are bare nerve endings.

B. True K^+ salts cause pain when applied to the base of an ulcer.

C. False   Pain receptors adapt very slowly; this protects the tissues against damage.

D. True   The sensitivity of pain receptors is increased by local tissue injury (hyperalgesia).

E. False   Damage to the gut wall by stimuli such as cutting or burning is painless.

297.

A. True   Both have highly organized actin and myosin filaments.

B. True   The iris is an example of multiunit smooth muscle.

C. True   Isolated hearts and gut segments show spontaneous activity in the organ bath.

D. True   Only the pace maker cells in the heart have unstable membrane potentials.

E. True   The Frank–Starling relationship describes this with respect to cardiac muscle.

298.

A. False   It is the membrane potential that would be required to balance the concentration gradient for that ion.

B. False   A positive membrane potential of about $+65$ mV is required to balance the Na^+ concentration gradient.

C. True   It can be calculated using the Nernst equation:
$E = 61.5 \log_{10} [I_o] [I_i].\text{valence}^{-1}$ at 37°C.

D. True   Membrane potential approaches $+65$ mV when freely permeable to Na^+.

E. True   From the Nernst equation ($\log_{10} 1 = 0$).

299.

A. False   This is sarcomere length and it shortens with contraction.

B. True   Its width is the length of the myosin molecule.

C. False   It is maximal when action and myosin overlap maximally and when adjoining actin molecules just fail to overlap.

D. True   This is where the transverse tubules penetrate the muscle fibre.

E. False   They are adjacent but are not directly connected.

300.

A. True   Wave amplitude is reduced also.

B. False   Surprisingly, muscle tone is low.

C. False   They are much more irregular.

D. False   It is inhibited during REM sleep.

E. True   Subjects woken at the end of REM sleep give vivid accounts of dreams.

Questions 301–307

301. Hemisection of the spinal cord at C7 on the right side would cause

A. Greater loss of pain sensation in the right foot than in the left foot.
B. Greater loss of motor power in the right leg than in the left leg.
C. Greater loss of conscious proprioception in the right than in the left leg.
D. Respiratory failure
E. Loss of the micturition reflex.

302. The ankle jerk reflex is exaggerated

A. When the arm muscles are voluntarily contracted.
B. Immediately after complete spinal cord transection at the cervical level.
C. On the left side some months after damage to the tracts in the right internal capsule.
D. In extrapyramidal system disorders such as Parkinsonism.
E. When cerebellar function is lost.

303. Delta (δ) wave activity in the electroencephalogram

A. Is low in frequency and amplitude.
B. Suggests that the patient is alert and concentrating.
C. When unilateral suggests a brain abnormality.
D. Is a feature of petit mal epilepsy.
E. Is more common in children than in adults while they are awake.

304. Increased intracranial pressure may cause

A. Cranial enlargement in children.
B. Squinting and loss of smell sensation in children.
C. Cupping of the optic disc.
D. An increase in cerebral blood flow.
E. Arterial hypertension.

305. Pain receptors in the gut and urinary tract may be stimulated by

A. Cutting through their wall with a sharp scalpel.
B. Distention.
C. Inflammation of the wall.
D. Acid fluid.
E. Vigorous rhythmic contractions behind an obstruction.

306. Signs of brainstem death include

A. Unconsciousness.
B. Loss of pupillary reaction to light.
C. Loss of tendon jerks in the arms and legs.
D. Loss of respiratory response to CO_2 in the absence of hypoxia.
E. Nystagmus in response to cold water in the external auditory canal.

307. Spasm of digital vessels in the hands in response to cold (Raynaud's phenomenon) may be relieved by

A. Cutting sympathetic nerves to the hand.
B. Stimulating parasympathetic nerves to the hand.
C. Alpha (α) adrenoceptor blockade.
D. Beta (β) adrenoceptor agonists.
E. Wearing gloves.

MCQ

Answers

301.

A. False   The left would be more affected; pain fibres cross the midline shortly after entering the cord.
B. True   The main motor tract to the right leg would be severed.
C. True   The fibres serving proprioception cross at the top of the spinal cord.
D. False   Diaphragmatic and some intercostal activity would remain intact.
E. False   The reflex centres for micturition are in the sacral cord.

302.

A. False   It is not exaggerated but contraction of arm muscles reinforces the reflex.
B. False   Immediately after cord transection, reflexes below the level of the lesion are lost in the stage of 'spinal shock'.
C. True   Muscle tone increases following contralateral internal capsular lesions.
D. False   Though muscle tone is increased, tendon jerks are not exaggerated.
E. False   Muscle tone is low following cerebellar damage and the knee jerk 'pendular'.

303.

A. False   Delta waves have slow frequency and large amplitude.
B. False   It is associated with deep sleep.
C. True   Delta waves may indicate brain damage as well as deep sleep.
D. False   This produces a characteristic spike and wave pattern in the EEG.
E. True   Delta wave activity is seen occasionally in the EEGs of normal awake children.

304.

A. True   Hydrocephaly occurs because the cranial bone sutures have not closed.
B. True   The cranial deformity in hydrocephalus may damage cranial nerves.
C. False   It causes papilloedema – bulging in the opposite direction.
D. False   Vessel compression may reduce cerebral flow severely.
E. True   This reflex response helps to maintain cerebral blood flow.

305.

A. False   The intestine may be cut painlessly during operations under local anaesthesia.
B. True   Stretch is an adequate stimulus for these receptors.
C. True   Chemicals released in inflammation lower the pain threshold (hyperalgesia).
D. True   As with a peptic ulcer.
E. True   This is the cause of the intermittent pain known as colic.

306.

A. False   Consciousness is a function of the cerebral cortical neurones.
B. True   The coordinating centres for pupillary reflexes are in the brainstem.
C. False   The reflex centres for tendon jerks are in the spinal cord.
D. True   Respiratory reflexes are coordinated in the brainstem.
E. False   Nystagmus is the normal reflex response of brainstem centres to this stimulus.

307.

A. True   Sympathetic nerves to digital vessels are tonic vasoconstrictor nerves.
B. False   The hand does not have a parasympathetic nerve supply.
C. True   Alpha receptors mediate sympathetic vasoconstriction.
D. False   Digital vessels have few beta receptors.
E. False   Raynaud's phenomenon is triggered by cold and wearing gloves may prevent cooling to the threshold temperature.

Questions 308–314

308. Muscle tone is reduced by
A. Curare-like drugs.
B. Lower motor neurone lesions.
C. Upper motor neurone lesions.
D. Cerebellar lesions.
E. Gamma efferent impulses to muscle spindles.

309. Effective treatments for severely raised intracranial pressure include
A. Removal of cerebrospinal fluid by lumbar puncture.
B. Reduction of extracellular fluid by diuretics.
C. Creating an anastomosis between a cerebral ventricle and a neck vein.
D. Creating an anastomosis between intracranial subdural space and the peritoneal cavity.
E. Placing the patient recumbent with the legs raised.

310. Disease of the extrapyramidal motor system in Parkinsonism causes
A. Tremor which is more obvious when the patient is performing skilled movements.
B. Muscle paralysis.
C. Increased muscle tone throughout the range of passive movement.
D. Increased involuntary facial movements during speech.
E. An unusual gait with small fast regular steps.

311. Lower motor neurone disease
A. Causes loss of voluntary movements but not of reflex movements.
B. Is a later stage of upper motor neurone disease.
C. Causes eventual wasting of the muscles concerned.
D. Does not affect ventilation of the lungs.
E. Is associated with involuntary twitchings of small fasciculi in the affected muscles.

312. Blockade of α (alpha) adrenoceptors is likely to cause a reduction in
A. Sweat production.
B. Bronchus diameter.
C. Gastrointestinal motility.
D. Total peripheral resistance.
E. Heart rate.

313. Bulging of the optic disc into the vitreous humour (papilloedema) is caused by
A. Raised intraoccular pressure (glaucoma).
B. Blockage of absorption of the aqueous humour.
C. A rise in intracranial pressure.
D. Inflammation of the optic nerve.
E. Interference with the venous drainage of the eye.

314. Atropine (which blocks muscarinic receptors) causes
A. Paralysis of accommodation for near vision in the eye.
B. Constriction of the pupil.
C. Constriction of the bronchi.
D. Diarrhoea.
E. Difficulty with micturition.

Answers

308.

A. True   These paralyse muscle by blocking transmission at neuromuscular junctions.
B. True   Lower motor neurones also paralyse skeletal muscle.
C. False   Loss of supraspinal influences results in spasticity of the affected muscles.
D. True   The cerebellum helps to maintain normal muscle tone.
E. False   These increase spindle sensitivity to stretch and hence muscle tone.

309.

A. False   This may cause fatal compression of the brainstem if the medulla is forced (coned) into the foramen magnum.
B. True   This reduces formation of cerebrospinal fluid.
C. True   This facilitates drainage of cerebrospinal fluid.
D. False   CSF is in the subarachnoid space.
E. False   This would increase intracranial pressure due to gravitational effects and impair CSF drainage by raising pressure in the venous sinuses.

310.

A. False   Parkinsonism causes tremor which is more obvious when the patient is at rest.
B. False   Paralysis is not a feature of the condition.
C. True   This is 'cogwheel' or 'lead pipe' rigidity.
D. False   The face is mask-like; there is poverty of facial movements.
E. True   The body's centre of gravity is shifted forward.

311.

A. False   The muscles are paralysed and not capable of voluntary or reflex movements.
B. False   It is totally independent of upper motor neurone disease.
C. True   It leads to 'disuse atrophy'.
D. False   Ventilation will be affected if the phrenic and intercostal nerves are involved.
E. True   'Fasciculation' is due to denervation hypersensitivity; muscles become ultra-sensitive to small amounts of acetylcholine released from the degenerating nerve terminals.

312.

A. False   Sweating is mediated by cholinergic nerves.
B. False   Bronchial smooth muscle has few alpha receptors; beta blockade tends to cause bronchoconstriction.
C. False   Stimulation of alpha or beta adrenoceptors inhibits the gut.
D. True   Alpha receptors mediate vasoconstriction.
E. False   The heart has few alpha receptors; beta receptor blockade slows the heart.

313.

A. False   Glaucoma causes depression ('cupping') of the optic disc.
B. False   This is a cause of glaucoma.
C. True   Papilloedema is an important sign of raised intracranial pressure.
D. True   Optic neuritis causes swelling of the optic disc.
E. True   This causes local oedema involving the disc.

314.

A. True   By paralysing the ciliary muscles.
B. False   It causes pupillary dilatation by paralysing circular muscle in the iris.
C. False   It tends to dilate the bronchi by blocking vagal effects.
D. False   It causes constipation by suppressing bowel activity.
E. True   Micturition depends on cholinergic nerves.

MCQ

Questions 315–320

315. Visceral pain
A. Is poorly localized compared with pain arising in skin.
B. Is often felt in the mid line.
C. May cause reflex contraction of overlying skeletal muscle.
D. May cause reflex vomiting.
E. May cause reflex changes in arterial blood pressure.

316. Posterior column damage in the spinal cord may impair
A. Vibration sense.
B. Pain sensation.
C. The flexor plantar response to stimulation of the sole.
D. Touch sensation.
E. The ability to stand steadily with the eyes closed.

317. Aphasia
A. Is an impairment of language skills without motor paralysis, loss of hearing or vision.
B. Implies impairment of consciousness.
C. Is called motor aphasia if the patient understands what the speech sounds and symbols mean but lacks the higher motor skills needed to express them.
D. Is called sensory aphasia if the patient does not understand the meaning of the words he hears, sees and uses.
E. Usually results from right-sided cortical damage.

318. Blockade of parasympathetic activity causes a reduction in
A. Sweat production.
B. Resting heart rate.
C. The strength of skeletal muscle contraction.
D. Salivation.
E. Intestinal motility.

319. Sensory disturbance consisting of
A. Pain, sensory loss and paraesthesiae in one leg suggests a spinal cord lesion.
B. Loss of pain, temperature but not touch sensation in the arms suggests a spinal cord lesion.
C. Loss of two-point discrimination but not touch sensation suggests a lesion in the thalamus.
D. Loss of all sensations on the left side suggests a right internal capsule lesion.
E. Loss of all sensations in a skin region suggests a peripheral nerve or posterior root lesion.

320. Damage to the cerebral cortex may cause loss of
A. Pain sensation on the opposite side of the body.
B. Reflex thermoregulatory activity.
C. Skilled movements in the absence of paralysis.
D. Ability to identify an object by its tactile characteristics.
E. Vision in one eye only.

Answers

315.

A.   True   This is characteristic of visceral pain.

B.   True   However pain from some viscera such as ureters and bile ducts is lateralized.

C.   True   In the abdomen this is seen as 'guarding'.

D.   True   Visceral pain is often associated with autonomic side effects.

E.   True   Another example of autonomic side effects, pressure may increase or decrease.

316.

A.   True   The fibres carrying this sensation travel in the posterior columns.

B.   False   The fibres carrying pain sensation travel in the spinothalamic tracts.

C.   False   The reflex does not depend on posterior column fibres.

D.   True   The fibres responsible for fine touch sensation travel in the posterior columns.

E.   True   Proprioceptive information is important in maintaining balance and it is carried in the posterior columns.

317.

A.   True   It is a cortical dysfunction.

B.   False   Level of consciousness is an independent entity.

C.   True   It may start with an inability to say the names of familiar objects but end up with loss of virtually all verbal communication skills.

D.   True   Patients with sensory aphasia tend to talk rubbish since they are unaware of the errors in their use of language.

E.   False   Language skills are carried in the left hemisphere in right and some left-handed people.

318.

A.   False   Sweat glands are innervated by sympathetic cholinergic nerves.

B.   False   Resting heart rate rises due to blockade of vagal tone.

C.   False   Parasympathetic nerves are not involved in skeletal muscle activity.

D.   True   Dryness of the mouth results from blockade of salivary secretion.

E.   True   Parasympathetic nerves are motor to intestinal smooth muscle.

319.

A.   False   Pain is uncommon with spinal cord lesions; the symptoms suggest irritation of a sensory root or peripheral nerve.

B.   True   The fibres carrying these sensations run in separate tracts in the spinal cord.

C.   False   It suggests a parietal cortex lesion where such sensory discriminations are made.

D.   False   It suggests right-sided brain-stem damage since pain is appreciated at subcortical level.

E.   True   Only peripheral nerves and posterior roots carry all modalities of sensation together from a circumscribed skin area.

320.

A.   False   The cerebral cortex is not involved in the conscious appreciation of pain.

B.   False   Reflex thermoregulation is organized in the hypothalamus.

C.   True   Such loss of skilled movements is called 'apraxia'.

D.   True   This 'asteriognosia' results from parietal cortex damage.

E.   False   Damage to the visual cortex causes loss of part of the visual field in both eyes.

Questions 321–326

321. In the hemiplegia following a right-sided cerebrovascular accident (stroke)
A. Left-sided muscle weakness is evident.
B. Muscles in the left side of the body are unable to contract.
C. Muscles which act on both sides of the body, such as respiratory muscles, tend to be spared.
D. Skilled movements are better preserved than unskilled movements.
E. Speech movements are better preserved than swallowing movements.

322. Characteristic features of cerebellar disease include loss of
A. Muscle tone.
B. Muscle strength.
C. Conscious muscle-joint sense.
D. Ability to make precise muscle movements.
E. Ability to fix the gaze steadily on an object.

323. Long-term consequences of transection of the spinal cord in the lower cervical region include
A. Loss of thermoregulatory sweat production in the legs.
B. Severe flexor spasms when the skin of the legs is stimulated.
C. Paralysis of bladder muscle.
D. Inability to regulate sympathetic tone in leg blood vessels in response to baroreceptor stimulation.
E. Inability to erect the penis and ejaculate semen.

324. Blockade of β (beta) adrenoceptors is likely to cause
A. Decreased intestinal motility.
B. Worsening of the condition in patients with bronchial asthma.
C. Worsening of the condition in patients in cardiac failure.
D. Inability to increase heart rate during exercise in patients with transplanted hearts.
E. Inability to increase blood flow to exercising muscles.

325. Cutaneous pain
A. Can be caused by overstimulation of touch receptors.
B. Can be caused by excitation of receptors by chemicals released in injured tissue.
C. Can be elicited more readily if the tissue has been injured recently.
D. Receptors adapt to stimulation more quickly than touch receptors.
E. Transmission at spinal cord level is facilitated by opening of potassium channels in the post-synaptic membrane.

326. Headache can be produced by
A. Dilatation of intracranial blood vessels.
B. Constriction of extracranial blood vessels.
C. Meningeal irritation.
D. Blood in the cerebrospinal fluid.
E. Loss of cerebrospinal fluid following lumbar puncture.

Answers

321.

A.	True	Voluntary movements such as making a handgrip are abnormally weak.
B.	False	Voluntary control is lost but the muscles can contract in reflex, synergistic and other involuntary movements.
C.	True	Perhaps because they have bilateral cortical representation.
D.	False	The most affected movements are those requiring high levels of cortical control.
E.	False	The vocal cord movements required for speech are more highly skilled than those required for swallowing.

322.

A.	True	Muscle tone depends in part on the integrity of the cerebellum.
B.	False	Muscle strength does not depend on the cerebellum.
C.	False	Cerebellar activity depends on unconscious, not conscious, proprioception.
D.	True	Loss of muscular coordination causes 'intention tremor'.
E.	True	The jerky eye movement in cerebellar disease when the gaze is fixed on an object is called 'nystagmus'.

323.

A.	True	Thermoregulatory control is coordinated through the sympathetic nervous system by centres in the hypothalamus.
B.	True	Due to exaggeration of the spinal withdrawal reflex.
C.	False	Both micturition and defaecation can occur reflexly (their reflex centres are in the sacral cord) but are no longer under voluntary control.
D.	True	This impairs the control of arterial blood pressure, especially in the erect position.
E.	False	These are spinal reflexes with centres in the lumbosacral region of the spinal cord.

324.

A.	False	Alpha and beta adrenoceptor stimulation in gut inhibits smooth muscle.
B.	True	By blocking the bronchodilatory action of adrenaline and noradrenaline.
C.	True	By several mechanisms including blocking the sympathetic drive to the heart.
D.	True	By blocking the chronotropic effect of circulating catecholamines.
E.	False	Increased flow in exercise depends on local metabolites, not beta adrenoceptors.

325.

A.	False	Pain is due to excitation of specific pain receptors.
B.	True	Such substances include histamine, bradykinin, 5-hydroxytryptamine, prostaglandins, nitric oxide and substance P.
C.	True	Chemicals released in the injured tissue reduce the stimulation threshold to cause hyperalgesia.
D.	False	Pain receptors adapt much more slowly than touch receptors.
E.	False	This would inhibit synaptic transmission and may explain how enkephalin and endorphin modulate transmission of pain impulses in the substantia gelatinosa.

326.

A.	True	Probably due to pain receptors in vessel walls stimulated by stretch.
B.	False	Dilatation of these extracranial vessels occurs in patients with throbbing migraine-type headaches that are relieved by certain vasoconstrictor agents.
C.	True	This causes the severe pain and neck stiffness in early meningitis.
D.	True	Surprisingly, blood also irritates the meninges to cause headache and neck stiffness.
E.	True	The brain tends to sag in the cranium and pull on pain receptors in the meninges.

Questions 327–330

327. Depressed brain function causes
A. Disorders of function which are independent of the cause of the depression.
B. Loss of unskilled movements before loss of skilled movements.
C. Restlessness and delirium before stupor and coma.
D. A progressive fall in the amplitude of waves in the EEG.
E. Depression of ventilation before loss of consciousness.

328. Loss of pain sensation in the
A. Feet may lead to skin ulceration.
B. Knee may lead to joint damage.
C. Ears and fingers usually precedes frostbite.
D. Leg follows surgical division of the spinocerebellar tracts in the spinal cord.
E. Face follows surgical division of the facial nerve.

329. Intracranial pressure tends to rise when
A. Cerebral venous pressure rises.
B. Forced expiration is made against a closed glottis.
C. There is a bout of coughing.
D. Cerebral blood flow increases.
E. Arterial P_{CO_2} falls below normal.

330. Severe pain may lead to
A. A fall in blood pressure due to a fall in vascular resistance in skeletal muscle.
B. A fall in heart rate due to an increase in cardiac vagal tone.
C. Vomiting through a reflex centre in the brainstem.
D. Profuse sweating due to activation of sympathetic nerves.
E. Suppression of cortisol secretion.

Answers

327.

A.	True	Alcohol, lack of oxygen, low blood sugar and hypothermia all impair cellular function in the brain and lead to a recognizable syndrome of neurological effects.
B.	False	Higher critical functions depending on cortical cells are first to go, e.g. driving ability.
C.	True	Coma implies that cellular depression has reached the less sensitive cells in the brainstem mediating consciousness.
D.	False	Amplitude increases initially to give delta waves in light coma before falling later.
E.	False	This brainstem function is preserved until the later stages of deep coma.

328.

A.	True	Probably because of failure to protect the foot and letting minor injury persist without attention.
B.	True	Again due to loss of the protective effects of pain.
C.	True	Nerve fibres stop conducting near freezing point so there is no further warning when freezing causes tissue damage.
D.	False	Pain sensation is blocked by surgical division of the spinothalamic tracts.
E.	False	It is lost following division of the sensory root of the trigeminal nerve.

329.

A.	True	This distends intracranial veins and hence raises pressure within the cranium.
B.	True	This (Valsalva) manoeuvre raises cerebral venous pressure.
C.	True	This also raises cerebral venous pressure.
D.	True	The vasodilation raises the volume of blood within the cranium.
E.	False	This constricts cerebral vessels and reduces cerebral blood volume.

330.

A.	True	This lowers total peripheral resistance.
B.	True	Consciousness may be lost if this is combined with muscle vasodilation in the 'vasovagal' syndrome.
C.	True	The vomiting centre is in the medulla oblongata.
D.	True	Sympathetic cholinergic nerves are motor to sweat glands.
E.	False	Severe pain increases cortisol secretion via the hypothalamus as part of the general response to trauma.

EMQs

Questions 331–340

EMQ Question 331

For each case of coma A–E, select the most appropriate option from the following list.

1. Hyperthermia.	2. Hypothermia.
3. Respiratory failure.	4. Hepatic failure.
5. Renal failure.	6. Diabetic ketoacidosis.
7. Hypoglycaemia.	8. Drug overdose.
9. Hypothyroidism.	10. Raised intracranial pressure.
11. Brainstem death.	12. Persistent vegetative state.

A.   A 70-year-old woman has been found in her kitchen unconscious when neighbours noted that she had failed to appear as usual for the second day running. On admission to hospital she is noted to have markedly cold skin but this is attributed to the current cold spell and not regarded initially as serious since the clinical thermometer shows only a slightly low body temperature at 35.5°C.

B.   A 5-year-old child admitted after a road traffic accident has been deeply unconscious since admission several days ago and is maintained on a ventilator. There is no response of the pupils to light and the corneal response is also absent. Instillation of ice-cold saline into the external auditory meatus produces no eye movements and there is no spontaneous breathing when ventilation is suspended (after pre-oxygenation) to allow the carbon dioxide level in arterial blood to rise to 50 per cent above normal.

C.   A 10-year-old child has been admitted in coma with a history of rapid deterioration with vomiting over the previous two days. Recently the child had lost weight and had been passing urine in large amounts more frequently than usual. Hyperventilation is noted. Laboratory investigations results include a pH of 7.1 and a bicarbonate level of 9 mmol per litre.

D.   A 35-year-old man known to ambulance personnel as a diabetic has been brought unconscious to hospital. His heart rate is 90 per minute and the pulse is strong, with blood pressure 150/50. Marked sweating is noted.

E.   A 30-year-old man was admitted to hospital in an 'intoxicated' state and with a history of vomiting a cupful of blood on the day of admission. He subsequently became drowsy and lapsed into coma, despite transfusion of blood. He is noted to have yellow discolouration of the skin and sclera.

Answers for 331

A. **Option 2** *Hypothermia.* 'Accidental' hypothermia tends to affect people of all ages when immersed in cold water or exposed on land to low temperatures without adequate insulation; it also occurs in elderly people during cold weather, usually when they have suffered an illness such as a stroke which means they lie poorly insulated in a relatively low temperature. Diagnosis requires a low reading thermometer, usually inserted rectally, since a clinical thermometer is shaken down to an initial temperature around 35–36°C and this may be taken as the temperature even though the True temperature is 5–10 degrees below this. The markedly cold skin is an important clue. Treatment of such patients is often unsuccessful since they have the damage produced by hypothermia added to the underlying condition such as a stroke in this case.

B. **Option 11** *Brainstem death.* This diagnosis is only made after careful repeated expert examination and after reversible causes such as Options 2, 8 and 9 have been excluded. Survival of the brainstem would be indicated by preservation of the brainstem corneal and pupillary reflexes, by the presence of nystagmus (jerky eye movements) provoked by stimulation of the vestibular system by the icy saline and by spontaneous breathing movements in the presence of a high carbon dioxide level. (The pre-oxygen fills the functional residual capacity with oxygen to prevent hypoxic damage during removal from the ventilator.)

C. **Option 6** *Diabetic ketoacidosis.* This is a typical history of childhood-onset of insulin-dependent diabetes mellitus. Lack of insulin's action leads to failure to assimilate absorbed glucose and other nutrients into the body cells, with resulting malnutrition and glycosuria leading to polyuria. In the absence of adequate intracellular glucose, energy production relies excessively on fat as a substrate and this leads to ketones and a huge excess of hydrogen ions (severe metabolic acidosis with pH 7.1 and bicarbonate down to about a third of normal due to buffering). This in turn leads to vomiting, coma and hyperventilation to compensate to some degree for the acidosis by lowering the carbon dioxide level. The blood glucose level would be 5–10 times normal.

D. **Option 7** *Hypoglycaemia.* This patient contrasts with the previous one in that he is known to be a diabetic and his condition suggests a low blood sugar. This is suggested by the hyperdynamic circulation, a compensation for hypoglycaemia (in contrast, ketoacidosis is associated with a weak pulse and circulatory failure). The sweating is also a sympathetic autonomic response to hypoglycaemia. The initial treatment is an intravenous injection of concentrated glucose. Such patients not uncommonly have repeated episodes of unconsciousness due to hypoglycaemia and become known to ambulance personnel.

E. **Option 4** *Hepatic failure.* The major clue here is the jaundice (yellow discolouration) which suggests a hepatic cause of coma. Hepatic failure often causes in the early stages a state similar to alcoholic intoxication and indeed the two could co-exist as excessive alcoholic consumption is a common cause of hepatic failure. However, in this case vomiting of blood has occurred (common in hepatic failure complicated by portal hypertension and oesophageal varices). It is likely that some of the blood lost will have been digested and the products of digestion absorbed from the gut. Digestion and absorption of this high protein load could cause hepatic coma to develop precipitated by toxic products of protein digestion which cannot be eliminated by the liver.

EMQ Question 332

For each case of neurological abnormality due to damage in the nervous system A–E, select the most appropriate option for the site of that damage from the following list of sites for the damaged area (lesion).

1. Lower motor neurones (peripheral).   2. Upper motor neurones (central).
3. Left cerebral hemisphere.   4. Right cerebral hemisphere.
5. Left half of spinal cord.   6. Right half of spinal cord.

A. A 40-year-old man has noticed that his right leg feels 'different', but he has not noticed any weakness. On testing, his right leg is not as good as the left at detecting a pin-prick or a cold metallic object.
B. An 80-year-old woman is found to have moderate weakness on one side of her body. She seems fairly aware of her surroundings but appears not to be able to speak.
C. A 20-year-old man was involved in a motor bike crash a month ago. He has weakness and clumsiness in his right arm but there is no abnormality of feeling. The thenar eminence on the right is flatter than that on the left. The biceps reflex on the right is weaker than that on the left.
D. A 70-year-old woman developed weakness in her right arm and leg a month ago and was admitted to hospital. The weakness is still present in her right arm and sensation is not as good as in the left. The biceps reflex on the right is stronger than that on the left.
E. A 30-year-old man in a wheelchair has severe weakness of both legs. The leg reflexes are brisker than normal.

EMQ Question 333

For each of the reflex systems A–E, select the most appropriate option for the anatomical location of the reflex centres from the following list.

1. Spinal cord.   2. Hypothalamus.
3. Cerebral cortex.   4. Cerebellum.
5. Brainstem.   6. Cervical spinal segments.
7. Thoracic spinal segments.   8. Lumbar spinal segments.
9. Sacral spinal segments.

A. Reflexes coordinating the activities of some pelvic organs.
B. Reflexes coordinating vascular tone in the skin, sweating and general skeletal muscle tone to maintain normal core temperature.
C. Reflexes coordinating the increases in peripheral vascular resistance that occur on changing from the lying down to the standing up position.
D. Reflexes coordinating the acts of swallowing and vomiting.
E. Reflexes coordinating the biceps and quadriceps jerks.

EMQ Question 334

For each physiological description A–E, select the most appropriate option from the following list of axons.

1. Small unmyelinated axons.   2. Large myelinated axons.
3. Small myelinated axons.   4. Large unmyelinated axons.
5. Motor axons.   6. Sensory axons.
7. Autonomic axons.   8. Somatic axons.

A. Axons which are concerned with reflex responses affecting cardiac function.
B. Axons which transmit motor impulses in the knee jerk reflex.
C. Axons which transmit sensory impulses in the knee jerk reflex.
D. Axons which transmit impulses around the lower end of the velocity range, around one metre per second.
E. Axons which transmit impulses by saltatory conduction at around the upper end of the velocity range, around 50 metres per second.

Answers for 332

A. **Option 5**   *Left half of spinal cord.* This man has impaired pain and temperature sensation in his right leg. These sensory modalities are conveyed in pathways which cross the mid line soon after entry to the spinal cord, so the lesion is in the left side, affecting the spino-thalamic tract.

B. **Option 3**   *Left cerebral hemisphere.* The age and symptoms are typical of a 'stroke'. We are not told the side of the weakness, but since the left cerebral hemisphere is concerned with speech in the great majority of people, the lesion is most likely to be in the left than the right hemisphere.

C. **Option 1**   *Lower motor neurones.* Weakness without sensory loss suggests a motor abnormality. Wasting and impaired reflexes are typical of a lower motor neurone lesion.

D. **Option 3**   *Left cerebral hemisphere.* Persisting weakness of an upper motor neurone type (brisk reflex), together with loss of sensation suggest the effects of a stroke affecting the brain on the opposite side.

E. **Option 2**   *Upper motor neurones.* This man has bilateral upper motor neurone weakness of the legs with typically increased reflexes. A common cause would be a spinal cord injury, in which case further testing should show serious sensory loss on both sides.

Answers for 333

A. **Option 9**   *Sacral spinal segments.* This region is like a minor accessory brain in co-ordinating micturition and defaecation and contributing to sexual reflexes.

B. **Option 2**   *Hypothalamus.* This is the region where responses to both hot and cold environments are coordinated. A hot environment favours vasodilation and sweating; a cold environment favours vasoconstriction and increased skeletal muscle tone.

C. **Option 5**   *Brainstem.* This is the region where the arterial baroreceptor reflexes are coordinated.

D. **Option 5**   *Brainstem.* This is also the site for the swallowing and vomiting reflexes.

E. **Option 1**   *Spinal cord.* The tendon reflexes in the limbs, such as the biceps and quadriceps jerks in response to striking their tendons, are spinal reflexes; they are not confined to any one region of the cord.

Answers for 334

A. **Option 7**   *Autonomic axons.* Cardiac function is modified by sympathetic and parasympathetic autonomic motor nerves. These responses are informed by autonomic sensory fibres, e.g. from baroreceptors. Though in general these are small unmyelinated axons, some of the preganglionic motor fibres are myelinated and a little larger.

B. **Option 2**   *Large myelinated axons.* The somatic tendon jerks involve very rapid responses, for which large myelinated axons (around 15 microns diameter) are required.

C. **Option 2**   *Large myelinated axons.* It is logical to have impulses carried at similar high speeds in both sensory and motor halves of the reflex arc.

D. **Option 1**   *Small unmyelinated axons.* Such axons (around 1 micron diameter) carry impulses where speed of response is low, as with slow pain and many autonomic responses.

E. **Option 2**   *Large myelinated axons.* The reason for the high speed is that saltatory conduction jumps the relatively long internodal distance in these axons at the speed of an electric current.

EMQ Question 335

For each paragraph on an aspect of pain A–E, select the most appropriate option from the following list.

1. Chemical mediators at site of pain.
2. Medium sized myelinated pain afferents.
3. Small unmyelinated pain afferents.
4. Gating of the pain pathway in the spinal cord.
5. Thalamus.
6. Endorphins and enkephalins.
7. Impulse spread to medullary reflex centre.
8. Impulse spread to vagal nuclei.

A. A pin prick to the foot gives rise to a sudden sharp sensation of pain and withdrawal of the affected limb.
B. A relatively crude non-specific sensation of pain is believed to be generated from the site of synapse of fibres in the spino-thalamic tracts.
C. Severe pain is usually treated with drugs which act on brain neuronal receptors for endogenous neurotransmitters believed to be released during severe exercise, especially when associated with mortal danger.
D. Patients who suffer the severe crushing pain of a myocardial infarction (heart attack) often vomit.
E. The pain of muscle and joint damage associated with a sports injury is often treated with drugs which inhibit the formation of prostaglandins.

EMQ Question 336

For each case of disordered movement A–E, select the most appropriate option from the following list of areas of neurological damage.

1. One cerebral hemisphere.
2. Extrapyramidal system.
3. Cerebellum.
4. Patchy areas throughout the central nervous system.
5. Motor neurones.
6. Sensory neurones.

A. The patient initially notices some weakness and clumsiness in one hand, with wasting of the thenar eminence. Twitching is noticed on the affected side. The weakness spreads over some months to both arms and legs so that walking is only possible with support.
B. The patient walks with a very unsteady, staggering gait. Speech is rather indistinct. When the patient fixes the gaze to one side, jerking movements of the eyes can be seen. When asked to touch the examiner's finger, the patient's finger moves irregularly and misses the target.
C. When the patient is sitting at rest, a tremor of the hand and slow 'vibration' of the foot is noticed. The patient has started to walk leaning forward and with small shuffling steps. On passive bending of the arm, increased resistance is noted.
D. The patient reports a variety of temporary disturbances, double vision and visual difficulties on both sides at different times, weakness and clumsiness in an arm or leg now and again. With time there has developed more constant difficulty and unsteadiness in walking.
E. The patient walks a little unsteadily, dragging one foot. Testing shows loss of power and impaired sensation in the arm and leg on that side.

Answers for 335

A. **Option 2** *Medium sized myelinated pain afferents.* These are the A fibres which conduct rapidly to give the initial sharp sensation of pain; they also initiate the rapid spinal withdrawal reflex in response to pain.

B. **Option 5** *Thalamus.* This is where the spino-thalamic tracts terminate and synapse. The general unpleasant sensation of pain is generated here, with cortical areas indicating the site of the pain.

C. **Option 6** *Endorphins and enkephalins.* These are the endogenous neurotransmitters on whose receptors the powerful opiate analgesics act to relieve severe pain. Their release during exercise may contribute to the mood-elevating effects of exercise. They may also account for temporary absence of severe pain as a result of injury on the battlefield.

D. **Option 7** *Impulse spread to medullary reflex centre.* The vomiting centre is in the medullar oblongata and can be activated by severe pain from a variety of causes (reflex vomiting).

E. **Option 1** *Chemical mediators at site of pain.* Prostaglandins are believed to be important mediators of persistent pain at a site of injury, particularly involving muscles and joints. Drugs which inhibit prostaglandin formation (NSAIDs: non-steroidal anti-inflammatory drugs) are often effective in this type of pain.

Answers for 336

A. **Option 5** *Motor neurones.* The symptoms are due to gradual destruction of motor neurones, with no suggestion of any sensory loss. Wasting and twitching suggest involvement of the lower motor neurones. The history is typical of motor neurone disease.

B. **Option 3** *Cerebellum.* The cerebellum smooths movements and makes them precise. The patient shows the opposite in the legs causing unsteadiness, in the muscles of speech causing slurring and in the eyes, causing nystagmus. 'Intention' tremors, i.e. shakiness during movements, are typical of cerebellar disease.

C. **Option 2** *Extrapyramidal system.* In contrast to the above, this patient has tremors at rest. The extrapyramidal system provides appropriate muscle tone and associated movements and these are impaired in the patient whose features are typical of Parkinsonism (an extrapyramidal disorder).

D. **Option 4** *Patchy areas throughout the central nervous system.* This patient has had a variety of temporary disturbances involving various scattered regions: optic nerves, nerves to the eye muscles, regions controlling arm and leg movements. The condition is intermittent but tends to lead gradually to permanent difficulties. This is typical of multiple sclerosis (MS).

E. **Option 1** *One cerebral hemisphere.* This patient has motor and sensory loss in one side of the body due to damage in the cerebral hemisphere on the other side. The features are typical of a patient with moderate recovery from one or more strokes affecting motor and sensory pathways in one cerebral hemisphere.

EMQ Question 337

For each physiological description A–E, select the most appropriate option from the following list of terms related to the autonomic nervous system.

1. Generalized sympathetic activity.
2. Generalized parasympathetic activity.
3. Cholinergic effect.
4. α alpha adrenergic effect.
5. β_1 beta one effect.
6. β_2 beta two effect.

A.   Following a painful injury, a person's heart rate abruptly falls from 100 to 50 beats per minute.

B.   In a period of excitement, a person's heart rate rises to 120 beats per minute and the person is aware of the heart pounding in the chest.

C.   After a large meal, a person retires to bed, feeling pleasantly relaxed and warm. Heart rate is 60 per minute, digestion of the meal is proceeding.

D.   A student with asthma inhales a medication which acts by stimulating receptors on bronchial smooth muscle and is relieved to find that the chest tightness and wheeze associated with breathing have disappeared.

E.   During strenuous sporting activity a 20-year-old has a heart rate of 200 beats per minute, is highly alert, has moderately dilated pupils and is sweating profusely.

EMQ Question 338

For each description related to muscle spindles A–E, select the most appropriate option from the following list of terms (fusal = spindle).

1. Sensory, non-contractile region.
2. Motor region.
3. Increased activity in sensory nerve supply.
4. Contraction of extra-fusal fibres.
5. Relaxation of spindle.
6. Relaxation of extra-fusal fibres.

A.   Striated region at each end of muscle spindles.

B.   A central region of the spindle specifically adapted to detecting distortion produced by stretching of the spindle.

C.   A reflex effect produced by increased sensory output from muscle spindles to the central nervous system.

D.   A direct effect on the spindle produced by contraction of muscles which antagonize the action of the muscle containing the spindle.

E.   A reflex effect both by increased motor activity to the spindle and by stretching of the muscle containing the spindle.

EMQ Question 339

For each kind of muscle described A–E, select the most appropriate option from the following list.

1. Muscle in the wall of the heart.
2. Muscle that moves the skeleton.
3. Muscle in the wall of the small intestine.
4. Muscle in the iris of the eye.

A.   This type of muscle is striated and has multiple peripherally-placed nuclei.

B.   This type of muscle is not striated and is not spontaneously active.

C.   This muscle is spontaneously active and is richly endowed with β_1 receptors.

D.   This muscle is not striated and is spontaneously active.

E.   This type of muscle is not spontaneously active and is richly endowed with receptors that respond to acetylcholine and are blocked by 'muscle relaxants'.

Answers for 337

A. **Option 3**   *Cholinergic effect.* Severe pain can lead to a burst of activity in cardiac vagal nerves; these parasympathetic nerves release acetylcholine at their terminals around the sinuatrial node to cause marked cardiac slowing.

B. **Option 5** β_1 *effect.* Tachycardia and increased force of cardiac contraction are specific cardiac sympathetic effects mediated through stimulation of β_1 adrenoceptors in the sinuatrial node and the myocardium respectively.

C. **Option 2**   *Generalized parasympathetic activity.* Relaxation is associated with parasympathetic activity and antagonized by sympathetic activity; warmth is associated with relatively high skin blood flow as sympathetic nerves are 'switched off'; a heart rate of 60, and digestive activity both require considerable parasympathetic activity to the heart (vagus nerves) and the gut.

D. **Option 6** β_2 *effects.* Stimulation of β_2 receptors mediates relaxation of bronchial muscle; such medication is a common inhalational treatment for asthma.

E. **Option 1**   *Generalized sympathetic activity.* A heart rate of 200 is the maximal predicted for a 20-year-old, it is produced by removal of vagal tone and a maximal level of sympathetic tone to the heart; increased alertness, dilated pupils and sweating are all indications of sympathetic activity.

Answers for 338

A. **Option 2**   *Motor region.* A spindle is a modified muscle fibre and the striated region at each end is due to actin and myosin arrangements which retain the ability to contact.

B. **Option 1**   *Sensory, non-contractile region.* This is the nuclear bag region which detects stretching of the spindle and sends information along fast-conducting fibres to the central nervous system.

C. **Option 4**   *Contraction of extra-fusal fibres.* This is the reflex response whereby stretching of the spindle leads to contraction of the muscle containing the spindle.

D. **Option 3**   *Increased activity in sensory nerve supply.* The antagonistic muscles stretch the muscle and its spindles and the direct effect on the spindle is stimulation of its sensory region and initiation of activity in the nerve endings supplying it.

E. **Option 4**   *Contraction of extra-fusal fibres.* Motor activity to the striated spindle ends makes them contract and stretch the central sensory region; stretching the muscle also stretches the spindles within it; in both cases the increased sensory output leads to reflex contraction of the extra-fusal fibres of the muscle containing the spindles.

Answers to 339

A. **Option 2**   *Muscle that moves the skeleton.* Skeletal muscle has an orderly arrangement of actin and myosin molecules that gives it a striated appearance under the microscope.

B. **Option 4**   *Muscle in the iris of the eye.* This type of muscle contains actin and myosin in a more random arrangement and so appears smooth rather than striated; it requires stimulation of autonomic nerves to make it contract; sympathetic stimulation contracts radial fibres to dilate the pupil, parasympathetic stimulation contracts circular fibres and dilates the pupil.

C. **Option 1**   *Muscle in the wall of the heart.* The heart beats spontaneously due to impulses from the sinuatrial node; sympathetic stimulation of beta one receptors increases the force of contraction.

D. **Option 3**   *Muscle in the wall of the small intestine.* This type of smooth muscle shows rhythmical contractions, even when removed from the body.

E. **Option 2**   *Muscle that moves the skeleton.* Skeletal muscle contracts only when stimulated by somatic motor nerves releasing acetylcholine; during general anaesthesia, muscle relaxation is often provided (e.g. during abdominal operations) by drugs which interfere with the action of motor nerves on the muscle fibres.

EMQ Question 340

For each statement A–E about a patient with a long established complete transection of the spinal cord at the lower cervical region, select the most appropriate option from the following list of physiological lesions/disturbances.

1. Somatic upper motor neurone lesion.   2. Somatic lower motor neurone lesion.
3. Loss of reflex centre.   4. Loss of sensory input.
5. Loss of sympathetic motor function.   6. Loss of parasympathetic motor function.

A. The patient has difficulty maintaining arterial blood pressure in the upright position because the total peripheral resistance cannot be appropriately increased.
B. The patient is unaware of damaging pressure on the lower limbs.
C. The patient has difficulty maintaining normal core temperature in a cool environment tolerated by other patients.
D. The patient's leg muscles are paralysed but can contract in response to striking the patellar tendon with a patellar hammer.
E. The patient has lost the normal sweating response in the legs to a hot environment.

EMQ

Answers for 340

A. **Option 5**   *Loss of sympathetic motor function*. Normally when upright we maintain arterial blood pressure by sympathetically induced vasoconstriction, particularly in the legs; otherwise blood tends to pool there giving postural hypotension.

B. **Option 4**   *Loss of sensory input*. There is no awareness of any sensation in the legs, so this warning of impending damage is lost.

C. **Option 5**   *Loss of sympathetic motor function*. Sympathetically induced vasoconstriction is also important in retaining core heat in a cool environment.

D. **Option 1**   *Somatic upper motor neurone lesion*. The motor tracts in the spinal cord are upper motor neurones with respect to the anterior horn cells which give rise to the axons of the lower motor neurones supplying the leg muscles; the knee jerk is a spinal reflex independent of upper motor neurones in long-established paraplegia.

E. **Option 5**   *Loss of sympathetic motor function*. Sweating is yet another activity which relies on an intact sympathetic motor pathway from the reflex centre to the sweat glands in the skin.

MCQs

Questions 341–347

341. The fovea centralis
A. Lies where the visual axis impinges on the retina.
B. Is not crossed by any major blood vessels.
C. Is the thickest part of the retina.
D. Has higher visual acuity than other parts of the retina.
E. Lies on the temporal side of the optic disc.

342. Endolymph
A. Is found within the membranous labyrinth.
B. Has a potassium concentration close to that of extracellular fluid.
C. Bathes the hair cells of the inner ear.
D. Is electrically negative with respect to perilymph.
E. Inertia is a factor in the stimulation of receptors in the semicircular canals during rotatory acceleration.

343. Olfactory cells
A. Are epithelial cells which synapse with olfactory nerves.
B. Generate impulses when stimulated which are relayed in the thalamus.
C. Are chemoreceptors.
D. Show little adaptation.
E. Are more important than taste in appreciating the flavour of food.

344. Adaptation for vision in poor light is
A. Complete after 2–3 minutes.
B. Due mainly to dilatation of the pupil.
C. Due to regeneration of rod but not cone pigments.
D. Faster if red goggles are worn before entering the dark environment.
E. More effective for peripheral than central vision.

345. The basilar membrane of the cochlea vibrates
A. At the same frequency as the applied sound.
B. With an amplitude which is proportional to the frequency of the applied sound.
C. With an amplitude which is proportional to the loudness of the applied sound.
D. Along more of its length when the applied sound has a high rather than a low frequency.
E. Mainly at the base of the cochlea for the sound frequencies commonly used in speech.

346. The cones in the retina differ from rods in that they are more
A. Numerous.
B. Concerned with colour vision.
C. Sensitive to light.
D. Concerned with high visual acuity.
E. Affected by vitamin A deficiency.

347. Increasing the salt concentration applied to a 'salt' taste bud increases
A. Its sensitivity to salt.
B. The amplitude of its generator potentials.
C. The amplitude of the action potentials generated.
D. Impulse traffic to the thalamus.
E. Impulse traffic up the ascending reticular formation.

Answers

341.
A. True   It detects objects in the centre of the field of vision.
B. True   There are no superficial structures to affect impinging light rays.
C. False It is relatively thin due to absence of superficial layers.
D. True   The above factors contribute to this.
E. True   It is marked by yellow pigment.

342.
A. True   Perilymph surrounds the membranous labyrinth.
B. False It is similar to that of intracellular fluid.
C. True   It bathes cochlear and vestibular hair cells.
D. False It is positive, of the order of +80 mV.
E. True   The inertia causes endolymph movements to lag those of the membranous laby-
          rinth and displace the hairs of the hair cells.

343.
A. False They are modified nerve cells in the nasal epithelium.
B. False Unlike other sensory inputs, olfactory impulses are not relayed in the thalamus.
C. True   They recognize certain molecular structures.
D. False It is the newcomer who recognizes the smell in the room.
E. True   In their absence, food loses much of its flavour.

344.
A. False It takes about 20 minutes.
B. False Dilatation of the pupil contributes but regeneration of bleached receptor pigments
          is the main factor.
C. False Regeneration of cone pigments plays a part.
D. True   Red light does not bleach rhodopsin.
E. True   Peripheral vision adapts better to dark conditions; rods predominate peripherally.

345.
A. True   Harmonics are also faithfully reproduced.
B. False Frequency and amplitude need not be related.
C. True   Hence very loud sounds can damage the basilar membrane.
D. False Low frequency vibrations travel further up the cochlea.
E. True   Speech frequencies (about 1000–3000 Hz) cause maximum vibration in this
          region.

346.
A. False There are about 6 million cones compared with 120 million rods.
B. True   Rods alone give achromatic vision.
C. False The rods are much more sensitive; their pigment is bleached in bright light.
D. True   Acuity is highest with foveal (cone) vision.
E. False Vitamin A is essential for rhodopsin synthesis for rod vision only.

347.
A. False It decreases; taste receptors adapt to stimuli applied to them.
B. True   Stronger stimuli lead to generator potentials of greater amplitude.
C. False There is an increase in impulse frequency, not amplitude.
D. True   All but olfactory impulses are relayed in the thalamus.
E. True   All sensory inputs send impulses via collaterals to this system.

Questions 348–353

348. On entering a darkened room, the
A. Threshold light intensity for the eye starts to rise.
B. First phase of retinal adaptation is mainly in the cones.
C. Final phase of retinal adaptation is mainly in the rods.
D. Adaptation is slower if a long period was spent in bright light beforehand.
E. Time course for pupillary dilatation is similar to that for dark adaptation.

349. Dilation of the pupil increases the
A. Amount of light entering the eye.
B. Refractive power of the eye.
C. Spherical aberration.
D. Depth of focus.
E. Field of vision.

350. The olfactory system can detect
A. 20–40 distinct odours.
B. Differences in odour between isomers of the same substance.
C. The direction from which an odour comes.
D. Small differences in the concentration of the substance responsible for the odour.
E. Odours better in old than in young people.

351. During accommodation for near vision
A. More light enters the eye.
B. The curvature of the cornea increases.
C. Chromatic and spherical aberration is decreased.
D. The depth of focus increases.
E. The visual axes of the two eyes converge.

352. Visual acuity is
A. A measure of the sensitivity of the retina to light.
B. Greater in a person with 6/12 (0.5) vision than in one with 6/9 (0.75).
C. Greater using central than using peripheral vision.
D. Greater using one eye than using both eyes.
E. Greater in normal than in colour-blind people.

353. The tympanic membrane
A. Modifies the frequencies of sound waves impinging on the ear.
B. Stops vibrating almost immediately after the sound stops.
C. Bulges outwards when the pharyngotympanic tube is blocked.
D. Transmits sound more effectively when the small muscles of the middle ear are contracted.
E. Cannot transmit sound waves if it is perforated.

Answers

348.

A. False   It begins to fall in the process of dark adaptation.
B. True   The initial adaptation is due more to cone adaptation.
C. True   Rods are slower to adapt but show more profound adaptation.
D. True   A previous long exposure would bleach most of the rhodopsin so more time would be needed for its resynthesis.
E. False   The pupil dilates almost immediately in the dark.

349.

A. True   This allows rapid adaptation for vision in poor light.
B. False   The iris has nothing to do with the refractive power of the eye.
C. True   By permitting light to pass through peripheral, and less perfect, parts of the lens.
D. False   As with a camera, a wide aperture tends to shorten the depth of focus.
E. False   Narrowing the aperture in a camera does not result in a smaller picture.

350.

A. False   It is thought that humans can differentiate between 2000 and 4000 different odours.
B. True   The receptors can detect small differences in molecular configuration.
C. True   Probably due to the different time of arrival of the odour at the two nostrils.
D. False   Though very low concentrations of odorous substances can be detected, differences in concentration of more than 30 per cent are needed to detect a difference in intensity.
E. False   Olfaction ability falls with age.

351.

A. False   Less light enters the eye as the pupils constrict.
B. False   The cornea is not involved in accommodation; the increase in refractive power in the eye is due to the increased convexity of the lens caused by contraction of the ciliary muscle.
C. True   The papillary constriction restricts light rays entering the eye to the centre of the lens where there is less chromatic and spherical aberration.
D. True   Due mainly to the improvement in optical characteristic mentioned in (C) above.
E. True   To allow the object to be focused on the two foveae.

352.

A. False   It is a measure of the ability to distinguish between (resolve) two points.
B. False   Acuity is expressed as the ratio of someone's reading distance compared with average normal.
C. True   Visual acuity is maximal at the fovea where cone receptors are predominant.
D. False   The two images reinforce each other.
E. False   Visual acuity does not depend on distinguishing colours.

353.

A. False   It faithfully reproduces the frequencies.
B. True   It is very nearly 'critically damped'.
C. False   It bulges inwards as middle ear air is absorbed.
D. False   Reflex contraction of these muscles protects by damping vibration transmission.
E. False   Small perforations cause about 5 decibels loss; complete destruction about 50.

Questions 354–359

354. In the refracting system of the eye
A. The cornea causes more refraction than the lens.
B. More refraction occurs at the inner surface of the cornea than at the outer surface.
C. The lens, by becoming more convex, can more than double the total refractive power of the eye.
D. The back surface of the lens contributes more to accommodation than the front.
E. Ageing reduces the maximum refractive power of the eye.

355. The hair cells in the semicircular canals are stimulated by
A. Movement of perilymph.
B. Linear acceleration.
C. Rotation at constant velocity.
D. Gravity.
E. Movement of endolymph relative to hair cells.

356. When light is shone into one eye, the pupil
A. Constricts even though its optic nerve has been cut.
B. Responds due to sympathetic nerve activity.
C. Does not respond if autonomic cholinergic nerves are blocked by local application of atropine.
D. In that eye constricts and the opposite pupil dilates.
E. Does not respond if there is brainstem death.

357. Light from an object to the right of the visual axis
A. Impinges on the retina in the right eye to the right of the fovea.
B. Impinges on the retina in the left eye to the left of the fovea.
C. Generates impulses which travel in the right optic tract.
D. Generates impulses which produce conscious sensation in the frontal lobe eye fields.
E. Forms an inverted image on the retina.

358. The tympanic membranes
A. Bulge inwards during descent in an unpressurized airplane.
B. Have an area about twice that of the oval window.
C. Prevent sound waves from reaching the oval and round windows at the same time.
D. Transmit only 10 per cent of applied sound energy to the cochlea for sound waves of 1000 Hz.
E. Transmit sounds in the 500–5000 Hz frequency range with the least loss of energy.

359. Utricles
A. Are gravity receptors.
B. Contain calcified granules.
C. Contain hair cells.
D. Contain endolymph which communicates with that in semicircular canals and cochlea.
E. Can initiate reflex changes in muscle tone.

Answers

354.

A.	True	This is because of the large change in refractive index from air to cornea.
B.	False	The outer interface is with air; cornea and aqueous have similar refractive indices.
C.	False	It can only increase total refractive power by about 15–20 per cent.
D.	False	During accommodation, the front of the lens bulges more than the back.
E.	True	As the lens stiffens, ability to increase convexity when ciliary muscles contract is diminished.

355.

A.	False	Perilymph is the fluid outside the membranous labyrinth.
B.	False	Their adequate stimulus is angular not linear acceleration or deceleration.
C.	False	A blindfold person is unaware of any sensation when rotated at constant velocity, e.g. as on the earth!
D.	False	Gravity produces linear acceleration.
E.	True	During angular acceleration or deceleration, the inertia of the endolymph causes it to move relative to the hair cells on the walls of the semicircular canals. The resulting movement of the hair cells generates afferent impulses that travel in the vestibular nerves.

356.

A.	False	The optic nerve is an essential part of the reflex pathway for the light reflex.
B.	False	It still constricts after the sympathetic nerves are cut.
C.	True	Atropine blocks this parasympathetic action.
D.	False	Both pupils constrict consensually.
E.	True	Failure of the pupils to respond to light is a sign of brainstem death.

357.

A.	False	It impinges to the left of the fovea.
B.	True	The retina of both eyes is stimulated in corresponding or homonymous areas.
C.	False	They travel in the left optic tract to the left occipital cortex.
D.	False	They enter consciousness in the left occipital cortex; frontal eye fields are concerned with eye movements.
E.	True	As in a camera.

358.

A.	True	Cabin pressure rises above middle ear pressure.
B.	False	Their area is about 20 times as great.
C.	True	This 'round window protection' prevents damping of vibrations in the inner ear.
D.	False	At this frequency, over half of the sound energy is transmitted.
E.	True	Impedance matching and auditory acuity are greatest at these frequencies which are those used in normal speech.

359.

A.	True	They respond to linear acceleration.
B.	True	The inertia of these otoliths enables utricles to respond to linear acceleration.
C.	True	These are stimulated by forces acting on the otoliths.
D.	True	They are all parts of the membranous labyrinth, filled with endolymph.
E.	True	Muscle tone is reflexly redistributed so that the body can withstand gravitational stresses.

Questions 360–365

360. The rods in the retina
A. Contain visual pigment which is more sensitive to red than to blue light.
B. Are rendered insensitive by ordinary daylight.
C. Are more widely distributed over the retina than are cones.
D. Reflect red light more than blue light.
E. Comprise about 20 per cent of foveal receptor cells.

361. Cones
A. Are found in the most superficial layer of the retina.
B. Show a graded depolarization in response to light.
C. Contain pigments which are more light-sensitive than the rod pigment.
D. Contain pigments which are most affected by yellow-green light.
E. Are absent in an individual with colour blindness.

362. The receptor cells serving taste
A. Are confined to the tongue.
B. Are stimulated when chemicals diffuse through the overlying epithelium to reach them.
C. Are primary sensory neurones.
D. Are histologically different for the four primary taste modalities.
E. For sweetness are more common at the tip than at the back of the tongue.

363. Sound waves
A. Are quantified on the decibel scale which is logarithmic.
B. With an intensity of 0 decibels are inaudible.
C. May have an intensity of minus 10 decibels.
D. With an intensity of 90 decibels are usually painful.
E. Are heard as a note one octave higher when their frequency increases eight-fold.

364. The frequency of impulses generated by receptors in a utricle is
A. Related to the orientation of the head.
B. Higher during travel at 100 than at 20 miles per hour.
C. Reduced in the weightless conditions in outer space.
D. Inversely related to the frequency being generated by the opposite utricle.
E. Related to the impulse frequency being generated by semicircular canal receptors.

365. Aqueous humour
A. Is produced by diffusion and active transport in the ciliary bodies.
B. Pressure is close to mean arterial pressure.
C. Formation depends on the enzyme carbonic anhydrase.
D. Is absorbed into veins at the junction of the iris and the cornea.
E. Is more easily absorbed when the pupil is widely dilated.

Answers

360.

A. False   Rhodopsin absorbs blue-green light with a wavelength around 500 nm.
B. True   Nearly all rhodopsin in broken down (bleached) in daylight.
C. True   The field of vision using rods is greater than that using cones.
D. True   Rhodopsin is a red pigment.
E. False   There are no rods in the fovea.

361.

A. False   They are in the layer furthest from the vitreous humour.
B. False   They hyperpolarize in response to light due to closure of Na^+ channels in the membrane.
C. False   Rhodopsin is the most sensitive of the pigments.
D. True   Cone pigments absorb light at wavelengths of 440, 535 and 565 nm; yellow-green light shows up relatively well in dim light.
E. False   Colour-blind individuals have cones but they lack one or more of the three cone systems that respond to the three primary colours.

362.

A. False   They are found also in the soft palate, pharynx and larynx.
B. False   The microvilli on top of receptors protrude through taste pores into the buccal cavity.
C. False   They are receptor cells which synapse with primary sensory neurones.
D. False   They look alike.
E. True   Sweet sensation is experienced at the front of the tongue; bitterness at the back.

363.

A. True   Loudness is related to the logarithm of sound intensity.
B. False   Zero decibels is the average threshold for hearing.
C. True   These sounds may be heard by people whose hearing ability is above average.
D. False   The threshold for pain is around 120 decibels.
E. False   They sound one octave higher when their frequency is doubled.

364.

A. True   This determines the plane of the gravitational pull on the otoliths.
B. False   The utricle is affected by acceleration, not velocity.
C. True   This can give rise to a form of travel sickness.
D. False   Often both respond in parallel.
E. False   The utricles and semicircular canals function independently; utricles respond to linear acceleration, semicircular canals to angular acceleration.

365.

A. True   Its crystalloid composition is not identical to that of plasma.
B. False   It is much lower. Above 20 mmHg is abnormal and suggests glaucoma.
C. True   Inhibitors of this enzyme reduce formation and are used in treatment of glaucoma.
D. True   This area with its overlying trabeculae is referred to as the canal of Schlemm.
E. False   The iris then blocks access to the canal of Schlemm.

Questions 366–371

366. Rhodopsin, the pigment of the rods is
A. A purple pigment.
B. Highly absorbent of red light.
C. Most sensitive to violet light.
D. Regenerated in the dark.
E. Least sensitive to red light.

367. In the visual field of the left eye, an object
A. In the upper temporal quadrant is detected in the lower nasal quadrant of the retina.
B. At the centre of the field of vision is detected in the optic disc.
C. Focused on the blind spot is in the nasal half of the visual field.
D. In the temporal half generates impulses which travel the left optic tract.
E. In the nasal half is more likely to be perceived in binocular vision than one in the temporal half.

368. The basilar membrane
A. Is broader at the base of the cochlea than at the apex.
B. Vibrations stimulate receptors to generate impulses at the frequencies of the applied sounds.
C. At the base of the cochlea vibrates only to incoming high frequency sounds.
D. In the apical region vibrates only to incoming sounds of low frequency.
E. Can be made to vibrate by pressure waves travelling through skull bone.

369. Taste receptors
A. For sour taste predominate at the sides of the tongue.
B. May respond to more than one modality of stimulus.
C. Give rise to a sour taste when stimulated by hydrogen ions.
D. Cannot detect small (<10 per cent) differences in the concentration of taste-evoking chemicals.
E. Respond more to substances in warm solutions than in cold ones even though the substance concentration is the same in both.

370. An audiogram
A. Is a plot of hearing loss (or hearing ability) against sound frequency.
B. Showing equal impairment of air and bone conduction suggests conductive deafness.
C. Showing hearing loss at low frequencies for air conduction suggests ear drum damage.
D. Showing loss at 8000 Hz for air and bone conduction suggests basal cochlear damage.
E. Showing hearing loss at the lower frequencies is common in elderly people.

371. Poor balance is more likely when there is
A. Semicircular canal rather than cochlear damage.
B. Impairment of basilar rather than carotid artery blood flow.
C. Spinothalamic tract rather than posterior column damage.
D. Dim rather than bright light.
E. Recent rather than long-standing destruction of one labyrinth.

Answers

366.

A.   False   It is red.
B.   False   It is red because it reflects red light selectively.
C.   False   It is most sensitive to blue-green light (around 500 nm).
D.   True   In the dark retinene and scotopsin combine to form rhodopsin.
E.   True   This is because it reflects the red light.

367.

A.   True   The image is inverted and reversed with respect to the object.
B.   False   The point focused upon is detected at the macula (fovea).
C.   False   The optic disc is medial to the fovea, so the blind spot is in the temporal part of the field of vision.
D.   False   Impulses related to the temporal region of the left field of vision cross to the right at the optic chiasma.
E.   True   The visual fields of the two eyes overlap, apart from the outer temporal areas.

368.

A.   False   The reverse is true.
B.   False   Nerves cannot transmit impulses at the top frequencies detectable by ear, about 20 000 Hz.
C.   False   At the base, the basilar membrane vibrates to high and low frequency sound waves.
D.   True   High frequency sounds are damped out before they reach the apex.
E.   True   This supplements the normal ossicular conduction, especially for loud sounds.

369.

A.   True   Receptors for bitter taste predominate on the posterior dorsum of the tongue.
B.   True   Recording from single taste receptors demonstrates that a single receptor can respond to more than one modality.
C.   True   All acids taste sour.
D.   True   Taste receptors are poor at discriminating between intensities; a concentration difference of more than 30 per cent is needed for discrimination.
E.   True   Food flavour is accentuated when hot; unpleasant medicine less offensive when cold.

370.

A.   True   It is obtained using an audiometer.
B.   False   In conductive deafness air conduction, but not bone conduction, is impaired.
C.   True   This is an example of conductive deafness.
D.   True   This can be caused by acoustic trauma, e.g. in heavy industry.
E.   False   Hearing loss in the elderly (presbycusis) particularly affects higher frequencies.

371.

A.   True   The cochlea does not contribute sensory information needed for balance.
B.   True   The basilar artery supplies brain stem areas particularly concerned with balance.
C.   False   The posterior columns transmit proprioceptive information needed for balance.
D.   True   Vision can compensate for loss of proprioception.
E.   True   Abrupt loss of input causes severe disturbance followed by gradual adaptation.

Questions 372–377

372. In someone with short-sightedness (myopia)
A. The eye tends to be longer than average from lens to retina.
B. A convex lens is required to correct the refractive error.
C. Close vision is affected more than distance vision.
D. The near-point is farther than normal from the eye.
E. A circular object tends to appear oval.

373. Colour blindness
A. Results from inability to detect one of the three primary light colours, red yellow and blue
B. Where red and green are indistinguishable is due to failure of red and green cone systems.
C. In which no colours can be detected is due to failure of all the cones systems.
D. Is more common in women than men.
E. Is a disability linked to the Y-chromosome.

374. Local application of atropine to the eye causes
A. Dilation of the pupil.
B. The near-point for clear vision to move closer to the eye.
C. Inability to focus on objects at infinity.
D. Reduced drainage of aqueous humour.
E. Difficulty in looking upwards.

375. In the middle ear
A. Destruction of the auditory ossicles abolishes hearing.
B. Paralysis of the auditory muscles makes sounds more faint.
C. Immobilization of the stapes causes greater deafness than removal of the ossicles.
D. Air pressure is normally atmospheric pressure.
E. The round window moves reciprocally with the oval window.

376. Interruption of the visual pathway in the
A. Left optic tract causes blindness in the right visual field (right homonymous hemianopia).
B. Optic chiasma causes blindness in the nasal half of each visual field (binasal hemianopia).
C. Left optic radiation causes loss of vision to the right.
D. Occipital cortex causes loss of the light reflex.
E. Occipital cortex causes loss of central vision with preservation of peripheral vision.

377. Squinting (strabismus) may result from
A. Poor vision in one eye in childhood.
B. A refractive error in childhood.
C. Central suppression of vision in one eye in childhood.
D. Damage to the cerebellum.
E. Damage to the internal capsule.

MCQ

Answers

372.

A. True   Hence distant objects are focused in front of the retina.
B. False A concave lens is required.
C. False It is distant objects that appear out of focus.
D. False Myopic people can focus on objects closer to the eye than normal people.
E. False This is caused by an asymmetrical cornea (astigmatism).

373.

A. True   One or more of the three types of cone fails to function.
B. False It is due to failure of one of the two systems.
C. False It is due to the presence of only one functioning cone system.
D. False It is 20 times more common in men.
E. False Its linkage to the X-chromosome explains its greater frequency in men.

374.

A. True   This paralyses the cholinergic constrictor fibres.
B. False The ciliary muscle needed for accommodation has cholinergic innervation.
C. False When focusing at infinity, the ciliary muscle is at rest.
D. True   The iris tends to obstruct the canal of Schlemm in the corneoscleral angle.
E. False Extraocular muscles are not affected by atropine.

375.

A. False Sound can still be transmitted by bone conduction.
B. False These muscles damp vibration of the ossicles reflexly in response to loud noises.
C. True   Immobilization prevents the oval window vibrating and causes severe deafness.
D. True   Air pressure is atmospheric, due to the patency of the pharyngotympanic tubes connecting the pharynx to the middle ear.
E. True   Fluid (endolymph) cannot be compressed; as the oval window moves in, the round window moves out.

376.

A. True   The left half of each retina is concerned with vision to the right and impulses from them travel in the left optic tract.
B. False The crossing fibres come from the nasal half of each retina and are responsible for temporal vision; bitemporal hemianopia results.
C. True   As with damage to the left optic tract.
D. False This is a brain stem reflex.
E. False The reverse is true because the fovea is bilaterally represented in the cortex.

377.

A. True   Poor vision in one eye impairs fixation of the eye concerned.
B. True   A refractive error impairs vision in the eye concerned to give poor fixation.
C. False Suppression of vision in one eye is a consequence, not a cause, of squint.
D. False Cerebellar damage may cause involuntary oscillatory movements (nystagmus) but not squinting.
E. True   Internal capsular damage may cause a paralytic squint due to damage to the oculomotor tracts.

Questions 378–384

378. Impairment of the sense of smell
A. May be confined to certain odours only.
B. May occur in hydrocephalus.
C. Is likely after thalamic damage.
D. Can be caused by inflammation of the nasal mucosa.
E. Is a recognized effect of temporal lobe tumour.

379. Involuntary oscillatory eye movements (nystagmus)
A. Do not occur in healthy people.
B. May result from cochlear disease.
C. Occur in cerebellar disease.
D. Occur when cold fluid is run into one external ear canal.
E. Do not affect acuity of vision.

380. Typical effects of ageing on the special senses include gradual loss of
A. Near vision.
B. Olfactory sensitivity (hyposmia).
C. 90 per cent of the accommodative power of the lens during the lifespan.
D. Hearing affecting bone and air conduction similarly.
E. Hearing affecting high and low frequencies similarly.

381. A child who focuses an object on the fovea of the left eye and on the temporal side of the fovea in the right eye is likely to have
A. A divergent squint.
B. A refractive error.
C. Suppression of vision in the left rather than in the right eye.
D. No suppression of vision in one eye if the left eye is covered for part of each day.
E. A lesser tendency to suppression of vision in one eye if given exercises requiring binocular vision.

382. In unilateral vestibular disease, typical features include
A. The sensation that the external world is revolving.
B. Prolonged nystagmus when cold water is placed in the external auditory meatus on the affected side.
C. A tendency to stagger when walking.
D. A tendency to fall in the dark.
E. Nausea and vomiting.

383. Impairment of visual acuity in bright light can be explained by
A. Random light scattering when there is deficient pigmentation of the eye due to albinism.
B. Random light scattering when there is asymmetrical corneal curvature due to astigmatism.
C. Random light scattering in the cornea when there is vitamin A deficiency.
D. Impairment of rod function when there is vitamin A deficiency.
E. Inability to alter the focal length of the lens when a cataract is present.

384. In long-sightedness (hypermetropia)
A. Objects at infinity cannot be focused sharply on the retina.
B. Objects at the usual near-point are focused behind the retina.
C. Ciliary muscle contracts more strongly to bring objects in mid-visual range into clear focus.
D. The range of unblurred vision (near-point to far-point) is greater than normal.
E. The near-point can be brought closer to the eye by the use of a biconcave lens.

Answers

378.

A.   True   If only some of the many receptor types involved in olfaction are lost.
B.   True   Due to damage to the olfactory nerves by distortion of the cranium.
C.   False   Smell pathways do not pass through the thalamus.
D.   True   This can prevent odours reaching the receptor cells.
E.   False   It may indicate a frontal lobe tumour.

379.

A.   False   They occur when a normal person stops rotating.
B.   False   Disease of the semicircular canals may cause nystagmus.
C.   True   Nystagmus is an ataxia of eye fixation.
D.   True   Due to cooling of fluid in the adjacent semicircular canal.
E.   False   The rapid eye movements tend to make vision blurred.

380.

A.   True   Recession of the near point is typical of the ageing eye (presbyopia); vision at 20–30 cm deteriorates.
B.   True   It affects over 70 per cent of elderly people.
C.   True   It falls from 10–15 dioptres in childhood to 5–10 at 30 and to about 1 dioptre at 70.
D.   True   It is a sensorineural deafness (presbycusis).
E.   False   High-pitched sounds are more affected.

381.

A.   False   The right eye is converging making it a convergent squint.
B.   True   Refractive errors are a common cause of squinting.
C.   False   Suppression of vision tends to occur in the non-fixing eye.
D.   True   Covering the 'good' eye helps to preserve vision in the non-fixing eye.

382.

A.   True   Unbalanced vestibular input causes this sensation (vertigo).
B.   False   In this 'caloric' test, reduction in nystagmus duration indicates vestibular abnormality.
C.   True   Due to inappropriate information affecting brain areas controlling balance.
D.   True   Compensating visual stimuli are then eliminated.
E.   True   Unbalanced, excessive or reduced vestibular inputs cause nausea and vomiting as seen in sea-sickness and space-travel sickness.

383.

A.   True   Normally absorption of light by dark pigment in the choroid prevents back-scattering of light into the retina.
B.   False   There is a refractive error but not random light scattering.
C.   True   Lack of vitamin A leads to keratin deposition in corneal epithelium (xerophthalmia).
D.   False   Rod function does not determine acuity in bright light.
E.   False   Impairment of acuity with cataract is due to random scattering by lens opacities.

384.

A.   False   This is true of shortsightedness (myopia).
B.   True   The eye is usually shorter than normal.
C.   True   This distance is closer than usual to the hypermetrope's near point.
D.   False   It is less than normal; the far point stays at infinity but the near point is further away.
E.   False   A convex lens is required to augment the power of the eye's refracting system.

EMQs

Questions 385–394

EMQ Question 385

For each term related to vision A–E, select the most appropriate option from the list below.

1. Normal vision.
2. Determined by the maximum convexity the lens can attain.
3. Usually involves contraction of the ciliary muscles.
4. Causes reflex contraction of circular smooth muscle in the iris.
5. Due to loss of lens elasticity with ageing.

A. Presbyopia.
B. Pupillary light reflex.
C. The near point.
D. Accommodation.
E. Emmetropia.

EMQ Question 386

For each visual term A–E, select the most appropriate option from the following list of descriptions.

1. Contain the least light-sensitive pigments in the retina.
2. The minimum amount of light that elicits light sensation.
3. The rate below which successive images are seen as separate images.
4. Contain rhodopsin.
5. Can be measured by use of Snellen letter charts.

A. Rods.
B. Visual threshold.
C. Cones.
D. Visual acuity.
E. Critical fusion frequency.

EMQ Question 387

For each visual disturbance A–E, select the most appropriate option from the following list.

1. A blind spot.
2. Inability to see in the dark.
3. Loss of vision.
4. A condition where visual images do not fall on corresponding retinal points.
5. Double vision.

A. Strabismus.
B. Diplopia.
C. Amblyopia.
D. Scotoma.
E. Nyctalopia.

Answers for 385

A. **Option 5**   *Due to loss of lens elasticity with ageing.* With increasing age, the lens loses its elasticity, so decreasing the ability of the eye to accommodate for near vision.

B. **Option 4**   *Causes reflex contraction of circular smooth muscle in the iris.* If light is shone on the retina, the circular ciliary muscles contract to decrease the size of the pupil so decreasing spherical aberration by the lens.

C. **Option 2**   *Determined by the maximum convexity the lens can attain.* The near point is the point nearest to the eye where the lens system can focus a sharp image. It depends on the elasticity of the lens and is nearest in infancy and recedes with age.

D. **Option 3**   *Usually involves contraction of the ciliary muscles.* Accommodation for near vision depends on contraction of the ciliary muscle to increase the convexity of the lens, convergence of the axes of the eyes and constriction of the pupils.

E. **Option 1**   *Normal vision.* Emmetropia is the term describing normal refraction in the eye. It contrasts with hypermetropia (long-sightedness) and myopia (short-sightedness).

Answers for 386

A. **Option 4**   *Contain rhodopsin.* Rhodopsin is responsible for vision in poor light. It (Visual Purple) is the most sensitive visual pigment with a peak sensitivity to light at 505 nm.

B. **Option 2**   *The minimum amount of light that elicits light sensation.* In dark adaptation the visual threshold falls.

C. **Option 1**   *Contain the least light-sensitive pigments in the retina.* The cones contain three colour sensitive pigments and are responsible for colour vision and vision in bright light.

D. **Option 5**   *Can be measured by use of Snellen letter charts.* The results are expressed as a fraction – 20/20 (or 6/6) being normal; a fraction less than unity, e.g. 10/20 indicates below normal acuity.

E. **Option 3**   *The rate below which successive images are seen as separate images.* Above that rate the images fuse to provide a continuous image.

Answers for 387

A. **Option 4**   *A condition where visual images do not fall on corresponding retinal points.* This is squint.

B. **Option 5**   *Double vision.* This is usually caused by problems in the control of the external ocular muscles which interfere with the ability of the eyes to form images on corresponding retinal points.

C. **Option 3**   *Loss of vision.* It may be partial or complete.

D. **Option 1**   *A blind spot.* Visual impairment with a scotoma depends on its location on the retina. Central scotomas are more disabling than peripheral scotomas.

E. **Option 2**   *Inability to see in the dark.* Night blindness is seen where there is a deficiency of Vitamin A that is needed for the production of rhodopsin.

EMQ Question 388

For each of the visual terms A–E, select the most appropriate option from the following list of definitions.

1. Blindness in half of the visual field.
2. Loss of central vision with normal peripheral vision.
3. Continuous jerky movements of the eyeballs.
4. People who can only distinguish between two primary colours.
5. Loss of peripheral vision with normal central vision.

A. Nystagmus.
B. Hemianopia.
C. Dichromats.
D. Central scotoma.
E. Macular sparing.

EMQ Question 389

For each of the structures concerned with sound transmission in the ear A–E, select the most appropriate option from the list below.

1. Bulges out when the oval window membrane bulges in.
2. Dampens vibration of the oval window membrane.
3. Dampens vibrations of the tympanic membrane.
4. Located in the foramen ovale.
5. Bulges in when the oval window bulges in.

A. Foot plate of stapes.
B. Tympanic membrane.
C. Tensor tympani muscle.
D. Stapedius muscle.
E. Round window.

EMQ Question 390

For each of the structures concerned with inner ear receptor organs A–E, select the most appropriate option from the list below.

1. The gelatinous partition of top of the crista that closes off the ampulla.
2. The sensory organ in the utricle.
3. The membrane structure overlying the receptor cells in the organ of Corti.
4. The sensory organ in the semicircular canals.
5. The hair processes on receptor cells in the inner ear.

A. Crista ampullaris.
B. Otolith organ.
C. Cupula.
D. Stereocilia.
E. Tectorial membrane.

Answers for 388

A.   **Option 3**   *Continuous jerky movements of the eyeballs.* These can occur normally (physiological nystagmus) but are exaggerated in certain diseases affecting the cerebellum.

B.   **Option 1**   *Blindness in half of the visual field.* Usually caused by a lesion in one optic tract. A lesion affecting one optic nerve causes total blindness in that eye.

C.   **Option 4**   *People who can only distinguish between two primary colours.* This is one form of colour blindness; healthy people (trichromats) can distinguish between the three primary colours.

D.   **Option 2**   *Loss of central vision with normal peripheral vision.* This is due to damage to the macula.

E.   **Option 5**   *Loss of peripheral vision with normal central vision.* This is often seen in patients with lesions affecting the occipital (visual) cortex.

Answers for 389

A.   **Option 4**   *Located in the foramen ovale.* It is embedded in the foramen ovale membrane.

B.   **Option 5**   *Bulges in when the oval window bulges in.* Tympanic membrane movements are transmitted by the auditory ossicles to the oval window.

C.   **Option 3**   *Dampens vibrations of the tympanic membrane.* This muscle is attached to the manubrium of the malleus and when it contracts reflexly in response to an incoming sound, it tightens the tympanic membrane and damps its movements.

D.   **Option 2**   *Dampens vibration of the oval window membrane.* The stapedius muscle is attached to the stapes and pulls on it reflexly to dampen its movements in response to incoming loud noise.

E.   **Option 1**   *Bulges out when the oval window membrane bulges in.* The round window lies where the scala tympani abuts on the middle ear and by bulging out when the stapes footplate bulges in reduces the pressure changes with incoming sounds in the inner ear.

Answers for 390

A.   **Option 4**   *The sensory organ in the semicircular canals.* Each semicircular canal has an ampulla whose sense organ is stimulated by movement of endolymph caused by rotary accelerations of the head in the three spatial planes in which the semicircular canals lie.

B.   **Option 2**   *The sensory organ in the utricle.* These sensory organs are stimulated by linear accelerations of the head that modify the pull of the otoliths on the hair cells of the otolith organ.

C.   **Option 1**   *The gelatinous partition of top of the crista that closes off the ampulla.* When there is movement of fluid in the semicircular canals it causes deflections of the cupula that alter the output of impulses from the underlying crista ampullaris.

D.   **Option 5**   *The hair processes on receptor cells in the inner ear.* These rod-shaped structures protrude from the hair cells and cause generator potentials when they are deformed by movement of endolymph.

E.   **Option 3**   *The membrane structure overlying the receptor cells in the organ of Corti.* This structure which overlies the organ of Corti may be involved in bending of hair cells when the basilar membrane is made to vibrate with incoming sound waves.

EMQ Question 391

For each of the structures concerned with hearing A–E, select the most appropriate option from the list below.

1. A centre for auditory reflexes.
2. Separates scala in the inner ear.
3. Equalizes middle ear with atmospheric pressure.
4. Responsible for bony conduction of incoming sound waves.
5. Important in air conduction of incoming sound waves.

A. The basilar membrane.
B. The skull.
C. The auditory ossicles.
D. The Eustachian tube.
E. Inferior colliculi.

EMQ Question 392

For each of the structures concerned with taste sensation A–E, select the most appropriate option from the list below.

1. Carries taste impulses serving the sensation of sweetness.
2. Associated with bitter taste sensation.
3. Carries taste impulses serving the sensation of bitterness.
4. Associated with sweet taste sensation.
5. Associated with salt taste sensation.

A. Taste buds at the back of the tongue.
B. Taste buds at the front of the tongue.
C. Taste buds at the side of the tongue.
D. The glossopharyngeal nerve.
E. The facial nerve.

EMQ Question 393

For each of the sensory pathways A–E, select the most appropriate option from the list below.

1. Third order sensory pathway from thalamus to the postcentral gyrus.
2. The tracts carrying proprioception impulses in first order sensory neurones to the nucleus gracilis and cuneatus.
3. A tract in the brainstem carrying sensory impulses to the thalamus.
4. A tract containing the second order sensory neurones carrying pain and temperature sensation.
5. A tract containing the ascending second order neurones carrying touch and pressure sensation.

A. Lateral spino-thalamic tract.
B. Thalamic radiation.
C. Medial (ventral) spino-thalamic tract.
D. Dorsal columns.
E. Medial lemniscus.

Answers to 391

A. **Option 2**   *Separates scala in the inner ear.* The basilar membrane on which the organ of Corti lies separates the scala media from the scala tympani.

B. **Option 4**   *Responsible for bony conduction of incoming sound waves.* If the middle ear is completely destroyed by disease, some hearing ability remains as sound waves can be conducted through the bone of the skull to the inner ear.

C. **Option 5**   *Important in air conduction of incoming sound waves.* The malleus, incus and stapes form a good lever system to transmit sound waves from the tympanic membrane to the round window without much attenuation.

D. **Option 3**   *Equalizes middle ear with atmospheric pressure.* The Eustachian tube connects the middle ear to the pharynx so that the pressure on either side of the tympanic membrane is about atmospheric.

E. **Option 1**   *A centre for auditory reflexes.* The cochlear nerve carries auditory impulses from the organ of Corti to the inferior colliculi, centres for auditory reflexes.

Answers for 392

A. **Option 2**   *Associated with bitter taste sensation.* The taste buds sensing bitter tastes are located in the vallate papillae in a V-shaped area on the back part of the upper surface of the tongue.

B. **Option 4**   *Associated with sweet taste sensation.* Taste buds that sense sweet stimuli are in the fungiform papillae on the dorsal surface towards the front of the tongue.

C. **Option 5**   *Associated with salt taste sensation.* The taste buds at the side of the tongue respond to salt and sour taste stimuli.

D. **Option 3**   *Carries taste impulses serving the sensation of bitterness.* The glossopharyngeal nerve carries impulses from the posterior third of the surface of the tongue and thus serves bitter taste sensation.

E. **Option 1**   *Carries taste impulses serving the sensation of sweetness.* The chorda tympani branch of the facial nerve carries sensory impulses from the anterior two-thirds of the tongue and thus serves the sensation of sweetness.

Answers for 393

A. **Option 4**   *A tract containing the second order sensory neurones carrying pain and temperature sensation.* These tracts carry pain and temperature impulses from receptors on the opposite side of the body to the thalamus.

B. **Option 1**   *Third order sensory pathway from thalamus to the postcentral gyrus.* In the postcentral gyrus the sensory impulses generate conscious sensation.

C. **Option 5**   *A tract containing the ascending second order neurones carrying touch and pressure sensation.* These tracts carry touch and pressure impulses from the opposite side of the body to the thalamus.

D. **Option 2**   *The tracts carrying proprioception impulses in first order sensory neurones to the nucleus gracilis and cuneatus.* These tracts carry impulses from muscle spindles and other receptors on the same side of the body that ascend in first order sensory neurones to the gracile and cuneate nuclei. From there second order neurones cross to the opposite side of the body in the sensory decussation to join the medial lemniscus and ascend to the thalamus.

E. **Option 3**   *A tract in the brainstem carrying sensory impulses to the thalamus.* This is the common sensory pathway in the brainstem carrying all sensory impulses to the thalamus.

EMQ Question 394

For each of the sensory disturbances A–E, select the most appropriate option from the list below.

1. The gradual loss of hearing ability with age.

2. The loss of ability to recognize objects by touch.

3. Absence of smell sensation.

4. Night blindness.

5. A refractive error due to the cornea having different refractive power in the horizontal and transverse planes.

6. A disorder of hearing where the patient complains of hearing abnormal noise.

A. Astereognosis.
B. Astigmatism.
C. Presbycusis.
D. Anosmia.
E. Tinnitus.

Answers for 394

A. **Option 2**   *The loss of ability to recognize objects by touch.* This ability is a cortical function and its loss suggests damage to the sensory cortex in the postcentral gyrus of the parietal lobe.

B. **Option 5**   *A refractive error due to the cornea having different refractive power in the horizontal and transverse planes.* This common refractive error is corrected by provision of cylindrical lenses that make refraction in the vertical plane equal refraction in the horizontal plane.

C. **Option 1**   *The gradual loss of hearing ability with age.* This affects about one third of people over seventy and is probably due to cumulative damage to the hair cells in the organs of Corti. It tends to be worse in people who have lived and worked in noisy environments.

D. **Option 3**   *Absence of smell sensation.* As with hearing, sensitivity to smell stimuli tends to decrease with age. Temporary anosmia is a feature of the common cold.

E. **Option 6**   *A disorder of hearing where the patient complains of hearing abnormal noise.* The noise is described as ringing, buzzing, roaring etc.

MCQs

Questions 395–400

395. Hydrostatic pressure in renal glomerular capillaries
A. Is lower than pressure in efferent arterioles.
B. Rises when afferent arterioles constrict.
C. Is higher than in most capillaries at heart level.
D. Falls by 10 per cent when arterial pressure falls by 10 per cent.
E. Falls along the length of the capillary.

396. Tubular reabsorption of a filtered substance is likely to be active rather than passive if its
A. Concentration in the tubular fluid is lower than in peritubular capillary blood.
B. Excretion is increased by cooling the kidney.
C. Renal clearance is lower than that of inulin.
D. Renal clearance rises at high plasma levels.
E. Urinary excretion rate:plasma concentration ratio is the same as for glucose.

397. The renal clearance of a substance
A. Is inversely related to its urinary concentration, U.
B. Is directly related to the rate of urine formation, V.
C. Is directly related to its plasma concentration, P.
D. Is expressed in units of volume per unit time.
E. Must fall in the presence of metabolic poisons.

398. In fluid in the distal part of the proximal convoluted tubule
A. Urea concentration is higher than in Bowman's capsule.
B. pH is less than 6 when the kidneys are excreting an acid urine.
C. Glucose concentration is similar to that in plasma.
D. Osmolality is about 25 per cent that of glomerular filtrate.
E. Bicarbonate concentration is lower than in plasma.

399. Renal tubules normally reabsorb
A. More water every hour than the entire plasma volume.
B. All filtered HCO_3^- in respiratory acidosis.
C. All filtered amino acids.
D. All filtered plasma proteins.
E. More K^+ than Cl^-.

400. As plasma glucose concentration rises above normal, glucose
A. Filtration increases linearly.
B. Transport maximum T_m increases linearly.
C. Clearance increases linearly.
D. Reabsorption increases and then levels off.
E. Excretion increases and then decreases.

Answers

395.

A.	False	It must be higher to maintain blood flow.
B.	False	The pressure drop across the afferent arterioles increases as they constrict.
C.	True	The afferent arterioles offer relatively little resistance.
D.	False	Redistribution of renal vascular resistance due to autoregulation tends to maintain glomerular hydrostatic pressure and hence filtration.
E.	True	Hydrostatic pressure falls due to vascular resistance; oncotic pressure rises due to loss of protein-poor filtrate; both these factors reduce filtration pressure along the length of the glomerular capillary.

396.

A.	True	This suggests transportation into the blood against a concentration gradient.
B.	True	Cooling impairs active metabolic processes.
C.	False	This indicates reabsorption but not whether it is active (e.g. glucose) or passive (e.g. urea).
D.	True	This suggests saturation of a carrier system.
E.	True	Anything filtered in glomeruli and having zero clearance must be actively reabsorbed.

397.

A.	False	It is directly related to urinary concentration.
B.	True	Clearance tends to fall at low urinary flow rates.
C.	False	It is inversely related to plasma concentration.
D.	True	Clearance $= UV/P$ in units of volume/unit time.
E.	False	It rises if the substance is normally reabsorbed by an active process.

398.

A.	True	Due to reabsorption of water.
B.	False	Acidification occurs mainly in the distal convoluted tubule.
C.	False	Most or all of the glucose is reabsorbed before the end of the proximal tubule.
D.	False	Osmolality changes little in the proximal convoluted tubule.
E.	True	Like glucose, HCO_3^- is usually completely reabsorbed in the proximal tubule.

399.

A.	True	About 99 per cent of the glomerular filtrate (about 8 litres/hour).
B.	True	This plus HCO_3^- manufactured in the kidney compensates the respiratory acidosis.
C.	True	These are filtered but do not appear in normal urine.
D.	True	Again some are filtered but do not appear in urine.
E.	False	About 20 times as much chloride as potassium is filtered (this is the ratio of their plasma concentrations).

400.

A.	True	Filtration rate is directly proportional to concentration.
B.	False	Transport maxima are constants.
C.	False	It remains at zero until the T_m is reached and then it rises linearly.
D.	True	It levels off after T_m glucose is reached.
E.	False	It is initially zero and then rises linearly.

Questions 401–406

401. A substance is being secreted by the renal tubules if its

A. Clearance rate is greater than 250 ml/minute.
B. Concentration is higher in arterial than in renal venous blood.
C. Excretion rate is increased by tubular enzyme poisons.
D. Concentration rises along the proximal convoluted tubule.
E. Concentration in urine is greater than in plasma.

402. In the nephron, the osmolality of fluid in the

A. Tip of the loop of Henle is less than that of plasma.
B. Bowman's capsules is less than that in the distal tubules.
C. Collecting duct rises when vasopressin is being secreted.
D. Proximal convoluted tubule rises along its length.
E. Medullary interstitium can exceed one osmole per litre.

403. Transport maximum (T_m) – limited reabsorption of a substance implies that its

A. Reabsorption is active.
B. Reabsorption is critically related to tubular transit time.
C. Reabsorption is complete below a certain threshold load.
D. Renal clearance falls with its plasma concentration.
E. Excretion rate is zero until its T_m value is reached.

404. When a patient's mean arterial blood pressure falls by 50 per cent

A. Renal blood flow falls by less than 10 per cent.
B. Glomerular filtration falls by about 50 per cent.
C. There is an increase in the circulating aldosterone level.
D. Renal vasoconstriction occurs.
E. Urinary output ceases.

405. The cells of the distal convoluted tubule

A. Reabsorb about 50 per cent of the water filtered by the glomeruli.
B. Secrete hydrogen ions into the tubular lumen.
C. Form NH_4^+ ions.
D. Reabsorb sodium in exchange for hydrogen or potassium ions.
E. Determine the final composition of urine.

406. If, during an infusion of para-aminohippuric acid, peripheral venous plasma PAH level is 0.02 mg/ml (not above renal threshold), urinary PAH level is 16 mg/ml and urinary flow rate 1 ml/min, then the

A. PAH level in renal venous blood must exceed 0.02 mg/ml.
B. PAH level in renal arterial blood must be about 0.02 mg/ml.
C. PAH level in glomerular filtrate must be about 0.02 mg/ml.
D. Renal plasma flow is nearer 800 than 1000 ml/minute.
E. Renal blood flow is nearer 1300 than 1500 ml/minute if the haematocrit is 0.40.

Answers

401.
A.   True   A clearance value above the glomerular filtration rate (about 140 ml/minute) indicates secretion.
B.   True   Some of the unfiltered fraction must have been secreted.
C.   False   This suggests that the substance is normally reabsorbed by an active process.
D.   False   This can be explained by water reabsorption.
E.   False   Again, this can be explained by a relatively greater reabsorption of water.

402.
A.   False   This fluid is hypertonic because of countercurrent concentration.
B.   False   Distal tubular fluid is hypotonic.
C.   True   Vasopressin (ADH) promotes water, but not salt, reabsorption in collecting ducts.
D.   False   The fluid remains isotonic with plasma.
E.   True   It can be about four times that of plasma.

403.
A.   True T_m limited reabsorption is one type of active tubular reabsorption.
B.   False   This applies to the other type of active tubular reabsorption, gradient-time limited reabsorption.
C.   True   As with glucose.
D.   False   Clearance is zero at all levels below the threshold.
E.   True   The concept applies also to amino acids and proteins.

404.
A.   False   Autoregulation cannot compensate for such large falls.
B.   False   It falls to about zero when glomerular capillary pressure falls below the sum of intracapsular pressure plus plasma oncotic pressure – around 30–40 mmHg.
C.   True   Due to release of renin and angiotensin formation, aldosterone is secreted.
D.   True   Reflex sympathetic vasoconstriction due to greatly decreased baroreceptor stimulation.
E.   True   When glomerular filtration stops, urinary output stops.

405.
A.   False   About 80 per cent of the filtered water is reabsorbed before it reaches the distal tubules.
B.   True   The rate is related to acid–base requirements.
C.   True   By conversion of glutamine to glutamate; NH_3 is a buffer for the H^+ being excreted.
D.   True H^+ secretion is related to the body's acid–base balance.
E.   False   Further modification takes place in the collecting ducts.

406.
A.   False   The renal venous blood level would be negligible.
B.   True   Since PAH is excreted only by the kidneys, the PAH level in peripheral venous blood determines the level entering the arterial system, and hence the renal arteries.
C.   True   Since PAH is freely filtered.
D.   True   Flow $=$ PAH clearance $=$ UV/P $= 16 \times 1/0.02 = 800$ ml/minute.
E.   True   Blood flow $=$ plasma flow/0.6 $= 1333$ ml/minute.

Questions 407–411

407. Renal blood flow falls
A. About 10 per cent when arterial pressure falls 10 per cent below normal.
B. About 5 per cent when metabolic activity in the kidney falls by 5 per cent.
C. During emotional stress.
D. After moderate haemorrhage.
E. Gradually from the inner medulla to the outer cortex per unit weight of tissue.

408. Urea
A. And glucose have similar molar concentrations in normal blood.
B. Concentration rises in tubular fluid as the glomerular filtrate passes down the nephron.
C. Is actively secreted by the renal tubular cells into the tubular fluid.
D. Concentration in blood may rise ten-fold after a high protein meal
E. Causes a diuresis when its blood concentration is increased.

409. Voluntary micturition
A. Depends on the integrity of a lumbar spinal reflex arc.
B. Is not possible after sensory denervation of the bladder.
C. Involves stimulation of the detrusor muscle in the bladder by autonomic sympathetic nerves.
D. Is normally accompanied by some reflux of bladder contents into the ureters.
E. Is inhibited during ejaculation.

410. The proximal convoluted tubules
A. Reabsorb most of the sodium ions in glomerular filtrate.
B. Reabsorb most of the chloride ions in glomerular filtrate.
C. Reabsorb most of the potassium ions in glomerular filtrate.
D. Contain juxtaglomerular cells which secrete rennin.
E. Contain the main target cells for antidiuretic hormone.

411. The renal clearance of
A. Inulin provides an estimate of glomerular filtration rate.
B. Chloride increases after an injection of aldosterone.
C. PAH falls when the PAH load exceeds the T_m for PAH.
D. Urea is lower than that of inulin.
E. Inulin is independent of its plasma concentration.

Answers

407.

A. False Due to autoregulation, flow changes little with small changes in perfusion pressure.
B. False Normal renal blood flow is vastly in excess of its metabolic requirements.
C. True Due to sympathetic vasoconstrictor nerves and circulating catecholamines.
D. True A reflex response to the fall in blood pressure so caused.
E. False Cortical flow is 10–20 times higher than medullary flow.

408.

A. True Both are around 5 mmol/litre.
B. True The urinary concentration of urea is many times that in plasma.
C. False 50 per cent of the filtered urea is passively reabsorbed; the rise in tubular concentration can be explained by the reabsorption of water.
D. False It rises but would not double in concentration.
E. True It causes an osmotic diuresis.

409.

A. False The reflex centres are in the sacral cord; their activity is modulated by higher centres.
B. True This breaks the reflex arc.
C. False Parasympathetic nerves are motor to the detrusor muscle.
D. False Valves where the ureters enter the bladder do not allow such reflux.
E. True During ejaculation, sympathetic activity constricts the bladder neck sphincter and prevents retrograde ejaculation of semen into the bladder.

410.

A. True More than half of the filtered sodium is actively absorbed in the proximal tubules.
B. True Negatively charged chloride ions follow the positively charged sodium.
C. True Most of the potassium is reabsorbed in the proximal tubule; some is re-excreted in the distal tubules in exchange for sodium.
D. False Rennin is an enzyme found in gastric juice that causes milk to clot. The juxtaglomerular cells that secrete renin are found where the distal tubule makes contact with the afferent arteriole.
E. False This hormone acts mainly on distal parts of the nephron.

411.

A. True Inulin is freely filtered but not reabsorbed or secreted in the tubules; therefore the amount excreted in the urine equals the amount filtered at the glomerulus.
B. False Aldosterone increases Na^+ and Cl^- reabsorption and so reduces their clearance.
C. True At high plasma levels, the T_m for PAH is exceeded and PAH is not completely cleared in one passage through the kidney.
D. True About 60 compared with 120 ml/minute; half the filtered urea is passively reabsorbed.
E. True The amount filtered is the amount excreted.

Questions 412–417

412. The collecting ducts in the kidney
A. Can actively transport water molecules into the urine.
B. Are the site of most of renal water reabsorption.
C. Are rendered impermeable to water by antidiuretic hormone (ADH).
D. Pass through a region of exceptional hypertonicity.
E. Determine to a large extent the final osmolality of urine.

413. Aldosterone
A. Is a steroid hormone secreted by the adrenal medulla.
B. Production ceases following removal of the kidneys and their juxtaglomerular cells.
C. Production decreases in treatment with drugs which block angiotensin-converting enzyme.
D. Secretion results in increased potassium reabsorption by the nephron.
E. Secretion results in a fall in urinary pH.

414. As fluid passes down the proximal convoluted tubule, there is a fall of more than 50 per cent in the
A. Concentration of sulphate ions.
B. Concentration of sodium ions.
C. Concentrations of amino acids.
D. Concentration of potassium ions.
E. Rate of filtrate flow in the tubules.

415. In normal healthy people, urinary
A. Specific gravity ranges from 1.010–1.020.
B. Osmolality ranges from 200–400 mosmol/litre.
C. Colour is due to small quantities of bile pigments.
D. pH falls as dietary protein rises.
E. Calcium excretion is increased by parathormone.

416. Aldosterone secretion tends to raise the volume of
A. Plasma.
B. Interstitial fluid.
C. Intracellular fluid.
D. Urine.
E. Cerebrospinal fluid.

417. The renal clearance of
A. Bicarbonate is similar to that of glucose.
B. PAH is nearer 600 than 1200 ml/minute in the average adult.
C. Creatinine provides an estimate of renal plasma flow.
D. Phosphate is decreased by parathormone.
E. Protein is normally zero.

Answers

412.

A.   False   Active transport of water has not been described in the body.
B.   False   More than half of the water in glomerular filtrate is reabsorbed in the proximal tubules.
C.   False   Conversely, they are rendered permeable to water by ADH which induces water channels in the collecting ducts.
D.   True   Osmolality in the inner medullary interstitium can exceed 1 osmol/litre.
E.   True   By determining the amount of water reabsorbed as the glomerular filtrate passes through the hypertonic medullary interstitium.

413.

A.   False   It is a steroid as its name suggests but is secreted by the adrenal cortex.
B.   False   Some aldosterone is secreted in response to ACTH secretion, high K^+ intake, heart failure, etc. in addition to activity in the renin/angiotensin system.
C.   True   ACE inhibitor drugs tend to reduce the level of angiotensin II which stimulates the adrenal cortex to produce aldosterone.
D.   False   It increases potassium secretion in exchange for sodium.
E.   True   It increases H^+ secretion also in exchange for sodium.

414.

A.   False   Sulphate concentration rises since relatively more water than sulphate is reabsorbed.
B.   False   It is little changed, since similar proportions of sodium and water are reabsorbed.
C.   True   These are completely reabsorbed by active transport.
D.   False   Potassium is reabsorbed in proportion to water.
E.   True   Due to reabsorption of about 80 per cent of the water.

415.

A.   False   It may range from 1.004 to 1.040.
B.   False   It may range from 100 to 1000 mosmol/litre.
C.   False   It is due to 'urochrome', a pigment of uncertain origin.
D.   True   Dietary proteins lead to acid residues such as sulphates and phosphates.
E.   True   More calcium is filtered due to the raised blood level, so more is excreted.

416.

A.   True   By retention of sodium chloride and water in the extracellular fluid compartment.
B.   True   This, like plasma, is a subcompartment of the extracellular fluid.
C.   False   The sodium chloride/water retention is confined to the extracellular compartment.
D.   False   It reduces it by retaining salt and water.
E.   False   CSF is a secretion classified as transcellular fluid; it is not a subcompartment of ECF.

417.

A.   True   Both are usually totally reabsorbed so their renal clearance is about zero.
B.   True   PAH clearance is a measure of renal plasma flow, not renal blood flow.
C.   False   It provides an estimate of the glomerular filtration rate since the amount filtered is close to the amount excreted.
D.   False   Phosphate clearance is increased by parathormone and lowers the blood phosphate level.
E.   True   Small amounts of protein are filtered but reabsorbed.

Questions 418–423

418. Potassium
A. Is actively secreted in the distal convoluted tubule.
B. Is reabsorbed in the proximal convoluted tubule.
C. Deficiency favours hydrogen ion secretion in the distal tubule.
D. Excretion is determined largely by potassium intake.
E. Blood levels tend to rise in patients with acute renal failure taking a normal diet.

419. Secretion of renin
A. Occurs in the stomach during infancy.
B. Is stimulated by the hormone angiotensin I.
C. Leads to raised levels of angiotensin II in the blood.
D. Is stimulated by a fall in extracellular fluid volume.
E. Inhibits ACTH secretion by the pituitary gland.

420. In chronic renal failure
A. Glomerular filtration rate may fall by 70 per cent before the condition gives rise to symptoms.
B. The specific gravity of the urine tends to be elevated, e.g. about 1.030.
C. Blood P_{CO_2} tends to be low.
D. Ionized calcium levels in the blood tend to be high.
E. Anaemia is common.

421. Diabetes insipidus (deficiency of antidiuretic hormone) causes a fall in the
A. Osmolality of the urine.
B. Reabsorption of water from the proximal tubules.
C. Extracellular but not intracellular fluid volume.
D. Extracellular fluid osmolality
E. Intracellular fluid osmolality.

422. The cystometrogram shows
A. A plot of bladder pressure on the ordinate axis against bladder volume on the abscissa.
B. Little rise in pressure with rise in volume at low bladder volumes.
C. A steep rise in pressure when volume rises above 100 ml.
D. That females generate higher pressures during micturition than males.
E. That patients with chronic urinary tract obstruction can generate higher than normal micturition pressures.

423. Treatment with an aldosterone antagonist causes a fall in
A. Urine volume.
B. Body potassium.
C. Body sodium.
D. Blood volume.
E. Blood viscosity.

Answers

418.

A.   True   In exchange for sodium ions.

B.   True   It is reabsorbed passively down the gradient created by Na^+ and H_2O reabsorption.

C.   True   Potassium and hydrogen compete for secretion in exchange for sodium.

D.   True   Thus potassium balance is maintained.

E.   True   In acute renal failure, the failure to excrete the potassium intake leads to high blood levels which can compromise the performance of the heart.

419.

A.   False   *Rennin* is the enzyme secreted by infant's gastric mucosa which curdles milk.

B.   False   Renin promotes angiotensin I formation from a circulating precursor.

C.   True   Angiotensin I is converted to angiotensin II by a converting enzyme in the lungs.

D.   True   Renin's action helps to restore this volume.

E.   False   There is no direct feedback between the two systems.

420.

A.   True   The kidneys have a large functional reserve.

B.   False   Renal ability to concentrate urine is impaired; the range of specific gravity decreases, converging towards that of protein-free plasma, 1.010.

C.   True   Poor excretion of acid residues causes metabolic acidosis which stimulates ventilation.

D.   False   Ionized calcium levels fall due to retention of phosphate ions and failure of renal activation of vitamin D.

E.   True   Due mainly to deficiency of erythropoietin.

421.

A.   True   Due to failure of the kidneys to reabsorb sufficient water.

B.   False   Reabsorption of water in proximal tubules is normal since it depends on the active reabsorption of sodium; reabsorption in the collecting ducts is affected.

C.   False   Both fluid compartments are depleted in volume.

D.   False   It rises due to depletion of water but not salt.

E.   False   Both compartments show the same raised osmolality; osmotic gradients are effective in moving water at cell membranes.

422.

A.   True   Bladder pressure is measured while known volumes of fluid are run into it.

B.   True   An example of receptive relaxation like that seen in the stomach.

C.   False   The deflection usually occurs when around 500 ml is introduced.

D.   False   The male urinary tract offers a higher 'peripheral resistance'.

E.   True   The increased work load causes muscular hypertrophy which allows generation of higher micturition pressures.

423.

A.   False   It increases due to increased salt and water loss.

B.   False   Body potassium rises since aldosterone normally increases its excretion.

C.   True   Due to decreased sodium reabsorption.

D.   True   Due to decreased extracellular fluid volume.

E.   False   The viscosity increases as the haematocrit increases.

Questions 424–429

424. Dialysis fluid used in the treatment of renal failure should contain the normal plasma levels of

A. Urea.
B. Potassium.
C. Osmolality.
D. Plasma proteins.
E. Hydrogen ions.

425. Long-standing obstruction of the urethra may cause

A. Enlargement of the prostate gland.
B. Hypertrophy of the bladder muscle.
C. Dilation of the ureters.
D. Reduction of the glomerular filtration rate.
E. An increase in residual volume in the bladder.

426. Emptying of the bladder may be less effective if

A. The sympathetic nerves carrying afferent information from bladder to spinal cord are cut.
B. The pelvic nerves are cut.
C. Anticholinergic drugs are administered.
D. Alpha-adrenergic receptor antagonists are administered.
E. Beta-adrenergic receptor agonists are administered.

427. Renal transplantation for chronic renal failure in adults should

A. Be covered by immunosuppression even when the donor is the recipient's identical twin.
B. Raise postoperative glomerular filtration rate to the 10–20 ml/minute level.
C. Correct abnormal calcium metabolism.
D. Correct anaemia.
E. Abolish the need for further renal dialysis.

428. Drugs which interfere with active transport of sodium in the proximal tubule tend to increase

A. Urine production.
B. Plasma osmolality.
C. Chloride excretion.
D. Interstitial fluid volume.
E. Plasma specific gravity.

429. A drug which inhibits carbonic anhydrase decreases

A. Bicarbonate formation and reabsorption in the kidney.
B. Plasma bicarbonate levels.
C. Blood pH.
D. Urinary loss of potassium ions.
E. Urinary volume and pH.

Answers

424.
A. False   It should be urea-free to provide a high concentration gradient for urea loss.
B. False   It should be lower to favour loss of potassium, which is elevated in renal failure.
C. False   It should be higher to reduce extracellular fluid volume and hence blood pressure.
D. False   Fluid transfer is governed by hydrostatic pressure and crystalloid osmolality gradients, not by colloid osmotic pressure gradients.
E. True   It should be buffered to prevent large pH changes.

425.
A. False   Prostatic enlargement is a cause, not a consequence, of urethral obstruction.
B. True   Due to the increased work it has to do.
C. True   Long-standing obstruction leads to urinary reflux when the uretero-vesical valves become incompetent.
D. True   Back-pressure in the ureters is transmitted to the nephrons and raises capsular pressure in the glomerulus.
E. True   This encourages urinary tract infection.

426.
A. False   Sympathetic trunks carry pain afferents, not stretch receptor afferents to the cord.
B. True   These carry the stretch receptor afferents from the bladder and parasympathetic motor fibres to the bladder; the micturition reflex is lost.
C. True   These block the parasympathetic motor fibres to the detrusor muscle.
D. False   Alpha receptor antagonists relax bladder sphincter muscle: they are used to facilitate bladder emptying in patients with benign prostatic hypertrophy.
E. True   They tend to relax the detrusor muscle.

427.
A. False   Donor and recipient have identical genes and immunological characteristics.
B. False   It should raise it to near normal, 120–150 ml/minute.
C. True   This reverses the tendency to demineralization of bone.
D. True   The transplanted kidney should supply the missing erythropoietin.
E. True   A healthy transplanted kidney should return all aspects of renal function to normal.

428.
A. True   By increasing salt and hence water loss.
B. False   This is regulated by ADH and the collecting ducts.
C. True   Chloride passively follows the sodium being excreted.
D. False   This falls with the loss of salt and water.
E. True   Due to concentration of the proteins by removal of water.

429.
A. True   Carbonic anhydrase in tubular cells catalyses the combination of CO_2 and H_2O to form H_2CO_3 which ionizes into H^+ and HCO_3^+ ions.
B. True   This is determined mainly by renal bicarbonate formation.
C. True   This falls as the plasma bicarbonate level falls.
D. False   More K^+ is secreted by the tubules in exchange for sodium since there are fewer H^+ ions to compete with K^+ in the sodium/potassium exchange pump.
E. False   Failure to reabsorb HCO_3 results in an osmotic diuresis of alkaline urine.

Questions 430–434

430. A patient with chronic renal failure usually has an increased
A. Blood urea.
B. Blood uric acid.
C. Creatinine clearance.
D. Acid–base disturbance when he or she vomits.
E. Acid–base problem on a high protein diet.

431. Cutting the sympathetic nerves to the bladder may cause
A. Difficulty in emptying the bladder.
B. Loss of tone in the internal sphincter of the bladder.
C. Loss of tone in the external sphincter of the bladder.
D. Loss of pain sensation in the bladder.
E. Infertility in the male.

432. Sudden (acute) renal failure differs from gradual (chronic) renal failure in that
A. Potassium retention tends to be more severe.
B. Blood urea levels tend to be higher.
C. Depression of bone marrow activity is unlikely to occur.
D. Metabolic acidosis is usually not a problem.
E. Dietary protein restriction is unnecessary.

433. In the treatment of someone with progressive renal failure
A. Protein should be excluded from the diet.
B. Water intake should be restricted to about 0.5 litre/day.
C. The diet should be potassium-free.
D. Adequate dietary iron intake prevents anaemia.
E. The calorific value of the diet should be gradually reduced.

434. A long-standing increase in arterial P_{CO_2} (respiratory acidosis) leads to an increase in
A. Renal bicarbonate formation.
B. Urinary ammonium salts.
C. Plasma potassium concentration.
D. The ratio of monohydrogen to dihydrogen phosphate in urine.
E. Urinary bicarbonate excretion.

Answers

430.

A. True   A high blood urea is usually the first sign of renal failure.
B. True   As with other end products of protein digestion.
C. False   Creatinine clearance, a measure of GFR, is reduced in proportion to the severity of the renal failure.
D. False   Loss of the acid vomitus would improve the typical acidosis.
E. True   Proteins are a major source of the acid residues and toxic substances which accumulate in renal failure.

431.

A. False   It may cause increased frequency of micturition.
B. True   Sympathetic activity tends to raise sphincter tone.
C. False   This sphincter is supplied by somatic nerves.
D. True   Afferent pain fibres run with the sympathetic nerves.
E. True   Sympathetic fibres are necessary for closure of the internal sphincter of the bladder during ejaculation to prevent reflux of seminal fluid.

432.

A. True   Potassium retention is one of the greatest hazards of acute renal failure and may cause death from myocardial depression.
B. False   The blood urea level is determined by the severity of the condition, not by its rate of progression.
C. False   Both may depress the marrow and lower RBC, polymorph and platelet counts.
D. False   Both impair renal bicarbonate production.
E. False   Protein restriction is advisable in both cases.

433.

A. False   A low protein diet is helpful but some protein is needed to provide essential amino acids for tissue maintenance.
B. False   This would not cover insensible loss plus urine volume; also in some stages of renal failure urine volume is increased.
C. False   Potassium intake is required to replace potassium lost in urine.
D. False   Anaemia is due to bone marrow depression, not iron deficiency.
E. False   Sufficient dietary intake is needed to prevent excessive tissue protein catabolism.

434.

A. True   This raises plasma bicarbonate to compensate for the raised P_{CO_2} in respiratory acidosis.
B. True   In acidosis, tubular cells excrete more to buffer the additional H^+ ions being secreted.
C. True   The increased secretion of H^+ ions in exchange for Na^+ results in decreased secretion of K^+ ions.
D. False   The ratio decreases as hydrogen ions are taken up by the phosphate buffer system.
E. False   The urine remains bicarbonate-free.

EMQs

Questions 435–444

EMQ Question 435

For each case of bladder abnormality A–E, select the most appropriate option from the following list.

1. Atonic bladder with overflow.　　　2. Stress incontinence.
3. Chronic prostatic obstruction.　　　4. Acute retention of urine.
5. Automatic bladder.　　　　　　　　6. Bladder diverticulum.

A. A 30-year-old woman with three children complains of wetting herself during coughing and sneezing.

B. A 20-year-old woman had a spinal injury two years ago as a result of diving into shallow water. She has lost normal control of the urinary bladder but can initiate micturition when the bladder is fairly full by pressing on the lower abdomen.

C. An 80-year-old man has been admitted to hospital as an emergency complaining of lower abdominal pain and inability to pass urine for 12 hours. In recent months he had noticed that the urinary stream was poor. On admission he has abnormal dullness to percussion over his lower abdomen and on rectal examination, enlargement of the prostate.

D. A 29-year-old man was admitted to hospital following a neck injury and paralysis of the legs. On the day after admission, knee and ankle jerks cannot be elicited and he is incontinent of urine.

E. A 75-year-old man complains of frequency of micturition and poor flow; his cystometrogram shows raised bladder pressures in the contracted state and an abnormally high residual volume.

EMQ Question 436

For each of the functional descriptions A–E, select the most appropriate option from the following list of regions of the nephron and urinary tract.

1. Proximal convoluted tubule.　　　2. Distal convoluted tubule.
3. Thin limb of loop of Henle.　　　　4. Thick limb of loop of Henle.
5. Collecting duct.　　　　　　　　　6. Ureter.
7. Bladder.　　　　　　　　　　　　8. Urethra.

A. The site of the final major adjustment of the pH of the filtered fluid.

B. A region where reabsorption is associated with the presence of microvilli on the luminal cell surface.

C. A region where the passage of a calculus (stone) is associated with severely painful smooth muscle contractions referred to one side of the lower part of the trunk.

D. The site of the final major adjustment of the ammonium content of the filtered fluid.

E. The site of the final major adjustment of the osmolality of the filtered fluid.

Answers for 435

A. **Option 2**   *Stress incontinence.* During coughing and sneezing intrathoracic and intra-abdominal pressure is raised. In the presence of impaired sphincter action at the bladder outlet, a common consequence of damage during delivery, the raised pressure can expel some urine from the bladder. Laughing may have a similar effect.

B. **Option 5**   *Automatic bladder.* The patient had a spinal injury which has led to loss of bladder control. Such injuries isolate the micturition centre in the sacral cord from higher centre control. In such patients the bladder can empty automatically when distended by means of the bladder stretch reflex centred in the sacral cord. Pressure on the abdomen can initiate the reflex at a convenient time before it occurs automatically.

C. **Option 4**   *Acute retention of urine.* In elderly men, prostatic enlargement leads to progressive compression of the prostatic urethra. This leads to increasing resistance to flow so that the urinary stream is poor. If the obstruction becomes complete so that micturition is impossible, the bladder becomes painfully distended.

D. **Option 1**   *Atonic bladder with overflow.* This is another case of spinal injury isolating the micturition centre in the sacral cord from higher centre control. However, in the acute phase that comes on immediately and lasts for some weeks after the injury, the patient usually shows a complete absence of spinal stretch reflexes below the level of the lesion spinal shock. The micturition stretch reflex is abolished so that the bladder loses tone, becomes distended and leaks uncontrollably due to the high pressure in the passively distended organ. Catheterization is important, to prevent damage to the bladder by such over-stretching.

E. **Option 3**   *Chronic prostatic obstruction.* This is another case of prostatic obstruction but without acute retention of urine. Gradual narrowing of the prostatic urethra raises the urethral resistance which the bladder must overcome. Hypertrophy of the bladder wall occurs (as in the left ventricle in systemic hypertension), hence bladder pressure during a micturating cystometrogram (record of bladder pressure versus volume) is increased. As in the failing heart, the bladder muscle fails to empty as completely as usual.

Answers for 436

A. **Option 2**   *Distal convoluted tubule.* Cells here have the ability to secrete hydrogen ions until the luminal pH has fallen to 4–5.

B. **Option 1**   *Proximal convoluted tubule.* This is the major site for reabsorption, which is facilitated by microvilli similar in many respects to those in the small intestine.

C. **Option 6**   *Ureter.* Passage of a calculus here is associated with the severe pain of renal colic, referred to one or other loin.

D. **Option 2**   *Distal convoluted tubule.* These cells form and secrete ammonia to buffer hydrogen ions secreted in the same region, especially when the rate of hydrogen ion secretion is high; this prevents luminal pH from falling below 4.

E. **Option 5**   *Collecting duct.* Depending on the circulating level of anti-diuretic hormone, the osmolality of the filtrate rises along the collecting duct, to a maximum about four times that of plasma.

EMQ Question 437

For each urinary solute A–E, select the most appropriate option from the following list of concentrations to be found in the urine of healthy people.

1. Always greater than in plasma.
2. Always less than in plasma.
3. Always the same as in plasma.
4. Can be less than or greater than in plasma.

A. Sodium.
B. Hydrogen ions.
C. Potassium ions.
D. Urea.
E. Para-aminohippurate (PAH).

EMQ Question 438

For each description A–E, related to glomerular filtration, select the most appropriate option from the following list of pressures.

1. 0 mmHg.
2. 5 mmHg.
3. 10 mmHg.
4. 15 mmHg.
5. 20 mmHg.
6. 30 mmHg.
7. 40 mmHg.
8. 50 mmHg.
9. 100 mmHg.

A. The pressure drop along the glomerular capillaries when the pressure at the end of the afferent arterioles is 60 mmHg and that at the start of the efferent arterioles is 40 mmHg.
B. The net filtration pressure from capillary lumen to Bowman's capsule when capillary pressure is 60 mmHg, the plasma protein oncotic pressure is 25 mmHg and the capsular pressure is 15 mmHg.
C. The net filtration pressure when capillary pressure is 35 mmHg, oncotic pressure 25 mmHg and capsular pressure 5 mmHg.
D. The capillary pressure which would exactly balance a plasma protein oncotic pressure of 20 mmHg.
E. A capsular pressure at which flow distally along the nephron would not occur.

EMQ Question 439

For each mechanism A–E related to renal handling of plasma solutes, select the most appropriate option from the following list of nephron functions.

1. Active tubular secretion.
2. Passive tubular secretion.
3. Active tubular reabsorption.
4. Passive tubular reabsorption.
5. Glomerular filtration.

A. The mechanism whereby healthy people avoid having glucose in the urine (glycosuria).
B. The mechanism whereby urea has a lower clearance than creatinine.
C. The mechanism whereby around 99 per cent of the filtered water is not lost in the urine.
D. The mechanism whereby the distal convoluted tubules eliminate excess hydrogen ions from the body.
E. The only mechanism whereby the ideal substance for measuring the glomerular filtration rate is eliminated from the body by the kidneys.

Answers for 437

A. **Option 4**   *Can be less than or greater than in plasma.* The plasma sodium level is around 140 mmol per litre; with a low sodium intake of 50 mmol per day and a urinary volume of one litre, the sodium concentration would be 50 mmol per litre; with a fairly high sodium intake of 250 mmol per day and the same urinary volume, the concentration would be 250 mmol per litre.

B. **Option 4**   *Can be less than or greater than in plasma.* Plasma pH is around 7.4; urinary pH can vary from less than 5 to around 8.

C. **Option 1**   *Always greater than in plasma.* The intakes and outputs of potassium are of a similar order to those given for sodium, so to maintain balance, the urinary concentrations are also similar to those of sodium; however the plasma potassium concentration is only about 4 mmol per litre.

D. **Option 1**   *Always greater than in plasma.* About 99 per cent of filtered water is reabsorbed, but only about half of the filtered urea.

E. **Option 1**   *Always greater than in plasma.* Not only is all the filtered PAH excreted (compare urea above), but, provided the tubular maximum is not exceeded, all the PAH reaching the kidney is also excreted.

Answers for 438

A. **Option 5**   *20 mmHg.* This is similar to the pressure drop along systemic capillaries when pressure at the arteriolar end is 35 mmHg and that at the venous end is 15 mmHg.

B. **Option 5**   *20 mmHg.* This would represent the situation at the proximal ends of the glomerular capillaries; further along the capillaries, their hydrostatic pressure falls, while the oncotic pressure rises as protein-poor fluid is filtered; both factors reduce the filtration pressure.

C. **Option 2**   *5 mmHg.* This would represent the situation in a patient with serious hypotension (due, for example, to haemorrhage), just before filtration pressure dropped to zero when no further urine could be formed (anuria).

D. **Option 5**   *20 mmHg.* With this capillary pressure, filtration would not occur; without any flow, capsular pressure would fall to near zero.

E. **Option 1**   *0 mmHg.* Like capillaries, nephrons need a pressure drop along them to permit flow distally.

Answers for 439

A. **Option 3**   *Active tubular reabsorption.* Reabsorption of glucose in the proximal convoluted tubules by a carrier mechanism relies on active reabsorption of sodium ions.

B. **Option 4**   *Passive tubular reabsorption.* Urea, like creatinine, is freely filtered, but, whereas virtually all the creatinine remains in the tubular lumen, about half the filtered urea passively diffuses back into the renal capillaries.

C. **Option 4**   *Passive tubular reabsorption.* Water follows absorbed solutes, particularly sodium and chloride ions, passively by osmosis, as they are reabsorbed into the capillaries.

D. **Option 1**   *Active tubular secretion.* An active pump exchanges absorbed sodium for secreted potassium and hydrogen ions.

E. **Option 5**   *Glomerular filtration.* The ideal substance for measuring glomerular filtration rate is freely filtered and neither absorbed from nor secreted into the tubules in any way; inulin and creatinine are close to the ideal.

EMQ Question 440

For each of the hormonal actions A–E related to the kidney, select the most appropriate option from the following list of hormones.

1. Aldosterone.
2. Antidiuretic hormone.
3. Cortisol.
4. Glucagon.
5. Insulin.
6. Parathormone.
7. Renin.
8. Erythropoietin.

A. An action that prevents glucose being lost in the urine of healthy people.
B. An action that decreases the renal clearance of sodium and thereby increases the extra-cellular volume.
C. An action that promotes the formation of angiotensin I.
D. An action that lowers extracellular phosphate by increasing the renal clearance of phosphate.
E. An action that tends to lower both intracellular and extracellular osmolality.

EMQ Question 441

For each aspect of the treatment of renal failure by haemodialysis or peritoneal dialysis A–E, select the best matching option from the following list of problems caused by renal failure.

1. Raised blood urea.
2. Abnormal arterial blood pressure.
3. Abnormal cardiac rhythms.
4. Hyperventilation.
5. Anaemia.
6. Impaired consciousness.

A. Removal of a variety of toxins, many unidentified, and correction of a variety of metabolic disturbances.
B. Dialysing with fluid with a potassium level well below the normal plasma value.
C. Manipulating pressures and osmolalities in the dialysis fluid to reduce or increase the patient's body fluid content.
D. Dialysing with fluid with a higher pH than the normal plasma level.
E. Dialysing to lower the osmolality of the body fluids, irrespective of any change in electrolytes.

EMQ Question 442

For each of the functional regions in the kidneys mentioned in A–E below, select the most appropriate option for the parts of the kidney associated with that function from the following list (outer medullary means beside the cortex and inner medullary means beside the renal pelvis).

1. Proximal convoluted tubule.
2. Distal convoluted tubule.
3. Thin limb of loop of Henle.
4. Thick limb of loop of Henle.
5. Collecting duct.
6. Outer medullary interstitial fluid.
7. Middle medullary interstitial fluid.
8. Inner medullary interstitial fluid.

A. A region where the osmolality is actively reduced to around one third of the plasma value.
B. A region where the osmolality is around twice the plasma value.
C. A region where the osmolality is around three to four times the plasma value.
D. A region where an energy substrate is reabsorbed by a carrier mechanism linked to active reabsorption of sodium ions, similar to that in the enterocytes of the small intestine.
E. A region where most of the filtered bicarbonate is 'reabsorbed'.

Answers for 440

A. **Option 5**   *Insulin.* Insulin, by favouring rapid entry of absorbed glucose into cells for conversion to glycogen, normally keeps the blood glucose level below the renal threshold for glucose excretion.

B. **Option 1**   *Aldosterone.* This hormone favours reabsorption of filtered sodium, thereby decreasing its clearance. The reabsorbed sodium is accompanied by chloride (following the electrical gradient) and water (following the osmotic gradient); all these are distributed mainly extracellularly, adding to the extracellular volume.

C. **Option 7**   *Renin.* This hormone acts on the circulating precursor, angiotensinogen to form angiotensin I.

D. **Option 6**   *Parathormone.* This hormone stimulates the release of calcium and phosphate from bone; it also increases phosphate clearance by decreasing the reabsorption of filtered phosphate from the tubules.

E. **Option 2**   *Antidiuretic hormone.* This hormone increases reabsorption of water from the collecting ducts; as water enters the extracellular fluid its osmolality decreases; the higher intracellular osmolality draws over half this water into cells, restoring osmotic equality of the intra- and extracellular fluids.

Answers for 441

A. **Option 6**   *Impaired consciousness.* Drowsiness and coma are related to a variety of disturbances; dialysis reduces toxins by creating a gradient for passive diffusion, it can also correct electrolyte and acid–base disturbances.

B. **Option 3**   *Abnormal cardiac rhythms.* Although these too are related to a variety of disturbances, a very high extracellular/plasma potassium level is the major cause.

C. **Option 2**   *Abnormal arterial blood pressure.* The pressure may be too high or too low; in both cases it may be corrected by increasing or decreasing extracellular and hence blood volume; this may be done by 'sucking' fluid out of the patient's blood by a raised dialysate osmolality or by lowering the dialysing equipment (or drainage bag with peritoneal dialysis) to remove fluid by gravity.

D. **Option 4**   *Hyperventilation.* Hyperventilation is a sign of serious acidosis, so the pH of the dialysate fluid should be increased.

E. **Option 1**   *Raised blood urea.* A raised urea raises total osmolality; as an extreme example, a rise of 30 mmol per litre would increase the normal osmolality (around 290 mosmol/kg) by just over 10 per cent; having the dialysate fluid free of urea allows a gradient for diffusion out of the patient's blood.

Answers for 442

A. **Option 4**   *Thick limb of loop of Henle.* This is where salt is actively pumped from the tubular lumen, without water following, so the tubular fluid becomes markedly hypotonic; in the absence of anti-diuretic hormone the fluid remains hypotonic as it enters the renal pelvis to become urine.

B. **Option 7**   *Middle medullary interstitial fluid.* The medullary interstitium shows a gradient normal osmolality to severe hyperosmolality across the medulla from renal cortex to pelvis.

C. **Option 8**   *Inner medullary interstitial fluid.* This is the last region the collecting ducts traverse, so if they are in a state of permeability to water due to the presence of antidiuretic hormone most of the water is drawn out of the duct lumen and the urine is very concentrated.

D. **Option 1**   *Proximal convoluted tubule.* In both gut and kidney the two key body requirements, glucose and sodium, are avidly absorbed/reabsorbed into the body.

E. **Option 1**   *Proximal convoluted tubule.* The major buffer, bicarbonate, is also conserved at this stage, by a fairly complex process involving active secretion of hydrogen ions into the lumen; the quotation marks are used because the bicarbonate entering the renal capillaries has been generated in the tubule cells; the secreted hydrogen ions join with the filtered bicarbonate to generate water and carbon dioxide molecules which are lost in the crowd.

EMQ Question 443

For each finding A–E related to renal transplantation, where both donor and recipient are adult, select the most appropriate variable related to that finding from the following list.

1. Glomerular filtration rate.	2. Renal plasma flow.
3. Brainstem death.	4. Persistent vegetative state.
5. Tissue compatibility.	6. Coma due to drug overdose.
7. Immunological rejection.	8. Erythropoietin.
9. Renin.	10. Aldosterone.

A. Prior to removal of the donor kidney, it had been established that the unconscious, artificially ventilated donor had persistently absent corneal and pupillary reflexes, there was no eye movement response to ice cold water in the external auditory meatus, nor was there any ventilatory response to carbon dioxide when the donor was temporarily disconnected from the ventilator.

B. A careful comparison of recipient and donor showed that their cells share an encouraging number of common antigens.

C. A month after transplantation the creatinine clearance is reported to be 85 ml/minute, which is regarded as satisfactory.

D. On the same occasion the para-aminohippurate clearance is reported to be 55 ml/minute, which does not seem compatible with the result reported in (C).

E. On a later occasion the patient is found to have a blood haemoglobin level of 143 g/litre, whereas prior to renal transplantation and while maintained satisfactorily on dialysis, the level was usually around 110 g/litre.

EMQ Question 444

For each aspect of renal function outlined A–E, select the most appropriate option from the following list of renal cellular contents or activities.

1. Carbonic anhydrase.	2. Renin.
3. Erythropoietin.	4. Active exchange of sodium for hydrogen
5. Passive Na^+/H^+ exchange.	ions.
6. Active sodium reabsorption.	7. Active chloride reabsorption.
8. Water channels.	

A. When a patient is deficient in both hydrogen and sodium ions due to vomiting gastric contents, renal function tends to make the alkalosis worse.

B. When a patient is deficient in extracellular fluid, adrenal cortical hormones help to restore its volume.

C. The loop of Henle contains cells which lead to a remarkably high osmolality in parts of the renal medulla.

D. Certain renal cells can sense the oxygen content of arterial blood and control the blood haemoglobin level.

E. A high level of antidiuretic hormone leads to a low urinary volume.

Answers for 443

A. **Option 3** *Brainstem death.* The reflex responses mentioned are all mediated through the brainstem and their persistent absence suggests death of the brain stem and hence of the brain since the brain stem is the least sensitive part of the brain; brainstem function is retained in the persistent vegetative state. Drug-induced coma is potentially reversible and organ donation is thus not considered.

B. **Option 5** *Tissue compatibility.* Tissue typing is analogous to but involves more factors than determining blood group; shared antigens reduce the risk of transplant rejection.

C. **Option 1** *Glomerular filtration rate.* Creatinine is freely filtered but not appreciably reabsorbed or secreted, so its clearance is a practical indicator of glomerular filtration rate. This result, over half the value for two normal kidneys, will provide excellent renal function. The value tends to rise in the weeks after transplantation, as the disturbances associated with the upheaval of transplantation settle down. In addition, the kidney tends to hypertrophy, as would happen in someone who had one kidney removed with the other one normal.

D. **Option 2** *Renal plasma flow.* Para-aminohippurate is normally completely eliminated from the circulation as it passes through the kidney, so indicates the renal plasma flow. With a normal haematocrit, the result would indicate a renal blood flow of 100 ml/minute, less than 10 per cent of normal and inconsistent with the above good creatinine clearance.

E. **Option 8** *Erythropoietin.* Dialysis can correct many disturbances of renal failure, but the lack of erythropoietin means the patient is subject to anaemia; the transplanted kidney provides adequate erythropoietin for a normal haemoglobin level.

Answers for 444

A. **Option 4** *Active exchange of sodium for hydrogen ions.* Stimulation of this pump to retain sodium also favours secretion of hydrogen ions, making the alkalosis worse. In addition, such patients are usually also short of potassium (lost with the vomited fluid) and this is made worse since potassium and hydrogen ions compete for the exchange. This condition is *hypokalaemic alkalosis* and the cure is to give intravenous sodium plus a safe supplement of potassium.

B. **Option 6** *Active sodium reabsorption.* As well as the above exchange, sodium absorption can be balanced electrically by chloride absorption; water follows by osmosis to restore the extracellular fluid volume.

C. **Option 7** *Active chloride reabsorption.* It has been shown that the loop of Henle actively reabsorbs chloride, which is balanced electrically by sodium (reverse of above); in this case water cannot follow, so the lumen becomes hypotonic and the interstitium hypertonic.

D. **Option 3** *Erythropoietin.* Active tubular cells become hypoxic when perfused with anaemic blood; this leads to synthesis of erythropoietin which stimulates the red bone marrow.

E. **Option 8** *Water channels.* Antidiuretic hormone induces these, so that the hypertonic renal medullary interstitium can osmotically draw water out of the collecting ducts, leaving a small volume of concentrated fluid to pass to the bladder.

MCQ

MCQs

Questions 445–450

445. In plasma, the half-life of
A. A hormone is half the time taken for it to disappear from the blood.
B. Insulin is between five and ten hours.
C. Thyroxine is longer than that of adrenaline.
D. Thyroxine is longer than that of triiodothyronine.
E. Noradrenaline is longer than that of acetylcholine.

446. During sleep there is a fall in the circulating level of
A. Cortisol.
B. Insulin.
C. Adrenaline.
D. Antidiuretic hormone.
E. Growth hormone.

447. Adrenocorticotrophic hormone (ACTH) secretion increases
A. When the median eminence of the hypothalamic is stimulated.
B. When aldosterone blood level falls.
C. When cortisol blood levels fall.
D. In bursts during the night as the normal hour of wakening approaches.
E. Following severe trauma.

448. Melatonin
A. Is produced mainly in the intermediate lobe of the pituitary gland.
B. Is synthesized in the body from serotonin (5-hydroxytryptamine).
C. Affects the level of pigmentation in human skin
D. Blood levels are highest during the night.
E. Influences the secretion rates of pituitary hormones.

449. Thyroid hormones, when secreted in excess, may cause an increase in the
A. Peripheral resistance.
B. Frequency of defaecation.
C. Energy expenditure required for a given workload.
D. Duration of tendon reflexes.
E. Heart rate when cardiac adrenergic and cholinergic receptors are blocked.

450. Aldosterone secretion is increased by an increase in plasma
A. Volume.
B. Osmolality.
C. Potassium concentration.
D. Renin concentration.
E. ACTH concentration.

Answers

445.

A.	False	It is the time it takes for the initial concentration to fall by half.
B.	False	It is much shorter (about five minutes); this allows more precise and continuous regulation of the blood glucose level.
C.	True	It is much longer since moment to moment regulation of its level is less critical.
D.	True	It is more highly protein-bound which appears to prolong its life.
E.	True	Acetylcholine is broken down almost immediately by cholinesterase.

446.

A.	True	The waking catabolic state changes to an anabolic state.
B.	True	Insulin secretion occurs mainly in association with meals.
C.	True	Adrenaline secretion is associated with stress.
D.	False	This rises as plasma osmolality rises; water is lost but not replaced during sleep.
E.	False	This increases, allowing growth and anabolic repair of tissue wear and tear.

447.

A.	True	The median eminence secretes corticotropin-releasing hormone (CRH), the releasing hormone for ACTH.
B.	False	Aldosterone secretion is regulated mainly by the renin/angiotensin system.
C.	True	This negative feedback helps to maintain the blood cortisol level.
D.	True	This is part of the circadian rhythm which produces high morning cortisol levels.
E.	True	Most forms of stress increase ACTH output by their neural input to the median eminence of the hypothalamus where CRH is formed.

448.

A.	False	Melanocyte-stimulating hormone is produced in the intermediate lobe of the pituitary; melatonin is produced mainly in the pineal gland.
B.	True	The necessary enzymes are in the pineal parenchymal cells.
C.	False	It has no role in regulation of human skin pigmentation.
D.	True	Melatonin secretion has a pronounced circadian rhythm, low during the day and high by night.
E.	True	Melatonin secreted in relation to prevailing conditions of light/darkness may adjust pituitary hormonal rhythms appropriately.

449.

A.	False	Increased metabolism leads to peripheral vasodilation.
B.	True	The frequency of defaecation increases in hyperthyroidism.
C.	True	Thyroid hormones uncouple oxidation from phosphorylation so that more energy appears as heat.
D.	False	The reverse is true.
E.	True	This suggests a direct action on cells in the sinoatrial node.

450.

A.	False	This reduces aldosterone secretion.
B.	False	This increases adrenocortical hormone (ADH) secretion.
C.	True	K^+ has a direct stimulatory effect on the adrenal cortex.
D.	True	This leads to formation of angiotensin II which stimulates the cortex.
E.	True	Though the main action of ACTH is on glucocorticoid secreting cells; it has some action on mineralocorticoid secreting cells.

Questions 451–456

451. Glucocorticoid injections lead to increases in
A. Lymph gland size.
B. Fibroblastic activity.
C. Anabolic activity in muscle.
D. Bone resorption.
E. Membrane stability in mast cell and lysosomes.

452. An intravenous infusion of noradrenaline differs from one of adrenaline in that it
A. Acts on alpha adrenoceptors.
B. Does not act on beta adrenoceptors.
C. Raises total peripheral resistance.
D. Increases cardiac output.
E. Decreases skin blood flow.

453. Growth hormone
A. Promotes positive nitrogen and phosphorus balance.
B. Secretion is under hypothalamic control.
C. Levels in the blood are higher in children than in adults.
D. Secretion surges during sleep.
E. Stimulates the liver to secrete somatomedins which regulate bone and cartilage growth.

454. Parathormone
A. Secretion is regulated by a pituitary feedback control system.
B. Acts directly on bone to increase bone resorption.
C. Decreases the urinary output of calcium.
D. Decreases phosphate excretion.
E. Promotes absorption of calcium from the intestines.

455. Antidiuretic hormone (vasopressin)
A. Is released from nerve endings in the posterior pituitary gland.
B. Tends to raise the osmolality of plasma rise.
C. Increases the permeability of the cells in the loop of Henle to water.
D. Secretion is little affected by changes in plasma osmolality of less than 10 per cent.
E. Secretion increases when plasma volume falls but osmolality is unchanged.

456. Pancreatic glucagon
A. Is produced by the beta cells of the islets of Langerhans.
B. Is a polypeptide.
C. Output is inversely proportional to the blood glucose level.
D. Has a half-life in the circulation of 3–4 hours.
E. Increases the breakdown of liver glycogen.

Answers

451.

A.   False   Glucocorticoids inhibit mitotic activity in lymphocytes.
B.   False   Glucocorticoids inhibit fibroblastic activity; this may allow chronic infections to spread since they are not walled off effectively by fibrous scarring.
C.   False   They are catabolic; released amino acids are converted to glucose.
D.   True   Decreased bone formation and increased resorption may cause osteoporosis.
E.   True   This blocks release of histamine and lysosomal enzymes in allergic responses.

452.

A.   False   Both act on alpha receptors but noradrenaline is the more potent stimulant.
B.   False   Both act on beta receptors but adrenaline is the more potent stimulant.
C.   True   Noradrenaline raises but adrenaline reduces it.
D.   False   Adrenaline raises but noradrenaline reflexly reduces it.
E.   False   Both constrict skin vessels due to their alpha receptor stimulant properties.

453.

A.   True   It is an anabolic hormone.
B.   True   Secretion in the pituitary is stimulated by growth hormone releasing factor and inhibited by somatostatin from the hypothalamus.
C.   False   Blood levels are similar in children and adults.
D.   True   Sleep is a time for anabolic activity.
E.   True   Somatomedins (insulin-like growth factors, IGF) from the liver inhibit the pituitary secretion of growth hormone and stimulate release of somatostatin from the hypothalamus.

454.

A.   False   It is regulated directly by the calcium level in the blood that perfuses it.
B.   True   It stimulates osteoclasts to resorb bone; excessive secretion causes cysts to form.
C.   False   The high blood calcium levels with parathormone and the resulting increase in calcium filtration in the glomeruli result in an increased calcium output in urine.
D.   False   It increases phosphate excretion by reducing renal phosphate reabsorption.
E.   True   It does this indirectly by stimulating 1,25-dihydroxycholecalciferol production.

455.

A.   True   It is formed in neurones whose cell bodies lie in the hypothalamus and whose axons transport it to the posterior pituitary gland.
B.   False   The water retention it induces makes plasma osmolality fall.
C.   False   It increases the permeability of the collecting ducts.
D.   False   Secretion is affected by 1 per cent changes in osmolality; the sensitivity of the hypothalamic receptors to osmolar change accounts for the constancy of plasma osmolality.
E.   True   Volume changes detected by vascular low-pressure receptors affect ADH secretion.

456.

A.   False   It is produced by the alpha cells.
B.   True   It is quite similar in structure to secretin.
C.   True   It normally prevents a serious fall in blood glucose.
D.   False   It is much shorter (5–10 minutes); this allows glucagon levels in the blood to adjust rapidly to changes in blood glucose levels.
E.   True   It also mobilizes fatty acids.

Questions 457–462

457. The concentration of ionized calcium in plasma is
A. The main regulator of parathormone secretion.
B. Less than the free ionized calcium concentration in intracellular fluid.
C. About 50 per cent of the total plasma calcium concentration.
D. Reduced when plasma pH rises.
E. Reduced when the plasma protein level rises.

458. Cortisol
A. Is bound in the plasma to an alpha globulin.
B. Is inactivated in the liver and excreted in the bile.
C. Injections lead to a rise in arterial pressure.
D. Inhibits release of ACTH from the anterior pituitary gland.
E. Is released with a circadian variation so that cortisol blood levels peak in the morning.

459. When secretory activity in the thyroid gland increases
A. The gland takes up iodide from the blood at a faster rate.
B. Its follicles enlarge and fill with colloid.
C. The follicular cells become more columnar.
D. The follicular cells ingest colloid by endocytosis.
E. The blood level of thyrotropin (TSH) increases.

460 Releasing hormones produced in the hypothalamus
A. Are secreted by cells in the median eminence.
B. Pass down nerve axons to reach the pituitary gland.
C. May control the output of more than one pituitary hormone.
D. Regulate the release of thyrotropin.
E. Regulate the release of oxytocin.

461. Adrenaline secretion from the adrenal glands increases the
A. Blood glucose level.
B. Blood free fatty acid level.
C. Blood flow to skeletal muscle.
D. Blood flow to the splanchnic area.
E. Release of renin in the kidneys

462. Thyroid-stimulating hormone (TSH) secretion is increased
A. After partial removal of the thyroid gland.
B. In infants born without a thyroid gland.
C. When metabolic rate falls.
D. In starvation.
E. When the diet is deficient in iodine.

Answers

457.

A.   True   Parathormone secretion is stimulated by a fall in the ionized Ca^{2+} level.
B.   False   It is more than 10^5 times higher.
C.   True   Most of the rest is bound to protein, mainly albumin.
D.   True   In alkalosis more calcium is protein-bound.
E.   False   The ionized calcium level is regulated independently.

458.

A.   True   It is bound to transcortin; free cortisol is released to replace that taken up by the tissues.
B.   False   The inactive products of cortisol degradation in the liver are conjugated with glucuronic acid and sulphate and excreted in the urine.
C.   True   Partly at least because of its mineralocorticoid effects.
D.   True   The negative feedback loop that maintains plasma cortisol levels constant.
E.   True   It is regulated through a hypothalamic 'clock'.

459.

A.   True   Iodide uptake is an index of activity.
B.   False   The follicles shrink as the colloid content falls.
C.   True   They change from cuboidal to columnar as their activity increases.
D.   True   Reabsorption lacunae form as thyroglobulin is broken down to release hormones.
E.   False   Negative feedback causes TSH levels to fall.

460.

A.   True   From there they travel to the anterior pituitary gland.
B.   False   They are carried in the hypophyseal-portal vessels from median eminence to anterior pituitary gland.
C.   True   For example, Gonadotrophin-releasing hormone (GnRH) controls pituitary secretion of follicle-stimulating hormone (FSH) and luteinizing hormone (LH).
D.   True   Thyrotropin-releasing hormone (TRH) controls thyrotropin release.
E.   False   Oxytocin is released from terminals of nerves running from the hypothalamus to the posterior pituitary gland.

461.

A.   True   By promoting glycogenolysis in the liver.
B.   True   By promoting lipolysis in the fat stores.
C.   True   By its predominant effect on beta-receptors in the smooth muscle of skeletal muscle arterioles.
D.   False   Splanchnic flow falls since alpha-receptors predominate in splanchnic arterioles.
E.   True   Juxtaglomerular cells respond to beta-receptor stimulation by releasing renin.

462.

A.   True   Due to a reduction in pituitary inhibition by circulating thyroxine.
B.   True   Due to absence of the normal pituitary inhibition by circulating thyroxine.
C.   False   TSH and thyroxine influence metabolic rate, not vice versa.
D.   False   The level falls, which tends to conserve energy.
E.   True   Due to inadequate manufacture of thyroxine, pituitary inhibition is reduced.

Questions 463–468

463. Insulin
A. Stimulates release of free fatty acids from adipose tissue.
B. Secretion tends to raise the plasma potassium level.
C. Facilitates entry of glucose into skeletal muscle.
D. Facilitates entry of amino acids into skeletal muscle.
E. Secretion is increased by vagal nerve activity.

464. The pituitary gland
A. Regulates activity in all other endocrine glands.
B. Output of prolactin is regulated by hypothalamic releasing factors.
C. Secretes antidiuretic hormone when blood osmolality falls.
D. Has an intermediate lobe which secretes melanotropin
E. Responds to nervous and hormonal influences from the brain.

465. Thyrocalcitonin
A. Is produced by the follicular cells of the thyroid gland.
B. Increases basal metabolic rate.
C. Reduces blood calcium in parathyroidectomized animals.
D. Secretion occurs when the blood phosphate level rises.
E. Stimulates osteoclast activity.

466. The thyroid gland
A. Takes up iodide against its electrochemical gradient.
B. Decreases in size when dietary iodine is deficient.
C. Is relatively avascular.
D. Contains enzymes which oxidize iodide to iodine.
E. Contains enzymes which iodinate tyrosine.

467. Adrenaline differs from noradrenaline in that it
A. Increases the heart rate when injected intravenously.
B. Is the main catecholamine secreted by the adrenal medulla.
C. Increases the strength of myocardial contraction.
D. Is a more potent dilator of the bronchi.
E. Constricts blood vessels in mucous membranes.

468. Growth hormone secretion
A. Is stimulated by somatostatin released from the hypothalamus.
B. Increases when the blood glucose level falls.
C. Has a lactogenic effect.
D. Increases the size of viscera.
E. Stimulates liver production of somatomedins.

Answers

463.

A.   False   It stimulates uptake of fatty acids by adipose tissue.
B.   False   It lowers it by promoting potassium uptake by cells.
C.   True   Thus lowering the blood sugar level.
D.   True   Thereby favouring anabolism.
E.   True   This mobilizes insulin at the beginning of a meal.

464.

A.   False   For example, parathyroid activity is not regulated by the pituitary.
B.   True   Output can be increased and decreased by the action of prolactin-releasing hormone (PRH) or prolactin-inhibiting hormone (PIH) respectively.
C.   False   ADH is secreted by the posterior pituitary in response to a *rise* in blood osmolality.
D.   True   This may stimulate melanin production in human melanocytes.
E.   True   The anterior pituitary is influenced by hormones arriving in portal-hypophyseal vessels and the posterior pituitary by impulses travelling in the hypothalamo-hypophyseal tract.

465.

A.   False   It is produced by 'parafollicular' cells in the thyroid thought to be derived from the ultimobranchial bodies.
B.   False   It does not affect basal metabolic rate.
C.   True   Its action is independent of the parathyroid glands.
D.   False   It is secreted when the blood calcium level rises.
E.   False   It stimulates bone deposition by osteoblasts.

466.

A.   True   It is taken up by an active process (the iodide pump).
B.   False   Hyperplasia due to TSH stimulation occurs to give goitre.
C.   False   It has one of the highest blood flow rates in the body; bleeding during surgery may be a problem.
D.   True   This is a stage in the formation of thyroxine.
E.   True   Iodination takes place in the colloid.

467.

A.   True   Noradrenaline injection causes reflex slowing of the heart.
B.   True   Adrenaline constitutes some 80 per cent of this secretion.
C.   False   Both increase the strength of myocardial contraction.
D.   True   It has stronger beta effects (including bronchodilation).
E.   False   Both vasoconstrict ('decongest') mucous membranes.

468.

A.   False   Somatostatin inhibits growth hormone secretion.
B.   True   This is the basis of a test of pituitary function.
C.   True   Prolactin and growth hormone are similar peptides.
D.   True   It stimulates growth of most tissues.
E.   True   These peptides mediate general stimulation of growth.

Questions 469–475

469. Vitamin D
A. Increases the intestinal absorption of calcium.
B. Is essential for normal calcification of bones in childhood.
C. Requires hepatic modification for activation.
D. Cannot be synthesized in the body.
E. Deficiency may result in hyperparathyroidism.

470. Prolactin
A. Has a similar chemical structure and physiological action to luteinizing hormone.
B. Is responsible for breast growth in puberty.
C. Release is inhibited by dopamine.
D. Secretion is stimulated by suckling of the breast.
E. Causes pre-formed milk to be ejected by the breast during suckling.

471. The level of ionized calcium in blood falls when
A. Blood phosphate levels fall.
B. Subjects hyperventilate.
C. The thyroid gland is perfused with a calcium-rich solution.
D. Plasma protein levels fall.
E. Sodium citrate is added to the blood.

472. Thyroxine
A. Is stored in the follicular cells as thyroglobulin.
B. Increases the resting rate of carbon dioxide production.
C. Is essential for normal development of the brain.
D. Is essential for normal red cell production.
E. Acts more rapidly than triiodothyronine (T_3).

473. Parathormone
A. Decreases the renal clearance of phosphate.
B. Mobilizes bone calcium independently of its actions on the kidney.
C. Depresses the activity of the anterior pituitary gland.
D. In the blood rises when the calcium level falls.
E. Stimulates the final activation of vitamin D (cholecalciferol) in the kidney.

474. The chemical structure of insulin
A. Contains a sterol ring.
B. Is identical in all mammalian species.
C. Is such that it is effective when taken by mouth.
D. Has been synthesized in the laboratory.
E. Can be synthesized by bacteria.

475. Hormones secreted by the adrenal cortex
A. Include cholesterol.
B. Are mostly bound to plasma proteins.
C. Include sex hormones.
D. Are excreted mainly in the bile after conjugation.
E. Are essential for the maintenance of life.

Answers

469.

A. True   This occurs mainly in the upper small intestine.
B. True   In its absence bones are weak and deformed (rickets).
C. True   Initial (25-) hydroxylation occurs here.
D. False   It can be produced in mammals by the action of ultraviolet light on 7-dehydrocholesterol in skin.
E. True   The low blood calcium level stimulates parathormone secretion.

470.

A. False   They are distinct hormones with different actions.
B. False   Breast growth depends on oestrogens and progestogens.
C. True   This mediates hypothalamic regulation of prolactin levels.
D. True   This is responsible for the maintenance of lactation in the puerperium.
E. False   Milk ejection is a consequence of oxytocin secretion.

471.

A. False   It rises since the product of $[Ca^+]$ $[PO_4^-]$ is constant.
B. True   Alkalosis increases calcium binding by plasma proteins.
C. True   Due to release of thyrocalcitonin.
D. False   But the total calcium level falls.
E. True   This binds calcium ions and prevents clotting.

472.

A. False   It is stored as thyroglobulin in the follicles.
B. True   By increasing the basal metabolic rate.
C. True   Deficiency in infancy causes mental retardation (cretinism).
D. True   Thyroxine deficiency can cause anaemia.
E. False T_3 acts within a day, thyroxine within 2–3 days.

473.

A. False   It increases it by depressing phosphate reabsorption.
B. True   It does so in the absence of the kidneys.
C. False   It does not affect the anterior pituitary.
D. True   Blood calcium level determines its rate of secretion.
E. True   From 25-hydroxy to 1,25-dihydroxycholecalciferol.

474.

A. False   It contains two peptide chains.
B. False   Minor differences occur but these differences do not affect insulin action.
C. False   Its peptide structure is broken down by digestive proteases in the gut.
D. True   In 1964 by Katsoyannis.
E. True   Using recombinant DNA.

475.

A. False   This is not a hormone.
B. True   For example, the globulin transcortin binds cortisol.
C. True   In both sexes they stimulate the growth of axillary and pubic hair.
D. False   After conjugation they are excreted mainly by the kidney.
E. True   Without replacement therapy, loss of adrenal cortical function results in death.

Questions 476–482

476. During an oral glucose tolerance test the
A. Subject is given 5–10 grams of glucose.
B. Plasma glucose should rise by less than 10 per cent from the fasting level.
C. Plasma insulin should rise by about 100 per cent from the fasting level.
D. Rise in plasma glucose is less than with intravenous administration.
E. Rise in plasma insulin is less than with intravenous administration.

477. Secretin differs from cholecystokinin-pancreozymin (CCK-PZ) in that it
A. Is formed by mucosal cells in the upper small intestine.
B. Stimulates the pancreas to secrete a juice which is rich in digestive enzymes.
C. Stimulates the pancreas to secrete a watery alkaline juice.
D. Has less effect on gallbladder smooth muscle.
E. Decreases gastric motility.

478. Inhibition of angiotensin-converting enzyme (ACE) decreases the
A. Formation of angiotensin II.
B. Plasma renin level.
C. Work of the heart.
D. Circulating level of angiotensin I.
E. Total body potassium.

479. The plasma level of adrenocorticotrophic hormone (ACTH)
A. Is normally maximal around midnight.
B. Is regulated mainly by the blood cortisol level.
C. Shows exaggerated circadian fluctuations with an adrenal tumour.
D. Is raised in the presence of complete adrenal failure.
E. Is reduced in patients on long-term high dosage glucocorticoids.

480. Possible consequences of hypothyroidism include having
A. A subnormal body core temperature.
B. A tendency to fall asleep frequently.
C. Increased body hair (hirsutism).
D. Moist hands and feet.
E. Prominent eyeballs.

481. Sudden complete loss of parathyroid function
A. Leads to skeletal muscle spasms.
B. May be fatal if treatment is not given to raise the blood level of ionized calcium.
C. Causes haemorrhagic disease due to lack of calcium for haemostasis.
D. May be treated in the short-term by slow intravenous injection of calcium ions.
E. May be treated in the long-term by regular doses of vitamin D.

482. When a patient with diabetes insipidus is treated successfully with anti-diuretic hormone the
A. Urinary flow rate should fall by about 50 per cent.
B. Urinary output should be reduced to around 5 ml/minute
C. Urinary osmolality should rise to between 100 and 200 mosmol/litre.
D. Salt intake should be carefully regulated.
E. Blood pressure should stabilize within the normal range.

Answers

476.

A.   False   50–100 grams of glucose are used.
B.   False   It normally rises by around 50 per cent.
C.   False   It rises about ten-fold from a very low fasting level.
D.   True   The rise is about half as great.
E.   False   Oral glucose stimulates much more release of insulin.

477.

A.   False   Both are formed by these cells.
B.   False   Secretin juice is poor in enzymes.
C.   True   Secretin juice is copious and rich in bicarbonate ions.
D.   True   'Cholecystokinin' implies stimulation of the gallbladder.
E.   True   CCK-PZ resembles gastrin and increases gastric motility.

478.

A.   True   The enzyme converts angiotensin I into angiotensin II.
B.   False   Plasma renin rises as the blood pressure falls.
C.   True   The fall in blood pressure it causes decreases the work of the heart and can be an effective treatment for some types of heart failure.
D.   False   It rises due to the increased renin and the inability to convert to angiotensin II.
E.   False   Due to the fall in aldosterone secretion, less potassium is excreted.

479.

A.   False   It is maximal around the time of awakening.
B.   False   This feedback system is over-ridden by the hypothalamic circadian rhythm.
C.   False   The level is high but the circadian rhythm is lost.
D.   True   Due to loss of negative feedback by cortisol.
E.   True   ACTH is suppressed by these exogenous glucocorticoids.

480.

A.   True   Due to the lowered metabolic rate.
B.   True   Due to the slowing of mental processes.
C.   False   Hair loss is characteristic of hypothyroidism.
D.   False   Decreased sweating is found in hypothyroidism.
E.   False   Prominent eyeballs are characteristic of the exophthalmos of hyperthyroidism.

481.

A.   True   This is a central feature of tetany.
B.   True   Due to severe convulsions.
C.   False   Calcium levels do not fall below the levels needed for haemostasis.
D.   True   This is the acute treatment of choice, e.g. calcium gluconate.
E.   True   This acts by increasing intestinal calcium absorption.

482.

A.   False   Typically it will be reduced by about 80 per cent.
B.   False   It should fall to the normal value of about 1 ml/minute.
C.   False   It should rise to about 600–900 mosmol/litre, 2–3 times normal plasma osmolality (300 mosmol/litre).
D.   False   ADH does not interfere with salt regulation.
E.   True   Due to greater stability of the body fluids.

Questions 483–489

483. Severe uncontrolled diabetes mellitus leads to a raised

A. H^+ ion concentration in body fluids.
B. Plasma K^+ concentration.
C. Urinary specific gravity and osmolality.
D. Blood volume.
E. Arterial P_{CO_2}.

484. Hyperthyroidism is associated with a

A. Positive nitrogen balance.
B. Decreased urinary excretion of calcium.
C. Clinical picture consistent with excessive beta adrenoceptor stimulation.
D. Diminished heat tolerance.
E. Rise in the level of thyroxine-binding protein in plasma.

485. An adrenal medullary tumour (phaeochromocytoma) may cause an increase in

A. Systolic blood pressure which may be transient or constant.
B. Tremor of the extended hand.
C. Basal metabolic rate.
D. Diastolic arterial pressure which does not respond to alpha adrenoceptor blocking drugs.
E. Urinary catecholamines.

486. Short stature is seen in adults who in childhood suffered from

A. Chronic malnutrition.
B. Castration.
C. Premature puberty.
D. Thyroid deficiency.
E. Adrenal deficiency.

487. Insulin

A. Requirements at night are similar to those during the day.
B. Half-life is usually reduced in patients with diabetes mellitus.
C. Is partly bound to proteins in the blood.
D. Requirements are increased in obesity.
E. Requirements are increased by exercise.

488. The risk of tetany is increased by

A. Sudden rises in plasma bicarbonate.
B. Sudden rises in plasma magnesium.
C. Removal of the anterior pituitary gland.
D. The onset of respiratory failure.
E. The onset of renal failure.

489. Destruction of the anterior pituitary gland causes

A. Amenorrhoea.
B. Diabetes insipidus.
C. Skin pallor.
D. Impaired ability to survive severe stress.
E. A fall in basal metabolic rate (BMR).

Answers

483.

A.   True   This is a prime feature of ketoacidosis.
B.   True   The excess H^+ ions compete with K^+ ions for excretion in the distal tubules.
C.   True   Due to the dissolved glucose.
D.   False   This falls due to osmotic diuresis and vomiting.
E.   False   Hyperventilation reduces P_{CO_2} to compensate the metabolic acidosis.

484.

A.   False   It is negative due to muscle wasting.
B.   False   It rises due to liberation of calcium from bone.
C.   True   Beta adrenoceptor blocking drugs relieve such features, e.g. tachycardia.
D.   True   Heat intolerance is due to the increased heat production.
E.   False   The protein levels are normal but they bind more thyroxine.

485.

A.   True   Due to phasic or tonic release of adrenaline and/or noradrenaline.
B.   True   Due to beta adrenoceptor stimulation by adrenaline.
C.   True   Due to release of adrenaline.
D.   False   α-receptor blockers typically lower the blood pressure.
E.   True   This is a diagnostic feature.

486.

A.   True   Early stunting cannot be compensated for later in childhood.
B.   False   This leads to increased height due to delayed closure of the epiphyses.
C.   True   The sex hormones promote early closure of the epiphyses.
D.   True   Thyroid hormones are essential for normal growth.
E.   True   Adrenal hormones also are essential for normal growth.

487.

A.   False   Insulin is required mainly in response to meals.
B.   False   The disease is not usually due to rapid insulin breakdown.
C.   True   Abnormal binding may occur in diabetes mellitus.
D.   True   Obese patients usually show increased insulin resistance.
E.   False   Exercise reduces insulin requirements.

488.

A.   True   In alkalosis, the calcium-binding power of the plasma proteins increases.
B.   False   Like calcium, magnesium ions tend to prevent tetany.
C.   False   The pituitary is not involved in calcium homeostasis.
D.   False   The acidosis in respiratory failure reduces calcium binding by protein.
E.   False   The acidosis in renal failure also reduces calcium binding by protein.

489.

A.   True   Due to absence of FSH and LH.
B.   False   ADH is released from the posterior pituitary.
C.   True   Due to loss of ACTH and melanocyte-stimulating hormone (MSH) actions.
D.   True   Due to loss of ACTH and failure of the cortisol surge in response to stress; loss of TSH and consequent hypothyroidism also contribute.
E.   True   BMR falls due to loss of TSH drive to the thyroid.

Questions 490–496

490. Removal of the thyroid gland (without replacement therapy) leads to an increased

A. Blood TSH level.
B. Blood cholesterol level.
C. Blood glucose level during an oral glucose tolerance test.
D. Response time for tendon reflexes.
E. Tremor of the fingers.

491. In severe diabetes mellitus, there may be a fall in

A. Extracellular fluid osmolality.
B. Appetite.
C. Blood volume.
D. Arterial blood pH to below 7.0.
E. Blood bicarbonate to half its normal value.

492. Excessive glucocorticoid production (Cushing's syndrome) causes an increase in

A. Skin thickness.
B. Bone strength.
C. Blood glucose.
D. Arterial pressure.
E. The rate of wound healing.

493. A pituitary tumour secreting excess growth hormone (GH) in an adult may lead to

A. A homonymous hemianopia.
B. Giantism.
C. Reduced levels of somatomedins in blood.
D. Enlargement of the liver.
E. A raised blood glucose level.

494. Hypoglycaemic coma differs from hyperglycaemic coma in that there is more likelihood of a

A. Rapid loss of consciousness.
B. Weak pulse.
C. Normal blood pH.
D. Glucose-free urine.
E. High acetone level in urine.

495. In adrenal failure there is likely to be a fall in the

A. Extracellular fluid volume.
B. Total red cell mass.
C. The sodium:potassium ratio in plasma.
D. Arterial blood pressure.
E. Blood urea.

496. In diabetic ketosis there is a decreased metabolic breakdown of

A. Ketones.
B. Glycogen.
C. Glucose.
D. Fat.
E. Amino acids.

Answers

490.
A. True   Due to loss of negative feedback to the pituitary.
B. True   Due mainly to a reduction in cholesterol excretion.
C. False The curve is flattened due to slow absorption of glucose.
D. True   The 'hung up' ankle jerk is a good example.
E. False Tremor is a feature of hyperthyroidism.

491.
A. False It rises due to excess glucose molecules plus water loss.
B. False It is increased due to loss of glucose in the urine.
C. True   Due to osmotic diuresis and vomiting.
D. True   This indicates life-threatening acidosis.
E. True   Bicarbonate is used up buffering the keto-acids.

492.
A. False Skin is thin due to protein catabolism; striae appear.
B. False Bones are weakened by breakdown of the protein matrix.
C. True   Due mainly to gluconeogenesis.
D. True   Due to the salt and water retention caused by gluco- and mineralocorticoids.
E. False Healing is slowed in this catabolic state.

493.
A. False Damage to the crossing nasal retinal fibres in the optic chiasma leads to bitem-
              poral hemianopia.
B. False After puberty when the epiphyses have closed, excess GH causes acromegaly.
C. False GH leads to increased production of somatomedins in the liver.
D. True   Body organs as well as the peripheries increase in size in acromegaly.
E. True   Growth hormone has 'diabetogenic' effects.

494.
A. True   Blood glucose can drop more rapidly than diabetic ketosis can develop.
B. False The pulse is usually strong in hypoglycaemic coma but weak in hyperglycaemic
              coma because of fluid depletion.
C. True   Hypoglycaemia does not affect the pH.
D. True   However, glucose may be present if urine containing glucose entered the bladder
              before the onset of hypoglycaemia.
E. False Usually acetone is absent in hypoglycaemic coma.

495.
A. True   Due to salt and water loss from lack of gluco- and mineralocorticoids.
B. False The haemoglobin level rises due to haemoconcentration.
C. True   It falls since loss of aldosterone leads to potassium retention.
D. True   Low blood volume may lead to hypotension and hypovolaemic circulatory fail-
              ure.
E. False It tends to rise due to the oliguria associated with the hypotension.

496.
A. False Breakdown continues normally but ketones accumulate due to rapid production.
B. False Insulin normally inhibits glycogenolysis.
C. True   Due to its impaired entry into the cells.
D. False Fat breakdown is increased to yield ketone bodies.
E. False Gluconeogenesis and amino acid catabolism increase.

Questions 497–501

497. A patient with severe diabetic ketoacidosis is likely to benefit from administration of

A. Intragastric fluids.
B. Intravenous insulin.
C. Isotonic glucose.
D. Isotonic sodium chloride.
E. Oxygen by breathing mask if hyperventilation is present.

498. Impaired growth hormone secretion

A. In children causes delayed puberty.
B. In children leads to short stature with more stunting of the limbs than the trunk.
C. Is associated with pale, fine and soft skin.
D. In adults leads to a reduction in the size of the viscera.
E. Can be treated effectively with bovine growth hormone.

499. Parathormone secretion is usually increased

A. In patients with chronic renal failure.
B. In people taking excessive amounts of vitamin D.
C. In patients with anterior pituitary tumours secreting excessive amounts of its hormones.
D. When blood phosphate levels fall.
E. When plasma protein levels fall.

500. An oral glucose tolerance test in a patient with

A. Diabetes mellitus shows a higher than normal fasting blood glucose level.
B. Diabetes mellitus shows glycosuria when blood glucose is three times the normal fasting level.
C. Diabetes mellitus shows a delayed return to the fasting blood glucose level.
D. An insulin-secreting tumour shows no rise in blood glucose level during the test.
E. Malabsorption syndrome shows a lower than normal peak level for blood glucose.

501. Surgical removal of the pituitary gland is likely to lead to a decrease in

A. Plasma osmolality.
B. Menstrual frequency.
C. Axillary hair.
D. Sexual desire (libido).
E. Breast size.

Answers

497.

A. False   Vomiting is likely so intravenous fluids are needed to correct the fluid deficit.
B. True   Insulin is needed to reverse the derangement of metabolism.
C. True   A water deficit is remedied by intravenous isotonic glucose.
D. True   This remedies the extracellular fluid deficit; the pH disturbance is corrected by restoring normal metabolism and fluid balance.
E. False   The hyperventilation is due to acidosis, not oxygen lack.

498.

A. False   Pituitary gonadotrophins, not growth hormone, determine the time of onset of puberty.
B. False   Pituitary dwarfs are usually normally proportioned.
C. True   In addition, body hair is normally sparse.
D. False   It has no detectable effect on organ size in adults.
E. False   Only the human form is effective.

499.

A. True   Phosphate retention results in a fall in the ionized calcium level in blood; this stimulates the parathyroid to produce more parathormone (secondary hyper-parathyroidism).
B. False   The increased level of ionized calcium in blood depresses parathyroid activity.
C. False   Pituitary hormones are not involved in the regulation of parathyroid activity.
D. False   This raises ionized calcium levels and depresses parathyroid activity.
E. False   This decreases the total blood calcium but not the ionized calcium level that regulates parathormone secretion.

500.

A. True   The level is higher due to impaired glucose homeostasis even in the fasting state.
B. True   The renal threshold for glucose is about twice the normal fasting level.
C. True   Due to impaired insulin response to the glucose stimulus.
D. False   Blood glucose rises but then falls to a low level due to excessive insulin secretion.
E. True   The curve is flattened due to impaired glucose absorption.

501.

A. False   Osmolality increases due to the induced diabetes insipidus.
B. True   Amenorrhoea is common due to loss of gonadotrophic hormones.
C. True   The adrenal androgens responsible for axillary hair are under ACTH control.
D. True   Libido is influenced by the sex hormones which are under gonadotrophic control.
E. True   The oestrogen and progesterone responsible for breast development are under gonadotrophic control.

EMQs

Questions 502–512

EMQ Question 502

For each action or function related to calcium and phosphate metabolism A–E, select the most appropriate option from the following list.

1. Increased blood calcium.
2. Decreased blood calcium.
3. Increased urinary phosphate excretion.
4. Decreased urinary phosphate excretion.
5. Increased alimentary absorption of calcium.
6. Decreased alimentary absorption of calcium.
7. Hydroxylation of cholecalciferol.

A. An action of parathormone which increases the likelihood of renal calculi by its effect on renal tubular function.
B. A hepatic function which is necessary for normal absorption of calcium from the gut.
C. An outcome of the action of parathormone on osteoclasts.
D. A renal function which is necessary for the absorption of calcium from the gut.
E. A consequence of vitamin D deficiency in childhood which can lead to softening and deformity of bones (rickets) due to inadequate mineral content.

EMQ Question 503

For each hormone A–E, select the best option from the following list of functions.

1. Causes milk ejection in the lactating breast.
2. Polypeptide growth factors secreted by the liver.
3. Stimulates sperm formation in the male.
4. Stimulates melanin formation in melanocytes.
5. Promotes water retention in the kidney.

A. MSH.
B. Somatomedins.
C. Oxytocin.
D. Vasopressin.
E. Luteinizing hormone.

EMQ Question 504

For each of the paediatric problems A–E, select the best option from the following list of causes.

1. Non-dysjunction of chromosome 21.
2. Adrenal cortical overactivity in children.
3. Pituitary deficiency.
4. Thyroid deficiency in children.
5. An XO chromosomal pattern.

A. Cretinism.
B. Precocious puberty.
C. Down's syndrome.
D. Ovarian agenesis.
E. Dwarfism.

Answers for 502

A.   **Option 3**   *Increased urinary phosphate excretion.* Parathormone liberates both calcium and phosphate ions from bone and in order not to exceed the solubility product for these ions it is necessary to excrete the excess phosphate. Parathormone favours this by inhibiting reabsorption of filtered phosphate. It thereby tends to raise the solubility product for these ions in urine, favouring development of renal calculi.

B.   **Option 7**   *Hydroxylation of cholecalciferol.* Cholecalciferol is ingested or synthesized in the skin under the influence of sunlight. To become an active hormone promoting absorption of calcium from the gut it must be converted into 1:25 dihydroxycholecalciferol. The first hydroxylation takes place in the liver.

C.   **Option 1**   *Increased blood calcium.* Parathormone stimulates osteoclasts to erode bone, thereby releasing calcium and phosphate. This raises the blood calcium level; the phosphate is excreted as discussed above.

D.   **Option 7**   *Hydroxylation of cholecalciferol.* The second hydroxylation necessary for activating vitamin D (cholecalciferol) takes place in the kidney under the influence of parathormone. Both hydroxylations (liver and kidney) are necessary before vitamin D can regulate total body calcium (mainly in bones) by stimulating its active absorption in the upper small intestine.

E.   **Option 6**   *Decreased alimentary absorption of calcium.* When vitamin D is deficient (dietary plus lack of adequate sunlight) the substrate for hydroxylation and activation is not available and absorption of calcium is deficient so that there is inadequate calcium for normal bone mineralization.

Answers for 503

A.   **Option 4**   *Stimulates melanin formation in melanocytes.* Melanocyte-stimulating hormone results in a darker pigmentation of the skin.

B.   **Option 2**   *Polypeptide growth factors secreted by the liver.* Their production is stimulated by the action of growth hormone on hepatic cells. Somatomedins interact with growth hormone and affect growth, cartilage and protein metabolism.

C.   **Option 1**   *Causes milk ejection in the lactating breast.* It is also important in causing the uterus to contract at parturition.

D.   **Option 5**   *Promotes water retention in the kidney.* Also known as antidiuretic hormone, vasopressin affects the permeability of certain parts of the renal tubule to allow greater reabsorption of water filtered in the glomerulus.

E.   **Option 3**   *Stimulates sperm formation in the male.* In the female, LH stimulates ovulation and luteinization of the corpus luteum.

Answers for 504

A.   **Option 4**   *Thyroid deficiency in children.* Such children are dwarfed, mentally retarded and pot bellied. Early treatment is urgent to prevent permanent mental retardation.

B.   **Option 2**   *Adrenal cortical overactivity in children.* The adrenal cortex can manufacture the sex hormones needed to initiate and maintain the secondary sexual characteristics of puberty. Disordered hypothalamic or pituitary function can also cause precocious puberty.

C.   **Option 1**   *Non-dysjunction of chromosome 21.* The non-disjunction of chromosome 21 during meiosis usually occurs in the ovary and increases in frequency with the age of the mother. Both of the chromosomes go to one of the daughter cells during meiosis.

D.   **Option 5**   *An XO chromosomal pattern.* In this condition (Turner's syndrome), the zygote does not receive a sex chromosome from one of the parents. The gonads are rudimentary or absent and the child develops female external genitalia. There is small stature and sexual maturation does not occur at puberty.

E.   **Option 3**   *Pituitary deficiency.* There are several causes of dwarfism but one of the causes is a hypothalamic or pituitary disorder that diminishes the secretion of growth hormone.

EMQ Question 505

For each substance A–E, select the best option for its functional description from the following list.

1. A 'mineralocorticoid'.
2. An androgen.
3. An alpha globulin that binds with cortisol.
4. A 'glucocorticoid'.
5. Causes breast development.

A. Corticosterone.
B. Progesterone.
C. Aldosterone.
D. Transcortin.
E. Dihydroepiandrosterone.

EMQ Question 506

For each item related to thyroid gland activity A–E, select the best option for its functional description from the following list.

1. The most active form of the thyroid hormones.
2. A disease caused by thyroxine deficiency in adults.
3. Protrusion of the eyeballs seen in patients with thyroid overactivity.
4. A pituitary gland hormone that stimulates the thyroid gland.
5. A glycoprotein stored in colloid in thyroid gland follicles.

A. Thyroglobulin.
B. Triiodothyronine (T_3).
C. TSH.
D. Myxedema.
E. Exophthalmos.

EMQ Question 507

For each item related to bone metabolism A–E, select the best option for its functional description from the following list.

1. Results in decalcification of bone in adults.
2. Results in bone formation.
3. Results in breakdown of bone matrix.
4. Results in impaired calcification of bone in children.
5. Results in inhibition of bone resorption.

A. Rickets.
B. Osteoblast activity.
C. Osteomalacia.
D. Osteoporosis.
E. Calcitonin.

Answers for 505

A. **Option 4**   *A 'glucocorticoid'.* Glucocorticoids promote protein catabolism, glucogene-
sis and gluconeogenesis.

B. **Option 5**   *Causes breast development.* Progesterone can be manufactured from preg-
nenolone in the adrenal cortex.

C. **Option 1**   *A 'mineralocorticoid'.* Aldosterone promotes fluid retention by facilitating
sodium retention by the renal tubules.

D. **Option 3**   *An alpha globulin that binds with cortisol.* Most circulating cortisol is bound
to transcortin and is inactive. Cortisol is freed and becomes physiologically active when
free cortisol levels fall.

E. **Option 2**   *An androgen.* This can cause 'virilization' in female patients with adrenocor-
tical tumours.

Answers for 506

A. **Option 5**   *A glycoprotein stored in colloid in thyroid gland follicles.* Thyroglobulin is
manufactured in the thyroid follicular cells and is secreted by exocytosis of granules into
the colloid for storage. The hormones remain bound to the colloid until they are secreted
into blood capillaries.

B. **Option 1**   *The most active form of the thyroid hormones.* T_4, which contains four iodine
molecules, is less physiologically active than T_3.

C. **Option 4**   *A pituitary gland hormone that stimulates the thyroid gland.* TSH secretion
from the anterior pituitary gland is controlled by the hypothalamic hormone, thyrotropin-
releasing hormone (TRF).

D. **Option 2**   *A disease caused by thyroxine deficiency in adults.* A disease characterized
by low basal metabolic rate, coarse hair and skin, poor cold tolerance and mental slow-
ness.

E. **Option 3**   *Protrusion of the eyeballs seen in patients with thyroid overactivity.* Due to
swelling of the external ocular muscles and other orbital tissues.

Answers for 507

A. **Option 4**   *Results in impaired calcification of bone in children.* Rickets is due to lack
of vitamin D in children. Poor calcium absorption in the gut results in bones with low
mineral content that are easily deformed.

B. **Option 2**   *Results in bone formation.* Osteoblasts are bone-forming cells that can lay
down collagen and other proteins for the bone matrix.

C. **Option 1**   *Results in decalcification of bone in adults.* Osteomalacia is due to lack of
Vitamin D in adults, usually childbearing women. It results in demineralization and de-
formation of the bones. When this affects pelvic bones, it may interfere with normal parturition.

D. **Option 3**   *Results in breakdown of bone matrix.* Osteoporosis is caused by loss of bony
matrix and the resulting bone weakness permits easy bone fracture to occur, especially in
the elderly.

E. **Option 5**   *Results in inhibition of bone resorption.* Calcitonin is a hormone secreted by
the parafollicular cells of the thyroid gland. It lowers the blood calcium level by inhibiting bone resorption.

EMQ Question 508

For each effect related to glucose metabolism A–E, select the best option for a possible cause from the following list.

1. Hypoglycaemia.	2. Metabolic acidosis.
3. Insulin deficiency.	4. Insulin.
5. Somatostatin.	

A.   Inhibition of insulin secretion.
B.   Increased potassium uptake by muscle.
C.   Negative nitrogen balance.
D.   Increased secretion of glucagon.
E.   Increased ventilation (Kussmaul breathing).

EMQ Question 509

For each endocrine disorder A–E, select the best option from the following list of effects.

1. Periodic episodes of severe hypertension.	
? Thirst, polyuria, obesity and tiredness.	3. Stones in the urinary tract.
	4. Tachycardia, sweating and heat intolerance.
5. Enlargement of the hands and feet and protrusion of the lower jaw.	

A.   Hyperparathyroidism.
B.   Thyrotoxicosis.
C.   Type 2 diabetes mellitus.
D.   Adrenal medullary overactivity.
E.   Acromegaly.

EMQ Question 510

For each endocrine disorder A–E, select the best option from the following list of effects.

1. Hypertension.	2. Polycythaemia.
3. Increased water and salt excretion.	4. Amenorrhoea.
5. Increased skin pigmentation.	

A.   Increased secretion of erythropoietin
B.   Decreased anterior pituitary secretion.
C.   Increased secretion of renin.
D.   Increased secretion of atrial natriuretic peptide (ANP).
E.   Decreased adrenal cortical activity.

Answers for 508

A. **Option 5**   *Somatostatin.* This is one of the effects of somatostatin secreted by the D cells of the islets of Langerhans.

B. **Option 4**   *Insulin.* Insulin increases both potassium and glucose uptake by muscle cells. Injections of glucose and insulin are sometimes given to lower potassium levels in blood when they are dangerously high.

C. **Option 3**   *Insulin deficiency.* This results from the increased breakdown of protein for gluconeogenesis in insulin deficiency.

D. **Option 1**   *Hypoglycaemia.* Glucagon acts to raise blood glucose by glycogenolysis and gluconeogenesis.

E. **Option 2**   *Metabolic acidosis.* The increase in ventilation with Kussmaul breathing results from stimulation of the respiratory system by the hydrogen ions liberated from keto-acids formed in severe diabetes.

Answers for 509

A. **Option 3**   *Stones in the urinary tract.* Excessive parathormone secretion in hyper-parathyroidism mobilizes calcium from bone. This calcium is excreted by the kidneys. Phosphate is also mobilized from the bones in hyperparathyroidism and excreted in the urine. When the calcium phosphate solubility product is exceeded, precipitation of calcium phosphate occurs and results in the formation of stones.

B. **Option 4**   *Tachycardia, sweating and heat intolerance.* The high metabolic rate in hyperthyroidism results in increased heat production and this is associated with tachycardia, sweating and heat intolerance.

C. **Option 2**   *Thirst, polyuria, obesity and tiredness.* The high blood glucose level in diabetes cause polyuria and consequential thirst. Obesity increases the tendency to develop type 2 diabetes.

D. **Option 1**   *Periodic episodes of severe hypertension.* Tumours in the adrenal medulla called phaeochromocytomas that release noradrenaline and adrenaline periodically can cause this.

E. **Option 5**   *Enlargement of the hands and feet and protrusion of the lower jaw.* Excessive growth hormone production in the adult after the epiphyses have closed results in thickening and enlargement of bones rather than their lengthening.

Answers for 510

A. **Option 2**   *Polycythaemia.* Erythropoietin acts on bone marrow cells to increase the production of erythrocytes.

B. **Option 4**   *Amenorrhoea.* This is due to loss of FSH and LH secretions that are responsible for maintaining the menstrual cycle.

C. **Option 1**   *Hypertension.* Renin from the kidneys causes hypertension by converting angiotensinogen to angiotensin I that is subsequently converted to angiotensin II that results in salt and water retention by the kidneys and an increase in peripheral resistance.

D. **Option 3**   *Increased water and salt excretion.* ANP is produced by atrial cells when they are stretched and causes increased loss of sodium and water by an action on the renal tubules.

E. **Option 5**   *Increased skin pigmentation.* One of the features of Addison's disease caused by loss of adrenal function is a bronze pigmentation of the skin. ACTH which is secreted in large amounts when adrenal cortical function is depressed, has some melanocyte-stimulating hormone (MSH) effect and this accounts for the skin pigmentation in Addison's disease.

EMQ Question 511

For each hormonal disturbance A–E, select the best option from the following list of effects.

1. Poor wound healing, thin skin and muscle wasting.
2. Raised arterial pressure, slow heart rate and raised peripheral resistance.
3. Glycogenolysis, gluconeogenesis and lipolysis.
4. Increased glycogen synthesis, potassium uptake, triglyceride deposition and hypoglycaemia.
5. Excessive thirst and urinary output.

A. Excessive secretion of glucagon.
B. Insufficient secretion of vasopressin.
C. Excessive secretion of glucocorticoids.
D. Excessive secretion of noradrenaline.
E. Excessive secretion of insulin.

EMQ Question 512

For each of the releasing or inhibiting hormones A–E, select the best option from the following list of effects.

1. An effect on somatomedin levels in the blood.
2. An effect on adrenal cortical activity.
3. An effect on lactation.
4. An effect on spermatogenesis.
5. An effect on thyroid-stimulating hormone (TSH) secretion.

A. Corticotrophin-releasing hormone (CRH).
B. Growth hormone-releasing hormone (GRH).
C. Prolactin-inhibiting hormone (PIH).
D. Thyrotropin releasing hormone (TRH).
E. Luteinizing hormone-releasing hormone (LHRH).

Answers for 511

A.   **Option 3**   *Glycogenolysis, gluconeogenesis and lipolysis.* These are some of the mechanisms by which glucagon raises the blood glucose level.

B.   **Option 5**   *Excessive thirst and urinary output.* Lack of vasopressin (ADH) secretion causes diabetes insipidus. In this condition there is reduced water reabsorption in the renal tubules and a consequential loss of body fluid that leads to thirst.

C.   **Option 1**   *Poor wound healing, thin skin and muscle wasting.* Glucocorticoids promote gluconeogenesis by the breakdown of protein in skin and muscle to form glucose.

D.   **Option 2**   *Raised arterial pressure, slow heart rate and raised peripheral resistance.* Noradrenaline constricts arterioles to raise arterial pressure and a consequential reflex slowing of the heart.

E.   **Option 4**   *Increased glycogen synthesis, potassium uptake, triglyceride deposition and hypoglycaemia.* These are some of the actions of insulin that lowers the blood sugar level.

Answers to 512

A.   **Option 2**   *An effect on adrenal cortical activity.* CRH from the hypothalamus stimulates the anterior pituitary gland to produce ACTH.

B.   **Option 1**   *An effect on somatomedin levels in the blood.* GRH stimulates the anterior pituitary gland to secrete GH (growth hormone), which in turn promotes somatomedin synthesis in the liver.

C.   **Option 3**   *An effect on lactation.* PIH is involved in prolactin secretion from the anterior pituitary gland. Reduction of PIH secretion seems to be the main factor in controlling prolactin secretion. Prolactin stimulates milk formation in the breasts.

D.   **Option 5**   *An effect on TSH secretion.* TRH (thyrotropin-releasing hormone) stimulates the anterior pituitary gland to secrete TSH (thyroid-stimulating hormone) that in turn increases activity in the thyroid gland.

E.   **Option 4**   *An effect on spermatogenesis.* LHRH (luteinizing hormone-releasing hormone) stimulates the anterior pituitary gland to secrete LH (luteinizing hormone) that in the male promotes spermatogenesis.

MCQs

Questions 513–519

513. In the normal menstrual cycle

A. Blood loss during menstruation averages around 100 ml.
B. The proliferative phase depends on oestrogen secretion.
C. Cervical mucus becomes more fluid around the time of ovulation.
D. Ovulation is followed by a surge in blood luteinizing hormone level.
E. Basal body temperature is higher after ovulation.

514. Fertilization of the human ovum normally

A. Occurs in the uterus.
B. Prevents further spermatozoa from entering the ovum.
C. Occurs 2–5 days after ovulation.
D. Occurs 5–7 days before implantation.
E. Leads to the secretion of human chorionic gonadotrophin (HCG) within two weeks.

515. Human spermatozoa

A. Contain 23 chromosomes.
B. Have enzymes in their heads which aid penetration of the ovum.
C. Are produced faster at 37 than at 32°C.
D. Are motile in the seminiferous tubules.
E. Are stored mainly in the seminal vesicles.

516. After a baby is born, there is normally a fall in

A. Its systemic vascular resistance.
B. Its pulmonary vascular resistance.
C. Direct flow from pulmonary artery to aorta.
D. Direct flow from right to left atrium.
E. Direct flow from right to left ventricle.

517. Secretion of testosterone

A. Depresses pituitary secretion of LH.
B. Causes the epiphyses of long bones to unite.
C. May lead to a negative nitrogen balance.
D. Stimulates growth of scalp hair.
E. Stimulates growth of body hair.

518. Human chorionic gonadotrophic hormone (HCG)

A. Is a steroid.
B. Acts directly on the uterus to maintain the endometrium.
C. Is formed in the anterior pituitary
D. Blood level rises steadily throughout pregnancy.
E. Can be detected in the urine as an early sign of pregnancy.

519. Compared with the adult, the newborn has less ability to

A. Excrete bilirubin.
B. Maintain a constant body temperature.
C. Tolerate brain hypoxia.
D. Manufacture antibodies.
E. Resist infection.

Answers

513.

A. False It varies widely but averages about 30 ml (one ounce).
B. True   This occurs in the first half of the cycle.
C. True   This mucus 'cascade' may facilitate sperm passage.
D. False The LH surge precedes and initiates ovulation.
E. True   Metabolic rate is raised by progesterone.

514.

A. False It occurs in the outer third of the uterine tube.
B. True   The zona pellucida becomes impermeable.
C. False The ovum remains viable for only about a day.
D. True   During this time the fertilized ovum travels along the uterine tube and spends several days free in the uterus.
E. True   This is necessary to maintain ovarian hormone production whose withdrawal causes endometrial necrosis.

515.

A. True   Half the complement of human somatic cells.
B. True   These are in the acrosome ('extremity body').
C. False Normal core temperature inhibits formation of spermatozoa.
D. False At this stage they are non-motile and cannot fertilize.
E. False They are stored in the epididymis.

516.

A. False This rises due to closure of the umbilical arteries.
B. True   Due to expansion of the lungs and their blood vessels.
C. True   Flow in the ductus arteriosus reverses due to (A) and (B).
D. True   Again due to reversal of the pressure gradient.
E. False Normally there is no opening in the intraventricular septum.

517.

A. True   This negative feedback keeps blood testosterone constant.
B. True   Sexual precocity can cause short stature.
C. False Testosterone is anabolic and leads to skeletal muscle hypertrophy.
D. False Scalp hair tends to recede.
E. True   This is a male secondary sexual characteristic.

518.

A. False It is a glycoprotein resembling luteinizing hormone (LH).
B. False It acts on the ovaries to maintain the corpus luteum.
C. False It is formed in the chorion of the developing embryo.
D. False It peaks in the first three months of pregnancy and then declines.
E. True   An immunological technique is used to identify it.

519.

A. True   'Physiological' jaundice is due to immaturity of the liver.
B. True   Temperature-regulating mechanisms are also immature.
C. False Fetal tissues are adapted to relative hypoxia.
D. True   Immunological competence develops around three months of age.
E. False Maternal antibodies (supplied via the placenta and breast) provide effective passive immunity.

Questions 520–526

520. Androgens are secreted in the
A. Testis by the seminiferous tubules.
B. Fetus in greater quantities than in early childhood.
C. In the female by the ovary.
D. In the male by the adrenal cortex.
E. In the male in decreasing quantities after the age of 30.

521. During pregnancy the
A. Uterine muscle enlarges due mainly to cell proliferation.
B. Uterus is quiescent until the onset of labour.
C. Breasts enlarge due mainly to the action of prolactin.
D. Haematocrit rises.
E. Basal metabolic rate rises by more than 10 per cent.

522. Males differ from females in that their
A. Pituitary glands secrete different gonadotrophic hormones.
B. Hypothalamus shows different patterns of hormone secretion.
C. Gonads produce gametes until later in life.
D. Blood gonadotrophin levels do not rise in later life.
E. Polymorphs show 'drumsticks' of chromatin on their nuclei.

523. Fetal haemoglobin
A. Is the only type identifiable in fetal blood.
B. Forms the bulk of total haemoglobin for the first year of life.
C. Has a higher oxygen-carrying capacity than adult haemoglobin.
D. Binds 2,3-DPI more avidly than does adult haemoglobin.
E. Has a higher affinity than the adult form for oxygen at low P_{O_2}.

524. For normal development and fertility of spermatozoa there must be
A. Secretion of testosterone.
B. Secretion of luteinizing hormone.
C. Secretion of follicle-stimulating hormone.
D. A testicular temperature of 37°C.
E. A sperm count of more than 10^{10}/ml.

525. In the mammary glands
A. Milk formation is stimulated by oestrogen and progesterone.
B. Milk formation can be depressed by hypothalamic activity.
C. Maintenance of lactation depends on suckling.
D. Lactation ceases if the anterior pituitary gland is destroyed.
E. Milk ejection ceases if the posterior pituitary gland is destroyed.

526. The male postpubertal state differs from the prepubertal in that
A. The gonads are responsive to gonadotrophic hormones.
B. There is a greater output of 17-ketosteroids in the urine.
C. Skeletal muscle is stronger per unit mass of tissue.
D. The circulating level of follicle-stimulating hormone is higher.
E. Hypothalamic output of gonadotrophin-releasing factors is greater.

Answers

520.

A. False They are secreted by the interstitial cells of the testis.
B. True   Fetal androgens control male sex organ development.
C. True   The ovaries secrete small amounts of androgen.
D. True   Adrenal androgens control pubic and axillary hair growth in both males and females.
E. True   There is a gradual fall, with no clear-cut 'climacteric'.

521.

A. False The enlargement is due more to an increase in the size of the muscle cells.
B. False Spontaneous uterine contractions occur during pregnancy.
C. False The enlargement is due mainly to oestrogen and progesterone.
D. False It falls due to the increase in plasma volume.
E. True   It increases by about one-third.

522.

A. False The gonadotrophic hormones are the same in males and females.
B. True   The female monthly cycle originates here.
C. True   Much later than the female menopausal age.
D. False Both sexes show a rise in FSH and LH levels.
E. False It is the female polymorphs that show this.

523.

A. False The adult type appears around mid gestation.
B. False It has almost disappeared by four months.
C. False They have similar oxygen capacities.
D. False It binds it less readily.
E. True   This aids oxygen transfer in the placenta.

524.

A. True   In its absence spermatogenesis is depressed.
B. True   This controls secretion of testosterone.
C. True   This also is required by the germinal epithelium.
D. False Testicular temperature should be maintained around 32°C.
E. False The normal value is around 10^8/ml.

525.

A. False These depress milk formation during pregnancy; prolactin stimulates milk formation.
B. True   By release of prolactin-inhibiting hormone (dopamine).
C. True   This causes prolactin secretion which initiates and maintains lactation after delivery.
D. True   Milk formation ceases due to loss of prolactin.
E. True   Due to loss of oxytocin in response to suckling.

526.

A. False They are responsive before puberty as well.
B. True   Due to greater production of sex hormones in the body.
C. True   This is one of the actions of testosterone.
D. True   This stimulates growth and function of the testes.
E. True   This initiates the various changes of puberty.

Questions 527–532

527. In the placenta
A. Fetal and maternal blood mix freely in the sinusoids.
B. The P_{O_2} in sinusoidal blood is similar to that in maternal arterial blood.
C. The barrier to oxygen diffusion is much greater than in alveoli.
D. Fetal blood in umbilical veins has a P_{O_2} within 10 per cent of that in maternal sinusoids.
E. Fetal blood becomes more than 50 per cent saturated with oxygen.

528. During pregnancy, there is an increase in
A. Maternal blood volume to twice the normal level.
B. Peripheral resistance.
C. Venous tone.
D. Ligament laxity.
E. Maternal parathormone secretion

529. In the fetal circulation the oxygen content of blood in the
A. Femoral artery is less than that in the brachial artery.
B. Superior vena cava is higher than that in the inferior vena cava.
C. Right ventricle is higher than that in the left ventricle.
D. Pulmonary artery is higher than that in the pulmonary veins.
E. Cerebral arteries is lower than in the maternal cerebral arteries.

530. Normal parturition depends on
A. An abrupt fall in placental secretion of oestrogen and progesterone.
B. Release of oxytocin from the posterior pituitary gland.
C. Activation of beta adrenoceptors in uterine muscle.
D. The presence of normal ovaries.
E. Innervation of the uterus.

531. The interstitial cells of the testis
A. Contribute to the volume of seminal fluid.
B. Are the source of the hormone inhibin.
C. Are stimulated to secrete by luteinizing hormone (LH).
D. Depend on hypothalamic activity to function properly.
E. Are non-functional unless the testis descends from the abdomen to the scrotum.

532. The size of the fetus at birth is likely to be smaller in
A. Small than in large mothers.
B. Multiple than in single fetus pregnancies.
C. Smoking than in non-smoking mothers.
D. Female than in male babies.
E. Firstborn than in subsequent babies.

Answers

527.

A.	False	The two circulations remain discrete.
B.	False	It is about half the arterial level in this sluggish flow.
C.	True	Due to a much thicker cellular barrier to diffusion.
D.	False	It is about 50 per cent lower due to the thick diffusion barrier.
E.	True	Due to its high affinity for oxygen.

528.

A.	False	It increases by about a third.
B.	False	It decreases (large uterine vessels, vasodilation).
C.	False	Venous tone decreases and varicose veins may develop in the legs.
D.	True	Due to relaxin, which helps the birth canal to dilate.
E.	True	Large amounts of calcium must be mobilized for the fetus.

529.

A.	True	Due to deoxygenated pulmonary arterial blood passing through the ductus arteriosus to the descending aorta.
B.	False	The IVC receives oxygenated blood from the placenta.
C.	False	Deoxygenated SVC blood streams to the right ventricle while oxygenated IVC blood streams via the foramen ovale to the left ventricle.
D.	True	Since the lungs are not ventilated, oxygen is lost rather than gained in its passage through the fetal lungs.
E.	True	Umbilical venous blood is only about 80 per cent saturated with oxygen and fetal arterial oxygen levels cannot exceed this; fetal tissues are adapted to survive in relative hypoxia.

530.

A.	False	Secretion is maintained at high levels until parturition.
B.	False	Birth can occur in the absence of the posterior pituitary.
C.	False	Beta activation may be used to delay onset of labour.
D.	False	Ovaries are not essential in late pregnancy and parturition.
E.	False	Parturition can occur with a denervated uterus; the cause of the onset of normal labour is unknown.

531.

A.	False	They secrete testosterone into the circulation.
B.	False	This hormone is produced by the seminiferous tubules.
C.	True	LH is the interstitial cell-stimulating hormone in the male.
D.	True	Gonadotropin releasing hormone from the hypothalamus is needed for LH secretion.
E.	False	Undescended testes can secrete testosterone.

532.

A.	True	Fetal size has some relationship to uterine capacity.
B.	True	Placental capacity per fetus is reduced.
C.	True	Excessive alcohol intake during pregnancy also reduces fetal size at birth.
D.	True	Males are on average about 200 grams heavier.
E.	True	On average later children are 200 grams heavier.

Questions 533–539

533. Testosterone secretion from the testis
A. Increases at puberty because LH levels increase.
B. Is responsible for the growth of facial hair.
C. Has a negative feedback effect on FSH secretion by the anterior pituitary gland.
D. Peaks in the early evening.
E. Is responsible for interest in the opposite sex.

534. The corpus luteum
A. Is essential for the secretory phase of the menstrual cycle.
B. Development is controlled by the pituitary gland.
C. Secretes hormones in early pregnancy when stimulated by pituitary gland hormones.
D. Is greyish-white in colour.
E. Begins to atrophy in the second month of pregnancy.

535. Erection of the penis
A. Cannot occur before puberty.
B. Is normally initiated by venoconstriction.
C. Depends on adrenergic sympathetic nervous activity.
D. Cannot occur after cervical spinal cord transection.
E. Is inhibited by ganglion blocking drugs.

536. The placenta
A. Contains villi which transport glucose into fetal blood.
B. Can convert glucose into glycogen.
C. Can store iron and calcium.
D. Actively transports oxygen into fetal blood.
E. Allows certain proteins to pass from maternal to fetal blood.

537. The ovaries
A. Begin to develop ova at puberty when acted on by FSH.
B. Are required for cyclical menstrual activity.
C. Must have double follicular rupture if identical twins are conceived.
D. Cease to respond to FSH after the menopause.
E. Secrete hormones which constrict uterine vessels.

538. The normal seminal ejaculate
A. Has a volume of about 5–10 ml.
B. Comes mainly from the seminiferous tubules and epididymis.
C. Contains fructose from the seminal vesicles.
D. Contains phosphate and bicarbonate buffers.
E. Contains prostaglandins.

539. The 21st day of the menstrual cycle differs from the seventh in that the
A. Endometrium is thicker and contains glands.
B. Blood level of progesterone is higher.
C. Blood is oestrogen free.
D. Blood level of FSH is at a maximum.
E. Endometrial glycogen content is higher.

MCQ

Answers

533.

A. True   LH secretion is controlled by hypothalamic GnRH (LH/FSH RH).
B. True   Females given testosterone may develop a beard.
C. False   Inhibin secreted by the testis has a negative feedback effect on FSH secretion.
D. False   It peaks around the time of awakening.
E. True   Castrates have little interest in sex.

534.

A. True   By its secretion of oestrogen and progesterone.
B. True   It depends on luteinizing hormone (LH).
C. False   It is controlled by human chorionic gonadotrophin (HCG) from the early placenta.
D. False   It is yellow; corpus luteum is Latin for 'yellow body'.
E. False   It is essential for the first three months of pregnancy.

535.

A. False   It is not uncommon in infants.
B. False   It is normally initiated by arteriolar dilatation.
C. False   It depends on parasympathetic cholinergic nerves; activity in sympathetic nerves is required for ejaculation.
D. False   It is based on a spinal reflex.
E. True   These block sympathetic and parasympathetic pathways.

536.

A. True   As in the intestinal villi.
B. True   This glycogen is stored in the placenta.
C. True   Also proteins and fat.
D. False   Oxygen transfer is accounted for by its pressure gradient.
E. True   For example, the gamma globulins concerned with passive immunity.

537.

A. False   The immature ova are formed before birth and no more are developed after birth.
B. True   Because of their secretion of oestrogen and progesterone.
C. False   Identical twins are derived from a single ovum.
D. True   Follicles disappear and are replaced by fibrous tissue.
E. False   Withdrawal of ovarian hormones leads to vasoconstriction.

538.

A. False   The normal volume is 2–5 ml.
B. False   These contribute only about 20 per cent of volume.
C. True   Seminal vesicles contribute about 60 per cent of seminal volume (prostate 20 per cent).
D. True   These help to neutralize acidic vaginal fluids.
E. True   Derived from seminal vesicles, prostaglandins may induce contractile activity in the female genital tract.

539.

A. True   The endometrium is in the secretory phase of the cycle.
B. True   It is very low on the seventh day.
C. False   Oestrogen remains high in the second half of the cycle.
D. False   The maximum is around the 14th day.
E. True   Conditions are optimal for implantation.

Questions 540–546

540. The newborn baby differs from the adult in that its
A. Urine has a lower maximum osmolality.
B. Urine has a lower minimum osmolality.
C. Blood–brain barrier is less permeable to bilirubin.
D. Temperature regulation is more efficient because of brown fat.
E. Blood has a greater affinity for oxygen at low oxygen pressures.

541. Changes in maternal physiology during pregnancy include a rise in
A. Nitrogen retention.
B. Mean arterial pressure of around 20 mmHg.
C. Arterial P_{CO_2}.
D. Tone in the urinary tract
E. The renal threshold for glucose.

542. Amniotic fluid is
A. Formed in early pregnancy by filtration from fetal skin capillaries.
B. Formed in late pregnancy by filtration from the gut mucosa.
C. Swallowed by the fetus.
D. Similar in electrolyte composition to plasma.
E. Inhaled and exhaled by the fetus.

543. Ejaculation of semen
A. Depends on a spinal cord reflex.
B. Depends on sympathetic nerve activity.
C. Involves rhythmic contractions of striated muscles.
D. Is accompanied by contraction of the cremasteric muscles.
E. Is followed by orgasm.

544. The fetus normally
A. Gains more weight in the last ten weeks of gestation than in the first 30 weeks.
B. Has a higher haemoglobin level at term than a normal adult.
C. Stores sufficient iron in the liver to last a year after birth.
D. Has a similar metabolic rate per metre^2 as an adult.
E. Passes rectal contents in the last three months of gestation.

545. Cessation of menstruation (secondary amenorrhoea) may occur because of
A. Psychological stress.
B. Severe weight loss.
C. Continuous administration of oestrogens.
D. An adrenal tumour.
E. Continuous administration of gonadotropin-releasing hormone (GnRH).

546. Development of secondary sexual characteristics before age nine could be
A. Due to abnormal secretion of adrenal cortical hormones.
B. Associated with short stature.
C. Due to a hypothalamic tumour.
D. Due to a pituitary tumour.
E. Present in a normal health child.

Answers

540.

A.   True   Its ability to concentrate urine is poor.

B.   False   Its ability to dilute urine is also poor.

C.   False   It is more permeable and brain damage can result with high blood bilirubin levels.

D.   False   Temperature regulation is poor in the newborn.

E.   True   Because of persisting fetal haemoglobin.

541.

A.   True   About 300 g nitrogen is retained, half by maternal tissues and half by fetal tissues.

B.   False   Blood pressure tends to fall, such a rise suggests disease.

C.   False   It tends to fall due to increased ventilation.

D.   False   Tone decreases and may lead to ureteric reflux and urinary infections.

E.   False   It falls, and glucose may appear in urine at normal blood glucose levels.

542.

A.   True   The non-keratinized skin is not waterproof.

B.   False   It is formed by the kidneys and excreted as urine in late pregnancy.

C.   True   Up to 0.5 litre/day is absorbed and excreted as urine.

D.   True   The protein content is, however, much lower.

E.   True   Surfactant from the lungs can be found in amniotic fluid in late pregnancy.

543.

A.   True   The centre is in the lumbosacral region.

B.   True   Stimulation of the hypogastric nerves in man can cause ejaculation.

C.   True   These compress the urethra.

D.   True   This causes elevation of the testicles.

E.   False   Ejaculation and orgasm coincide.

544.

A.   True   Fetal growth is exponential.

B.   True   Around 170–200 grams/litre.

C.   False   The stores last only a few months.

D.   False   It is about twice as great due to rapid growth.

E.   False   Passage of meconium before birth is a sign of distress.

545.

A.   True   Psychological stress affects hypothalamic activity.

B.   True   Amenorrhoea is common during starvation.

C.   True   Continuous progesterone administration can have the same effect.

D.   True   Androgens from the tumour may oppose the effects of female sex hormones on the endometrium.

E.   True   Normally GnRH secretion is pulsatile; thus interference with the normal hormone rhythms can cause amenorrhoea and infertility.

546.

A.   True   Adrenal androgens may lead to precocious puberty.

B.   True   Sex hormones cause closure of the epiphyses.

C.   True   If it secretes a gonadotropin-releasing hormone.

D.   True   If gonadotropins are produced.

E.   True   There is a wide scatter in the normal distribution of the age of onset of puberty.

Questions 547–552

547. The fetal
A. Blood in umbilical veins contains more amino acid than maternal blood in uterine veins.
B. Aorta has a higher rate of blood flow than the distal pulmonary artery.
C. Aortic blood pressure is lower than pulmonary arterial pressure.
D. Systemic resistance is higher than its pulmonary resistance.
E. Heart rate suggests fetal distress if it exceeds 100 beats/minute.

548. Lack of pulmonary surfactant
A. Is unlikely in infants born after 30 weeks gestation.
B. Can be diagnosed by examining the fetal amniotic fluid.
C. Increases the effort required for expiration.
D. Decreases the surface tension forces in the lungs.
E. Leads to poor oxygenation of the blood before birth.

549. A child whose sex chromosome pattern is
A. XY develops into a normal female.
B. XO shows incomplete sexual maturation at puberty.
C. XXX develops exaggerated female secondary sexual characteristics.
D. XXY develops into a true hermaphrodite.
E. XX is less likely to have haemophilia than one with XY.

550. The diagnosis of pregnancy is supported by finding
A. Conjugated progesterone in the urine.
B. Human chorionic gonadotrophin in the urine.
C. Viscous cervical mucus plugging the cervical canal.
D. Enlargement of the sebaceous glands in the mammary areolae.
E. A hardening of the cervical tissue.

551. The neonatal
A. Liver stores sufficient vitamin K for the first few months of life.
B. Blood volume is closer to 750 than 250 ml.
C. Blood glucose level fluctuates more than the fetal level.
D. Gut usually lacks certain enzymes needed for digestion of milk.
E. Peripheral vascular resistance is higher than that of the adult.

552. After a child is born
A. Its haemoglobin level rises steadily during the first year.
B. There should be a delay in clamping the umbilical cord so that blood from the placenta can drain into the fetus.
C. It should increase its weight by 10 per cent at four months.
D. Its brain can tolerate a lower blood glucose level than that of an adult.
E. Its brain can tolerate a lower oxygen level than that of an adult.

Answers

547.

A. True   Amino acids are actively transported from maternal to fetal blood in the placenta.
B. True   Due to high flow through the ductus arteriosus to the aorta.
C. True   Blood flows from the pulmonary artery to the distal aorta.
D. False   Distal aortic flow is greater than distal pulmonary artery flow and the pressure is lower (resistance = pressure/flow).
E. False   It is normally about 140/minute; below 100 suggests distress.

548.

A. False   Its formation starts around the 35th week.
B. True   Fetal breathing movements wash it into this fluid.
C. False   It increases the work of inspiration.
D. False   Without surfactant the surface tension forces are great; these forces must be overcome during inspiration.
E. False   The lungs are not used for gas exchange before birth; lack of surfactant causes poor oxygenation in the neonate.

549.

A. False   He develops into a normal male.
B. True   The gonads fail to develop (Turner's syndrome).
C. False   Abnormalities do not result.
D. False   He develops as a male with abnormal testes and a high risk of mental retardation (Klinefelter's syndrome).
E. True   Haemophilia is an X-linked recessive condition.

550.

A. False   This is normally present in the childbearing period.
B. True   This is not otherwise present.
C. True   Progesterone increases the viscosity of cervical mucus.
D. True   These are known as Montgomery's tubercles.
E. False   The cervix softens during pregnancy.

551.

A. False   Vitamin K is not stored and deficiency at birth is common.
B. False   It would be about 240 ml in a three-kilogram neonate.
C. True   The neonatal liver is less mature than the maternal liver.
D. False   It can usually deal adequately with the nutrients in milk.
E. True   The AV pressure gradient is almost as great as in the adult and flow is much smaller (resistance = pressure gradient/flow).

552.

A. False   It falls from around 170–200 g/litre to around 110 g/litre.
B. True   The placenta contains about half as much blood as the fetus; some can be transferred by uterine contraction.
C. False   Its weight should be doubled at this stage and trebled at one year.
D. True   It can tolerate about 25 per cent of the normal adult fasting level.
E. True   Fetal tissues are adapted to survive moderate hypoxia.

MCQ

Questions 553–558

553. Removal of the testes in the adult causes
A. A rise in the pitch of the voice.
B. Loss of libido.
C. Loss of the ability to copulate.
D. Hot flushes, irritability and depression.
E. A fall in the blood levels of LH and FSH.

554. Administration of oestrogens and progestogens to women
A. Prevents menstruation if given daily throughout the year.
B. Tends to cause salt and water retention.
C. Depresses secretion of pituitary gonadotrophins.
D. Decreases the likelihood of ovulation.
E. Tends to accentuate acne vulgaris.

555. Secondary sexual characteristics do not develop in children
A. Who have been castrated.
B. Whose seminiferous tubules, but not interstitial cells, have been damaged by radiation.
C. Suffering from severe malnutrition.
D. With dwarfism.
E. Lacking pituitary hormones.

556. Methods of reducing fertility include
A. Confining intercourse to the period from the 10–20th day of the menstrual cycle.
B. Bilateral ligation and division of the uterine tubes.
C. Bilateral ligation and division of the vas deferens.
D. The use of agents which prevent the fertilized ovum from implanting.
E. Mechanical barriers (condoms and caps) which are the most effective methods.

557. Infertility usually occurs
A. When the sperm count is reduced to 10 per cent of normal.
B. When posterior pituitary function is lost.
C. When one uterine tube is blocked.
D. In males with undescended testes.
E. Because of a reproductive disorder in the female partner.

558. Maternal blood loss in the first 24 hours after delivery
A. Is considered abnormal if it exceeds 600 ml.
B. Is greater after a short than after a long labour.
C. Is increased if part of the placenta is retained.
D. May justify transfusion of unmatched AB Rh-positive blood.
E. May, if excessive, impair anterior pituitary function.

Answers

553.

A.	False	Laryngeal changes induced by testosterone are permanent.
B.	True	Testosterone secretion increases libido.
C.	False	The sexual reflexes persist in the absence of testosterone.
D.	True	Rather like menopausal symptoms.
E.	False	These rise due to loss of feedback inhibition.

554.

A.	True	Withdrawal causes menstruation.
B.	True	Possibly due to structural affinity with mineralocorticoids.
C.	True	By a negative feedback mechanism.
D.	True	By suppressing pituitary gonadotrophins.
E.	False	Oestrogens antagonize the effect of androgens on sebaceous glands and improve acne.

555.

A.	True	Gonadal hormones are essential for their development.
B.	False	Testosterone promotes secondary sexual characteristics even if the germ cells cannot develop.
C.	False	They are delayed but appear eventually.
D.	False	In most cases they develop.
E.	True	These are required to stimulate the gonads to produce the essential sex hormones.

556.

A.	False	This is the maximally fertile period.
B.	True	This is difficult to reverse.
C.	True	An interval is necessary before infertility can be assumed.
D.	True	Intrauterine devices (IUDs) act in this way.
E.	False	Oral contraceptives and intrauterine devices are more effective.

557.

A.	True	Even though only one sperm ultimately fuses with the ovum.
B.	False	Vasopressin and oxytocin are not needed for fertilization.
C.	False	This would only reduce fertility moderately.
D.	True	The higher temperature in the abdomen impairs function in the spermatogenic epithelium.
E.	False	Male and female causes are about equally common in infertile couples.

558.

A.	True	This is the threshold for post-partum haemorrhage.
B.	False	After a long labour, the uterine contractions which normally close off the maternal sinusoids may be less efficient.
C.	True	This also hinders sinusoidal compression.
D.	False	Blood group O Rh-negative (universal donor) may be used.
E.	True	This is a recognized complication (Sheehan's disease).

Questions 559–565

559. Failure to ovulate in a given cycle is likely if

A. Pregnanediol appears in the urine in the second half of the cycle.
B. Basal body temperature is constant throughout the cycle.
C. Unilateral abdominal pain is experienced at mid-cycle.
D. Cervical mucus showed evidence of unopposed oestrogen action in the second half of the cycle.
E. The endometrium shows proliferating glands in the second half of the cycle.

560. Features indicating poor physical condition in the newborn include

A. A blue rather than a pale grey colour.
B. A steadily rising heart rate.
C. Spontaneous limb movements.
D. Relaxed muscles with low tone.
E. A grimace rather than a cough when the pharynx is stimulated.

561. Premature labour is associated with a greater

A. Risk of maternal complications.
B. Risk of cerebral haemorrhage in the fetus.
C. Fat content of the baby's skin.
D. Fetal head to body size ratio.
E. Need to feed the baby with milk.

562. Following the menopause, the

A. Vaginal secretions become more acid.
B. Myometrium decreases in bulk.
C. Libido may increase.
D. Lack of sex hormones may produce general body changes.
E. Level of pituitary gonadotrophins falls markedly.

563. Women having their first child after the age of 35 have a greater

A. Average blood loss than younger women.
B. Incidence of ineffective uterine contractions during labour.
C. Compliance of the perineum and vagina.
D. Incidence of fetal abnormalities.
E. Risk of spontaneous abortion.

564. Infertility in the male can be explained by observations that

A. There are no motile sperms in semen 15 minutes after ejaculation.
B. 50 per cent of the sperms in the semen are abnormal.
C. The sperm count is 10^8/ml.
D. The sperm count is 50 per cent below average.
E. There is widespread autonomic neuropathy.

565. Pregnant women with five or more previous deliveries have a greater risk of having

A. Anaemia.
B. An unfavourable presentation of the baby in the pelvis.
C. Complications due to rhesus incompatibility.
D. Serious loss of blood after delivery.
E. Involuntary urination while coughing (stress incontinence).

Answers

559.

A.   False   This is a normal derivative of progesterone which dominates the second half of the cycle.
B.   True   Normally there is a rise in the second half of the cycle.
C.   False   This is a sign of ovulation (mittelschmerz).
D.   True   Progesterone would normally prevent this effect ('ferning' due to salt crystals) in the second half of the cycle.
E.   False   Proliferating glands are normally present at this stage.

560.

A.   False   The pale grey colour suggests circulatory failure.
B.   False   This suggests recovery from vagal slowing.
C.   False   These are a good sign.
D.   True   This suggests severe hypoxia.
E.   True   This indicates depressed reflexes.

561.

A.   False   The fetus is smaller and is delivered more easily.
B.   True   Due to the greater fragility of cerebral veins at this stage of maturity.
C.   False   The skin tends to be brick red due to lack of fat.
D.   True   The body 'catches up' in late pregnancy.
E.   False   Milk is less well digested by premature infants.

562.

A.   False   They become less acid; infection is more likely.
B.   True   The uterus decreases in size.
C.   True   It may increase or decrease.
D.   True   Including osteoporosis and coronary artery disease.
E.   False   It rises due to loss of sex hormone negative feedback.

563.

A.   True   Uterine contraction is less effective in stopping bleeding.
B.   True   Again, due to deteriorating uterine function with age.
C.   False   It is less; Caesarean section is more often needed.
D.   True   Down's syndrome is one example of the genetic problems.
E.   True   Fetal abnormalities may be an important cause of this.

564.

A.   True   The sperms should be motile for at least one hour.
B.   True   This indicates a serious defect in sperm formation.
C.   False   This is the normal value.
D.   False   The count must be below 10–20 per cent to cause infertility.
E.   True   This neuropathy can affect the sexual reflexes.

565.

A.   True   Due partly to depletion of iron stores.
B.   True   Due to flabby uterine and abdominal wall muscles.
C.   True   There have been more opportunities for sensitization.
D.   True   Again due to deteriorating uterine function.
E.   True   Due to pelvic damage.

Questions 566–567

566. Secretion of androgens in the adult female
A.   Is abnormal.
B.   In large amounts can cause enlargement of the clitoris.
C.   Does not affect the voice.
D.   May lead to growth of facial hair.
E.   May result in amenorrhoea.

567. Fetal death is likely to result from serious impairment of fetal
A.   Liver function.
B.   Alimentary tract function such as obstruction.
C.   Renal function.
D.   Cerebral function.
E.   Cardiac function.

Answers

566.

A.	False	Adrenal androgen secretion is normal.
B.	True	It may grow to resemble a small penis.
C.	False	The voice deepens due to permanent laryngeal enlargement.
D.	True	As in the male.
E.	True	By suppressing the normal endometrial cycle.

567.

A.	False	The maternal liver can compensate.
B.	False	Fetal nutrition depends on the placenta.
C.	False	The maternal kidneys can compensate.
D.	False	Fetal survival does not depend on normal brain function.
E.	True	Fetal circulation is needed to harness maternal support systems to supply fetal needs.

EMQs

Questions 568–576

EMQ Question 568

For each aspect A–E, of multiple pregnancy (twins, triplets etc), select the most appropriate option from the following list of obstetrical terms.

1. Individual fetal mass.
2. Total mass of all fetuses.
3. Fetal prematurity.
4. Neonatal mortality.
5. Placental adequacy.
6. Assisted reproduction.
7. Perinatal mortality.

A. A mother with multiple pregnancies is more likely to have an inappropriately early (premature) onset of labour.

B. Since there is always a risk of loss of the fetus in early pregnancy, starting with two or more embryos increases the chance of at least one reaching maturity.

C. Multiple pregnancies decrease the likelihood of delayed labour due to inadequate size of the birth canal.

D. Multiple births are associated with an increased risk of neonatal jaundice and, more seriously, difficulty in overcoming surface tension forces during inspiration (respiratory distress syndrome).

E. The chances of surviving problems in the weeks before and after birth are less for a twin than a single birth, less still for a triplet and even less for a quadruplet.

EMQ Question 569

For each case of reduced fertility A–E, select the most appropriate option from the following list of aspects of the male and female reproductive systems.

1. Ovulation.
2. Spermatogenesis.
3. Transport in the uterine tube.
4. Transport in the vas deferens.
5. Erection of the penis.
6. Ejaculation.
7. Implantation.

A. A couple's infertility is attributed to medication with a drug which interferes with relaxation of vascular smooth muscle in the reproductive system.

B. Contraception is provided by a combination of oestrogen and progesterone given for 21 consecutive days in each month.

C. Contraception is provided by an intrauterine device.

D. A couple's infertility is attributed to the man's wearing a tight-fitting garment which holds the testes close to the trunk.

E. Infertility is attributed to surgery which has damaged sympathetic nerves in the pelvis.

EMQ

Answers for 568

A. **Option 2**   *Total mass of all fetuses.* Despite each fetus being small for its age, the total mass is exceptionally large, exaggerating the likelihood of labour before completion of the usual nine months of gestation.

B. **Option 6**   *Assisted reproduction.* Insertion of early embryos into the uterus as a means of treating infertility is a common cause of multiple birth; such embryos are at increased risk of abortion, so it is usual to insert several.

C. **Option 1**   *Individual fetal mass.* Each fetus of a multiple set is smaller than average at the time of labour, so is less likely to be hindered by a relatively small birth canal.

D. **Option 3**   *Fetal prematurity.* The more premature the fetus, the less mature is its liver, and the less able is it to conjugate the bilirubin load after birth; more seriously, it is also much more likely not to have developed the capacity to produce adequate surfactant to reduce the otherwise punishing effect of surface tension forces in the newborn lung.

E. **Option 7**   *Perinatal mortality.* This term refers to the risk of death in late pregnancy and early infancy; it mounts dramatically with the number of fetuses because of the combined effects of placental inadequacy, prematurity, and the problems of dealing with multiple infants at one delivery.

Answers for 569

A. **Option 5**   *Erection of the penis.* Erection depends on relaxation of smooth muscle in arterioles supplying the erectile tissue of the penis; its failure is described as impotence, in which condition ejaculation is not possible.

B. **Option 1**   *Ovulation.* The contraceptive pill leads to feedback inhibition of release of the gonadotrophins follicle-stimulating hormone and luteinizing hormone which control maturation and release of the ovum.

C. **Option 7**   *Implantation.* The intrauterine device interferes with implantation of the fertilized ovum.

D. **Option 2**   *Spermatogenesis.* This type of garment can raise the testicular temperature to a level where spermatogenesis is considerably impaired, leading to reduced fertility.

E. **Option 6**   *Ejaculation.* Ejaculation depends on sympathetic nerves for expulsion of seminal fluid into the urethra, and also for contraction of the bladder neck to prevent retrograde ejaculation into the bladder.

EMQ

EMQ Question 570

For each aspect A–E of the male and female reproductive systems, select the most appropriate option from the following list of hormones.

1. Follicle-stimulating hormone.
2. Gonadotrophin-releasing hormone.
3. Inhibin.
4. Luteinizing hormone.
5. Oestradiol.
6. Progesterone.
7. Testosterone.

A. A peptide hormone formed in testes and ovaries which acts as a local growth factor and also gives negative feedback to the hypothalamic–pituitary axis.

B. A steroid hormone formed in the testes which is necessary for normal spermatogenesis.

C. A peptide hormone formed in the hypothalamus which is necessary for normal spermatogenesis.

D. A steroid hormone which accounts for the rise in metabolic rate in the second half of the menstrual cycle.

E. A peptide hormone which plays a major role in both ovulation and the activity of the interstitial (Leydig) cells in the testis.

EMQ Question 571

For each effect of pregnancy A–E, select the most appropriate option from the following list of physiological terms.

1. Smooth muscle relaxation.
2. Smooth muscle constriction.
3. Brainstem reflex.
4. Sacral spinal cord reflex.
5. Decreased metabolic rate.
6. Increased metabolic rate.

A. The pregnant woman feels excessively hot in quite cool conditions; she dresses more lightly than most people and is keen to have windows opened for ventilation.

B. The pregnant woman has suffered several episodes of urinary frequency with a burning sensation on passing urine; this has been attributed to urinary infection, from which she has not previously suffered.

C. The pregnant woman suffers frequently from a burning sensation referred to the mid line of the chest; she didn't have it before pregnancy, it is not related to taking exercise, but indigestion tablets seem to help.

D. The woman in early pregnancy feels severely nauseated and quite frequently vomits, particularly first thing after getting up.

E. Despite eating more than usual, the pregnant woman suffers from decreased frequency and difficulty in defaecation.

EMO

Answers for 570

A. **Option 3**   *Inhibin.* This hormone (like many others) exists in several forms sometimes referred to as the inhibins; in the testis it is formed by Sertoli cells which nurture spermatozoa, so are a marker for spermatogenesis, completing the feedback loop.

B. **Option 7**   *Testosterone.* Among its widespread effects, testosterone, which is formed by interstitial cells of the testis, is responsible for spermatogenesis in the seminiferous tubules.

C. **Option 2**   *Gonadotrophin-releasing hormone.* This key hormone is required for the release of follicle-stimulating and luteinizing hormones in both sexes, so is responsible for all sexual activity; control by the hypothalamus allows the complicated control which is different in the two sexes, so that, while male sexual activity shows no regular fluctuation, female sexual activity follows the monthly cycle, which can be modified by nutritional and psychological factors.

D. **Option 6**   *Progesterone.* As implied by its name, this hormone is particularly associated with gestation; in the second half of the cycle it stimulates development in the endometrium which favours implantation of a fertilized ovum.

E. **Option 4**   *Luteinizing hormone.* A surge of this hormone is the precursor of ovulation and it also acts in the testis, giving it the secondary name of interstitial cell-stimulating hormone; note that, as in the body generally, hormones are either peptide or steroid based; in the reproductive system the peptides tend to be common to male and female, whereas the steroids make the difference.

Answers for 571

A. **Option 6**   *Increased metabolic rate.* These symptoms are like those of hyperthyroidism; in both cases the resting metabolic rate is increased; this leads to a parallel increase in heat production, so a cooler environment is needed for thermoneutrality.

B. **Option 1**   *Smooth muscle relaxation.* The hormones of pregnancy induce smooth muscle relaxation in many parts of the body; loss of tone in the bladder hinders complete emptying and favours reflux into the ureters; the urinary stasis favours infection.

C. **Option 1**   *Smooth muscle relaxation.* This time the muscle involved is the cardiac sphincter; loss of tone favours reflux of acid from the stomach into the oesophagus where the very low pH causes burning pain – 'heartburn of pregnancy'.

D. **Option 3**   *Brainstem reflex.* 'Morning sickness' is a classical sign of early pregnancy; the vomiting reflex is stimulated, possibly by the sudden change in hormonal levels, sharp rise in chorionic gonadotrophin, and rises in oestrogen and progesterone.

E. **Option 1**   *Smooth muscle relaxation.* Again this is the problem, this time affecting the lower bowel so that emptying of the rectum is inefficient.

EMQ Question 572

For each aspect of labour A–E, select the most appropriate option from the following list of muscle activities.

1. Smooth muscle relaxation.   2. Smooth muscle contraction.
3. Skeletal muscle relaxation.   4. Skeletal muscle contraction.

A. The onset of the first stage of labour is when regular spasms of abdominal pain begin (labour pains).
B. The onset of the second stage of labour is when the uterine cervix becomes fully dilated.
C. During the second stage of labour the mother is encouraged to make powerful bearing down/pushing actions to help deliver the baby.
D. After the third stage of labour which ends with the expulsion of the placenta, the mother may be given oxytocin, or encouraged to put the infant to the breast.
E. During the first stage of labour, the mother is encouraged to avoid bearing down actions and breath-holding so that the baby is not forced against an incompletely dilated cervix.

EMQ Question 573

For each description of a phase in the menstrual cycle A–E, select the most appropriate option for the following list of days.

1. Day 0.   2. Day 4.
3. Day 7.   4. Day 14.
5. Day 21.   6. Day 27.

A. Vaginal secretions are at their most fluid; the endometrium has regenerated but is not yet optimal for implantation.
B. The endometrium has undergone ischaemic necrosis (death due to lack of blood flow) and external discharge has been noted.
C. The level of luteinizing hormone is around its peak, the level of oestradiol is medium, and that of progesterone relatively low.
D. The menstrual discharge has just ended.
E. The level of progesterone is around its peak.

EMQ Question 574

For each aspect of spermatogenesis and the seminal ejaculate A–E, select the most appropriate option from the following list of components of the male reproductive system.

1. Leydig cells.   2. Sertoli cells.
3. Seminiferous tubules.   4. Epididymis.
5. Seminal vesicles.   6. Prostate gland.
7. Vas deferens.

A. At their site of formation, the spermatozoa acquire the haploid number of chromosomes.
B. Testosterone, which is essential for normal spermatogenesis, is produced by cells stimulated by follicle-stimulating hormone.
C. Spermatozoa are stored for some 2–4 weeks, while their motility and ability to fertilize steadily increase.
D. Most of the volume of the seminal ejaculate consists of a slightly alkaline fluid rich in fructose.
E. The spermatozoa in the seminal ejaculate leave the scrotum because of powerful contraction of smooth muscle cells.

Answers for 572

A. **Option 2**   *Smooth muscle contraction.* Labour begins when the state of uterine quiescence is replaced by regular, painful, contractions of the uterine smooth muscle.

B. **Option 1**   *Smooth muscle relaxation.* Full relaxation of the smooth muscle in the uterine cervix sets the stage for passage of the baby; in the body generally, expulsion is achieved by contraction behind and relaxation in front of what is being expelled; in the heart expulsion of contents takes place on a very short time scale, in the bladder and rectum it is longer, and in the uterus the time scale is relatively very long.

C. **Option 4**   *Skeletal muscle contraction.* This is a form of the Valsalva manoeuvre, where abdominal skeletal muscle contracts to favour expiration against a closed glottis; this manoeuvre helps expulsion of abdominal contents when the relevant orifice is open as well as in delivery of the baby, the manoeuvre has a part is speeding micturition and defaecation, and in producing vomiting.

D. **Option 2**   *Smooth muscle contraction.* Oxytocin favours powerful contraction of the uterine smooth muscle which helps to limit bleeding after delivery (post-partum haemorrhage); stimulation of the breast by the baby leads to release of endogenous oxytocin from the posterior pituitary.

E. **Option 3**   *Skeletal muscle relaxation.* The mother cannot influence the uterine contractions, but can favour relaxation of the abdominal muscles by avoiding the Valsalva manoeuvre, usually expressed as 'not pushing down', but rather breathing shallowly.

Answers for 573

A. **Option 4**   *Day 14.* This is the middle of the cycle, when ovulation is just occurring; fluid vaginal secretions favour passage of spermatozoa; if the ovum is fertilized it will be ready to implant in about a week when the endometrium will be at its most receptive.

B. **Option 1**   *Day 0.* The menstrual cycle is timed from when the patient first notices the menstrual discharge.

C. **Option 4**   *Day 14.* The sudden peaking of the level of luteinizing hormone initiates ovulation; at this stage the level of oestradiol is falling from its initial peak in the proliferative phase; the level of progesterone is about to start rising steeply.

D. **Option 2**   *Day 4.* The menstrual discharge lasts around four days on average.

E. **Option 5**   *Day 21.* At this stage progesterone is having its maximal effect and the endometrium is at its most receptive; in the absence of a fertilized ovum the progesterone level will fall leading to menstruation; if an ovum implants, the gonadotrophic hormone it produces will stimulate the corpus luteum to maintain and increase secretion of progesterone so maintaining the endometrium and the pregnancy.

Answers for 574

A. **Option 3**   *Seminiferous tubules.* This is where the spermatozoa originate and begin their development.

B. **Option 1**   *Leydig cells.* These are the interstitial cells between the seminiferous tubules.

C. **Option 4**   *Epididymis.* This is the main storage and maturation site.

D. **Option 5**   *Seminal vesicles.* These contribute about two-thirds of the ejaculate volume; the alkalinity protects the sperm against vaginal acidity and the fructose is a source of energy.

E. **Option 7**   *Vas deferens.* This transports the spermatozoa under the influence of sympathetic stimulation of the smooth muscle in its wall.

EMQ Question 575

For each stage of pregnancy A–E, select the most appropriate option from the following list of months.

1. Month one.	2. Month two.
3. Month five.	4. Month eight.

A. The levels of oestradiol and progesterone are around their maximum; the level of chorionic gonadotrophin is submaximal.
B. Morning sickness is relatively mild, if present; joint discomfort is not usually a problem either.
C. The levels of oestradiol, progesterone and chorionic gonadotrophin are all rising rapidly.
D. The level of chorionic gonadotrophin is approaching its maximum; the levels of oestradiol and progesterone are well below their maximum.
E. Heartburn from regurgitation of gastric acid to the oesophagus is favoured by a marked loss of smooth muscle tone in the lower oesophagus and by a marked rise in intra-abdominal pressure.

EMQ Question 576

For each of the phases of the female life cycle A–E, select the most appropriate option from the following list of ages.

1. 10–15 years.	2. 15–20 years.
3. 20–25 years.	4. 30–35 years.
5. 40–45 years.	6. 50–55 years.
7. 60–65 years.	

A. The risk of having a baby with the major genetic abnormality of Down's syndrome is around its maximum.
B. Fertility is at its maximum and the complications of pregnancy at a minimum.
C. The chances of natural conception are almost zero; the level of gonadotrophic hormones is around its maximum.
D. Secondary sexual characteristics usually begin to appear at this age.
E. The risk of coronary artery disease is now close to the male level; bone density is likely to have decreased markedly.

Answers for 575

A. **Option 4**   *Month eight.* In the last trimester (3-month period) of pregnancy, the hormones sustaining pregnancy are having their maximal effect; the maximal level of chorionic gonadotrophin occurs in the first trimester when it is maintaining the corpus luteum.

B. **Option 3**   *Month five.* The middle trimester tends to have the least discomfort; morning sickness has usually subsided and the physical effects of a relatively huge uterus in the last trimester are not yet marked.

C. **Option 1**   *Month one.* The gonadotrophin rises rapidly to produce the corpus luteum essential in the first trimester, and the corpus luteum rapidly increases its activity to initiate the major changes of pregnancy via oestradiol and progesterone.

D. **Option 2**   *Month two.* The middle of the first trimester is the mirror image of the last trimester in terms of these hormones.

E. **Option 4**   *Month eight.* Regurgitation is favoured by relaxation of the lower oesophageal sphincter, particularly by progesterone and by the concomitant surge in uterine size and intra-abdominal pressure; both of these effects subside dramatically on delivery of the baby, and so does the heartburn.

Answers for 576

A. **Option 5**   *40–45 years.* This is the last epoch with a moderate fertility; by this time the primordial ova are four decades old.

B. **Option 3**   *20–25 years.* In both sexes most physical characteristics are around the optimal.

C. **Option 6**   *50–55 years.* A minute number of conceptions take place around the age of 50; nearly all women have reached the menopause with its surge of gonadotrophins directed at the senescent gonads.

D. **Option 1**   *10–15 years.* Changes in fat and hair distribution, the onset of menstruation (menarche) and the adolescent growth spurt usually begin in this epoch.

E. **Option 7**   *60–65 years.* Some 15 years after the menopause these changes are associated with withdrawal of oestrogens and progesterone; many women take hormonal replacement therapy during this period; it relieves hot flushes and other symptoms which may be related to the surge in gonadotrophins; some protection against coronary artery disease and osteoporosis can be balanced against adverse long-term effects.

MCO

MCQs

Questions 577–582

577. Ultrafiltration
A. Separates the colloidal contents of a solution from the crystalloid contents.
B. Is involved in the movement of water and electrolytes across cell membranes.
C. Is involved in the formation of tissue fluid by the capillaries.
D. Is involved in the formation of glomerular filtrate by the kidneys.
E. Is involved in the formation of cerebrospinal fluid by the choroid plexuses.

578. The Fick principle enables
A. Blood flow through an organ to be calculated if organ uptake (U), arterial concentration (A) and venous concentration (V) are known for a given substance.
B. Cardiac output to be calculated by injecting an indicator into the pulmonary artery and monitoring its concentration downstream in a systemic artery.
C. Renal plasma flow to be calculated using PAH as the substance measured.
D. Cardiac output to be estimated using the lungs as the organ and carbon dioxide as the substance measured.
E. Cerebral blood flow to be measured using nitrous oxide as the substance taken up by the brain.

579. Mitochondria
A. Have membranes similar to the cell membrane.
B. Are the chief site for protein synthesis.
C. Are the chief sites for generation of ATP.
D. Are more numerous in brown than in white fat cells.
E. Are absent near the membranes of actively secreting cells.

580. Sleep is associated with
A. An alpha rhythm in the electroencephalogram.
B. Increased activity in the reticular activating system.
C. A high level of vagal tone to the heart.
D. Grinding movements of the teeth.
E. A rise in central body temperature.

581. During the Valsalva manoeuvre (forced expiration with glottis closed)
A. Pressure rises in the urinary bladder.
B. The initial rise in arterial pressure coincides with a fall in the rate of venous return.
C. Cardiac output rises.
D. Heart rate slows.
E. Peripheral resistance rises.

582. Jejunal mucosal cells are similar to proximal convoluted tubular cells in that both
A. Absorb glucose by a process linked with sodium absorption.
B. Absorb chloride ions actively.
C. Absorb amino acids actively.
D. Are rich in mitochondria.
E. Possess microvilli on their luminal border.

Answers

577.

A.   **True**   It depends on pore size and hydrostatic pressure gradients; colloids are larger particles than crystalloids.

B.   **False**   Substances cross cellular walls by active transport or down electrochemical gradients; hydrostatic pressure gradients are not involved.

C.   **True**   An outward hydrostatic pressure gradient exists at the arterial end of the capillary.

D.   **True**   The pressure gradient across glomerular capillary walls is greater than that in other capillaries.

E.   **True**   But active secretion is also involved in the formation of CSF.

578.

A.   **True**   From the principle, $U = F(A - V)$, so $F = U/(AV)$.

B.   **False**   This method is related to the indicator dilution rather than the Fick principle.

C.   **True**   Uptake = urine volume × urine concentration, V = zero; the formula is then the same as for PAH clearance.

D.   **True**   Either oxygen or carbon dioxide can be the substance measured.

E.   **True**   The Kety method to measure cerebral blood flow uses the Fick principle.

579.

A.   **True**   Both membranes have the same lipid bilayer structure.

B.   **False**   This applies to the ribosomes.

C.   **True**   ATP is formed by oxidative phosphorylation.

D.   **True**   Brown fat cells can generate energy, and hence heat, more rapidly.

E.   **False**   They are concentrated where most energy is required.

580.

A.   **False**   The alpha rhythm disappears during sleep.

B.   **False**   Activity decreases; increased activity is associated with alertness.

C.   **True**   This maintains a slow heart rate during sleep.

D.   **True**   Teeth-grinding is associated with REM sleep and is called *bruxism*.

E.   **False**   This tends to drop during the early hours of sleep.

581.

A.   **True**   Due to the rise in intra-abdominal pressure.

B.   **True**   Both result from the sudden initial rise in intrathoracic pressure.

C.   **False**   It falls due to the reduced venous return.

D.   **False**   It rises to compensate for a falling arterial pressure.

E.   **True**   Another reflex compensatory mechanism to restore arterial pressure.

582.

A.   **True**   In both cases, glucose absorption is blocked by phlorhizin.

B.   **False**   In both, these follow passively the absorption of sodium.

C.   **True**   Again the process requires active absorption of sodium.

D.   **True**   Both expend considerable energy.

E.   **True**   The two types of cell have very similar functions.

Questions 583–589

583. Exercise which doubles the metabolic rate is likely to at least double the

A. Oxygen consumption.
B. Cardiac output.
C. Stroke volume.
D. Arterial P_{CO_2}.
E. Minute volume.

584. The endoplasmic reticulum

A. Is a complex system of intracellular tubules.
B. Is a component of the Golgi apparatus.
C. Has a membrane structure similar to the cell membrane.
D. Is associated with ribonucleoprotein.
E. Is well developed in secretory cells.

585. In bone

A. Osteoclasts are responsible for bone resorption.
B. Osteoclasts are inhibited by parathyroid hormone.
C. Maintenance of normal calcium content depends on exposure to mechanical stress.
D. Strontium ions may substitute for calcium ions.
E. The width of the epiphyseal plate is an index of its growth rate.

586. The standard deviation of a series of observations

A. Is related to the scatter of the observations.
B. Is such that about 95 per cent of observations lie within one standard deviation of the mean.
C. Should be calculated only if observations are normally distributed.
D. Is a measure of the significance of the observations.
E. Is a more valid expression of scatter than is the absolute range for small numbers of observations, e.g. less than five.

587. Human circadian (24-hour) rhythms

A. Are triggered totally by external (exogenous) factors.
B. Depend more on the integrity of the cerebral cortex than of the hypothalamus.
C. Adapt within 48 hours on changing from day to night shift work.
D. For melatonin secretion produce high night-time and low day-time levels of the hormone.
E. For the eosinophil count produce peak values around midday.

588. The mammalian cell membrane

A. Is seen as an optically dense line using light microscopy.
B. Consists mainly of protein.
C. Is more permeable to fat- than to water-soluble particles.
D. Contains enzymes.
E. Contains the receptors for steroid hormones.

589. During early inspiration there is an increase in

A. Heart rate.
B. Central venous pressure.
C. Intrapulmonary pressure.
D. Abdominal girth.
E. Afferent impulse traffic in the vagus nerves.

Answers

583.

A.   **True**   Oxygen consumption is directly related to metabolic rate.
B.   **False**   This rises more slowly than metabolic rate because tissue O_2 extraction increases.
C.   **False**   Since heart rate rises, stroke volume does not rise in proportion to metabolic rate.
D.   **False**   This is little changed.
E.   **True**   This rises proportionately more than metabolic rate.

584.

A.   **True**   It is analogous to the sarcoplasmic reticulum in muscle cells.
B.   **False**   The Golgi apparatus differs in structure, function and location in the cell.
C.   **True**   As do mitochondria.
D.   **True**   RNA is found in the ribosomes which are attached to the cytoplasmic side of the tubules in rough endoplasmic reticulum and are responsible for protein synthesis.
E.   **True**   It is the site of hormone and enzyme synthesis.

585.

A.   **True**   They contain an acid phosphatase.
B.   **False**   They are stimulated to resorb bone with release of calcium ions.
C.   **True**   Calcium is released from bone during bed rest and inactivity.
D.   **True**   This may subject bones to increased radioactivity.
E.   **True**   The epiphyseal plate is relatively wide during childhood.

586.

A.   **True**   It increases as scatter increases.
B.   **False**   This is true for two standard deviations; for one standard deviation it is 66 per cent.
C.   **True**   Otherwise (B) above does not hold.
D.   **False**   It is only a description of the scatter of observations.
E.   **False**   It should not be calculated for very small numbers of observations.

587.

A.   **False**   External triggers modulate an endogenous clock.
B.   **False**   The hypothalamus is thought to be the location of the endogenous clock.
C.   **False**   Adaptation takes about a week or longer.
D.   **True**   Melatonin given at bedtime has been used to allay the circadian rhythm disturbances of sleep with jet-lag.
E.   **False**   The peak is at night when cortisol level is minimal.

588.

A.   **False**   It is beyond the resolution of the light microscope.
B.   **False**   It consists mainly of lipid.
C.   **True**   Fat-soluble particles dissolve easily in the lipid matrix.
D.   **True**   These are involved in active transport.
E.   **False**   Steroid hormones cross the membrane and act intracellularly.

589.

A.   **True**   This is part of the cycle of respiratory sinus arrhythmia.
B.   **False**   It decreases due to expansion of the great veins.
C.   **False**   It falls due to expansion of the thoracic cage.
D.   **True**   Due to descent of the diaphragm.
E.   **True**   From stretch receptors in the lung mediating the Hering–Breuer reflex.

Questions 590–596

590. Lysosomes

A. Are membrane-bound organelles in the cytoplasm.
B. Contain enzymes known as lysozyme.
C. Are present in serous salivary glands.
D. Enable neutrophil granulocytes to digest phagocytosed material.
E. Can digest cellular contents.

591. On lying down there is a decrease in the

A. Central venous volume.
B. Total systemic peripheral resistance.
C. Ventilation/perfusion ratio in lung apices.
D. Vital capacity.
E. Rate of formation of urine.

592. One mole of calcium ion

A. Is equivalent to two osmoles of calcium.
B. Has the same mass as two equivalents of calcium ion.
C. Is present in one litre of a normal solution of calcium ions.
D. Weighs 40 grams.
E. Depresses the freezing point of water to the same extent as one mole of sodium ion.

593. The Valsalva manoeuvre is followed by a decrease in

A. Intrapleural pressure.
B. Intra-abdominal pressure.
C. Cardiac output.
D. Arterial blood pressure.
E. Heart rate.

594. Carbonic anhydrase has a role to play in the formation of

A. HCl by the parietal cells of the stomach.
B. Carbaminohaemoglobin.
C. Cerebrospinal fluid in the choroid plexuses.
D. Bicarbonate by the pancreas.
E. Aqueous humour by the ciliary bodies.

595. Sinus arrhythmia

A. Refers to the cyclical changes in blood pressure that accompany the respiratory cycle.
B. Can be observed in normal people.
C. Has a greater amplitude in old than in young people.
D. Is mediated mainly through sympathetic nerves to the heart.
E. Can be used as an index of autonomic nerve function.

596. Membrane ion channels

A. Consist mainly of carbohydrate and lipid.
B. Have a specific structure for each ion species.
C. For sodium may be blocked by tetrodotoxin.
D. May be opened by a given change in transmembrane potential.
E. Remain open as long as the activating signal is present.

Answers

590.

A. True   They are present in most cells.
B. True   Lysozyme breaks down organic structures.
C. True   Lysozyme in saliva helps to destroy ingested bacteria.
D. True   The granules are examples of lysosomes.
E. True   This is responsible for decomposition of tissues after death.

591.

A. False   Volume expands as blood shifts from veins in the lower extremities to the chest.
B. True   A reflex response to an increased central blood volume.
C. True   Apical perfusion increases during recumbency.
D. True   Due to vascular distension in the lungs and pushing up of the diaphragm.
E. False   An increase in central blood volume results in increased urine formation.

592.

A. False   One mole of any ion in solution exerts one osmole of osmotic pressure.
B. True   Because calcium is divalent.
C. False   A normal solution has one equivalent weight of ion per litre.
D. True   This is the atomic weight in grams.
E. True   1 osmole of a substance in 1 litre of water depresses the freezing point by 1.86°C.

593.

A. True   It returns to its normal negative value.
B. True   It also returns to normal.
C. False   It rises as blood surges back to the central circulation.
D. False   It rises due to the great increase in cardiac output.
E. True   A reflex response to the surge in arterial pressure.

594.

A. True   It facilitates H^+ and HCO_3^- formation from H_2O and CO_2 and H^+ is secreted.
B. False   Carbaminohaemoglobin is formed when CO_2 combines directly with amino groups of the globin component of haemoglobin.
C. False   Blockade of the enzyme does not affect CSF formation.
D. True   It facilitates H^+ and HCO_3^- formation from CO_2 and H_2O and HCO_3^- is secreted.
E. True   Blockade of the enzyme reduces the rate of formation of aqueous humour. It may be used to lower intraocular tension in patients with glaucoma.

595.

A. False   It refers to the cyclical changes in heart rate that accompany the respiratory cycle.
B. True   It is a normal, harmless phenomenon.
C. False   It decreases in amplitude with age.
D. False   It is mediated by vagal nerves and abolished by vagal blockade with atropine.
E. True   It is impaired in vagal autonomic neuropathy.

596.

A. False   They are usually proteins.
B. False   There is usually a family of channels for each ion species.
C. True   This toxin from the puffer fish specifically blocks sodium channels.
D. True   These channels are 'voltage-gated' channels; 'ligand-gated' channels are opened by chemical substances such as acetylcholine.
E. False   They close automatically after a certain interval.

Questions 597–603

597. The hydrogen ion concentration in a solution
A. Equals the hydroxyl ion concentration at pH 7.
B. Rises with increasing acidity.
C. Of pH 5 is 100 times greater than that in a solution of pH 7.
D. Is inversely related to the hydroxyl ion concentration.
E. Is approximately doubled if the pH falls by 0.3 units.

598. The human cell nucleus
A. Has a membrane which is permeable to nucleic acid.
B. In somatic cells contains 44 chromosomes.
C. Stores its genetic material in the nucleolus.
D. Has a skeleton of fine filaments.
E. Is essential for cell division.

599. Athletic training leads to an increase in the
A. Ratio of lean body mass to body fat.
B. Resting vagal tone.
C. Resting stroke volume.
D. Maximal oxygen consumption.
E. Blood lactate level for a given level of work.

600. The total osmotic pressure of human plasma is
A. About 25 mmHg.
B. Similar to that of 0.9 per cent saline.
C. Similar to that of 0.9 per cent glucose solution.
D. Opposing the tendency of fluid to leave capillaries.
E. Equal to that of intracellular fluid.

601. With increasing age there is a fall in the
A. Arterial pulse pressure.
B. Ability to detect smells.
C. Ability of the kidneys to concentrate urine.
D. Residual volume of the lungs.
E. Fasting blood glucose concentration.

602. Ingestion of protein
A. Raises metabolic rate more than ingestion of equally calorific amounts of fat or carbo-hydrate.
B. Tends to lower the pH of urine.
C. Permits the body to synthesize the essential amino acids.
D. Yields more toxic metabolites than fat or carbohydrate.
E. Should exceed 2 g/kg body weight/day to satisfy normal body requirements.

603. Drinking a litre of water
A. Increases secretion of antidiuretic hormone.
B. Reduces the plasma sodium concentration.
C. Causes more osmolar change in portal venous than in systemic venous blood.
D. Causes body cells to shrink.
E. Decreases the specific gravity of the body.

Answers

597.

A.   **True**   This is the neutral pH of water.
B.   **True**   The pH falls.
C.   **True**   pH is minus $\log_{10}$ hydrogen ion concentration.
D.   **True**   The product of these ionic concentrations is constant.
E.   **True**   Log $2 = 0.301$.

598.

A.   **True**   Messenger RNA crosses the nuclear membrane.
B.   **False**   The total is 46; i.e. $44 + XX$ or XY.
C.   **False**   The nucleolus is a condensation of RNA; the genetic material is in chromosomes.
D.   **True**   These are attached to the nuclear membrane.
E.   **True**   For example, red blood cells cannot divide.

599.

A.   **True**   Skeletal muscle bulk increases with activity more than fat.
B.   **True**   This explains the slow pulse rate seen in athletes.
C.   **True**   This maintains resting cardiac output with the slower heart rate.
D.   **True**   This is a good index of physical fitness.
E.   **False**   Due to greater capacity to deliver oxygen to muscle, the reverse is true.

600.

A.   **False**   It is about 5500 mmHg (25 mmHg is the colloid osmotic pressure).
B.   **True**   Both have an osmolality around 290 mosmol/litre.
C.   **False**   It is similar to 5 per cent glucose which contains about the same number of particles.
D.   **False**   The colloid osmotic pressure does this; the crystalloids pass capillary walls freely and exert no effective pressure gradient across the capillary wall.
E.   **True**   Intracellular and extracellular fluid have the same osmolality.

601.

A.   **False**   It rises with loss of arterial elasticity.
B.   **True**   The condition is called hyposmia.
C.   **True**   Due to a fall in maximal renal medullary osmolality.
D.   **False**   It increases as small airways collapse more readily.
E.   **False**   It rises as glucose homeostasis loses efficiency.

602.

A.   **True**   Due, perhaps, to the additional metabolic work in processing protein in the body.
B.   **True**   Protein is the main dietary source of the acidic residues excreted by the kidney.
C.   **False**   Essential amino acids cannot be synthesized in the body.
D.   **True**   These metabolites, normally detoxified in the liver, may cause hepatic encephalopathy in hepatic failure.
E.   **False**   One gram per kilogram is adequate.

603.

A.   **False**   It suppresses secretion of antidiuretic hormone.
B.   **True**   Osmolality is reduced in all the body fluid compartments.
C.   **True**   The water is absorbed via the portal vein.
D.   **False**   They swell as water is drawn in osmotically.
E.   **False**   It moves it upwards from its value of less than 1.0.

Questions 604–610

604. The Golgi apparatus is
A. Found in all eukaryotic cells.
B. A collection of complex tubules and vesicles.
C. Well developed in cells with secretory activity.
D. Associated with endoplasmic reticulum.
E. Not conspicuous in neurones.

605. An acid–base buffer system
A. Can be a mixture of a weak acid and its conjugate base.
B. Can be a solution of sodium and bicarbonate ions.
C. Prevents any change in pH when acid is added.
D. Works best when acid and base are equal in concentration.
E. With pK = 4 would be a better blood buffer than one with pK = 6.

606. Rapid eye movement (REM) sleep is
A. Associated with EEG waves of high amplitude.
B. Less common after a period of sleep deprivation.
C. Associated with a high level of general muscle tone.
D. Ineffective in relieving fatigue.
E. A more frequent component of sleep in the elderly than in the young.

607. From childhood to old age
A. There is a steady decrease in total sleeping time per day.
B. Deep (stage 4) sleep increases as a percentage of total daily sleep.
C. Brain mass steadily decreases.
D. Body water decreases as a percentage of body mass.
E. Sleep becomes less aggregated into a single sleeping period.

608. Immersion of an upright adult to chest level in water increases the
A. Water pressure on the feet to nearer 100 than 20 mmHg.
B. Thoracic blood volume.
C. Total peripheral resistance.
D. Sodium excretion in the urine.
E. Transmural pressure in the blood vessels of the feet.

609. In the days following a major surgical operation there is
A. An increase in plasma cortisol level.
B. A negative nitrogen balance.
C. Potassium retention.
D. A negative sodium balance.
E. A decreased tendency for the blood to clot.

610. The graph of body mass (ordinate) versus age
A. Normally steepens from birth to five years.
B. Normally steepens during secondary sexual development.
C. Steepens earlier than usual with precocious puberty.
D. Is parallel for males and females.
E. Deviates towards the normal curve with successful treatment of a child with dwarfism.

Answers

604.

A.	True	Usually close to the nucleus.
B.	False	It is a collection of about six flattened, membrane-enclosed sacs stacked together.
C.	True	Secretions are packaged into vesicles in the Golgi apparatus.
D.	True	Proteins formed by the granular endoplasmic reticulum fuse with the membranes of the Golgi sacs before being packed into vesicles and released into the cytoplasm.
E.	False	Neurones are secretory cells.

605.

A.	True	Or a mixture of a weak base with its conjugate acid.
B.	False	It can be a mixture of carbonic acid and bicarbonate ions.
C.	False	It minimizes, but does not prevent, pH change.
D.	True	$pH = pK + \log$ [base]/[acid]; $\log 1 = 0$.
E.	False	pK should be near blood pH, which is 7 4.

606.

A.	False	The waves are of high frequency and low amplitude.
B.	False	REM sleep increases proportionately after sleep deprivation.
C.	False	General muscle tone is reduced.
D.	False	Fatigue is poorly relieved if REM sleep is prevented.
E.	False	It occurs less frequently in the elderly.

607.

A.	True	The elderly seem to need less sleep.
B.	False	This percentage also falls steadily.
C.	False	It increases markedly in early childhood.
D.	True	From over 80 per cent in the fetus to less than 50 per cent in old age.
E.	True	Though aggregation increases in infancy, it later declines steadily.

608.

A.	True	100 mmHg is equivalent to 1.36 metres of H_2O.
B.	True	Due to pressure on capacity vessels in the lower body.
C.	False	Increased central blood volume reflexly lowers resistance.
D.	True	Increased central blood volume causes diuresis, perhaps via atrial natriuretic hormone.
E.	False	It decreases transmural pressure and so protects the vessels against distension due to gravitational forces.

609.

A.	True	This is essential for normal recovery.
B.	True	Cortisol breaks down protein to form glucose.
C.	False	Potassium excretion increases.
D.	False	There is a positive sodium balance.
E.	False	The clotting tendency increases for about ten days.

610.

A.	False	It becomes less steep over this period.
B.	True	This is the adolescent growth spurt.
C.	True	Sex hormones produce an early adolescent growth spurt.
D.	False	Females show an earlier adolescent growth spurt.
E.	True	The faster than normal growth rate is an important sign of appropriate treatment.

MCQ

Questions 611–616

611. Obesity can be treated successfully by
A. Diuretic drugs.
B. Supplementing the normal diet with slimming foods.
C. Confining the diet to foods of low calorific value.
D. Increasing exercise without increasing food intake.
E. Reducing food intake relative to energy expenditure.

612. An injection of atropine typically produces a decrease in
A. Resting heart rate.
B. Skeletal muscle strength.
C. Salivary flow.
D. Mucus secretion in the airways.
E. Impulse transmission at autonomic ganglia.

613. In percentage terms, arterial P_{CO_2} is more affected than arterial O_2 content by
A. Carbon monoxide poisoning.
B. Anaemia.
C. A 20 per cent fall in inspired P_{O_2}.
D. Ascent to 2000 metres (about 6500 feet) above sea level.
E. Increasing the oxygen pressure in the air breathed to three atmospheres.

614. Polycythaemia is caused by
A. Lung disease which causes a fall in oxygen saturation in arterial blood.
B. Heart disease which causes a right to left shunt.
C. Chronic renal failure.
D. Pregnancy.
E. High doses of vitamin B_{12}.

615. When kept afloat by a life jacket, survival time in water at 15°C is
A. Usually 12–24 hours.
B. Limited by muscular fatigue.
C. Extended if many layers of clothing are worn.
D. Extended by swimming gently rather than floating motionless.
E. More prolonged in fat than in thin persons.

616. An organ transplant is less likely to be rejected if the recipient
A. Is given glucocorticoid treatment.
B. Has previously received a skin graft from the same individual.
C. Is an infant.
D. Is an identical rather than a non-identical twin of the donor.
E. Has the same blood group as the donor.

Answers

611.
A. **False** This reduces body water but not body fat.
B. **False** This makes the person fatter.
C. **False** This is ineffective unless the total energy intake is reduced.
D. **True** Energy expenditure increases; energy intake is unchanged.
E. **True** This is the only effective long-term treatment.

612.
A. **False** It increases due to blocking of acetylcholine's action at the sinus node.
B. **False** Atropine does not block acetylcholine's action on skeletal muscle.
C. **True** Salivation is stimulated by cholinergic autonomic nerves.
D. **True** This may be useful during surgical operations.
E. **False** This cholinergic transmission is resistant to atropine.

613.
A. **False** Pressure is little affected but content is decreased.
B. **False** Pressure is normal but content decreased.
C. **True** Arterial P_{O_2} is reduced but content falls by only 3 per cent or so because of the shape of the oxygen dissociation curve.
D. **True** This causes a fall of about 20 per cent in inspired oxygen pressure.
E. **True** This causes a huge rise in P_{O_2} but a relatively small increase in arterial oxygen content since the haemoglobin is almost fully saturated when breathing oxygen at 100 mmHg pressure.

614.
A. **True** A fall in the O_2 content of arterial blood stimulates production of erythropoietin.
B. **True** This also reduces the oxygen content of arterial blood.
C. **False** Anaemia is common in chronic renal failure due to damage to the erythropoietin-producing cells.
D. **False** The increase in plasma volume causes a fall in red cell count.
E. **False** This prevents megaloblastic anaemia but does not raise red cell concentration above normal.

615.
A. **False** It is usually under two hours.
B. **False** It is limited by hypothermia.
C. **True** This improves insulation by trapping layers of water around the body to form a stable microclimate.
D. **False** Swimming increases heat loss by disturbing the microclimate.
E. **True** Due to better thermal insulation by the superficial fat.

616.
A. **True** This suppresses immune reactions.
B. **False** This would sensitize the immune response.
C. **True** The immune system is less well-developed in infants.
D. **True** Only identical twins have identical genes and hence identical tissue antigens.
E. **True** However, blood group compatibility is not a reliable index of tissue compatibility.

Questions 617–622

617. Obesity
A. Is associated with reduced life expectancy.
B. Is one cause of diabetes mellitus.
C. In parents is associated with obesity in their children.
D. Is usually due to an endocrine disorder.
E. May be treated by surgical removal, or bypass, of part of the small intestine.

618. Sudden exposure to an atmospheric pressure of 100 mmHg (13 kPa), as might occur with loss of aircraft cabin pressure at around 15 000 m altitude, causes
A. Rupture of the eardrums by outward bulging.
B. The appearance of gas bubbles in joints and lungs.
C. No serious fall in the alveolar oxygen pressure if the person is breathing pure oxygen.
D. Expansion of gas in closed spaces in the body.
E. Gradual loss of consciousness in 10–15 minutes due to hypoxia.

619. Restoration of the blood volume after haemorrhage is aided by
A. Contraction of venous reservoirs.
B. A fall in capillary pressure in certain vascular beds.
C. Arteriolar vasoconstriction.
D. Mobilization of intracellular fluid into the circulation.
E. An increase in the osmotic pressure of the plasma proteins.

620. A transplanted kidney is
A. Able to maintain the recipient's blood urea at normal levels.
B. Able to correct the anaemia of chronic renal failure.
C. Probably being rejected if the glomerular filtration rate is falling rapidly.
D. Probably being rejected if there is a sharp rise in body temperature in the absence of infection.
E. Probably being rejected if the urinary volume is low and the osmolality high.

621. Helium is used to replace nitrogen in gas breathed by divers because it
A. Is more soluble in body fluids.
B. Diffuses through the tissues more rapidly.
C. Causes less depression of cerebral function.
D. Diminishes the work of breathing relative to nitrogen.
E. Combines less readily with haemoglobin.

622. Someone who has received an electric shock causing ventricular fibrillation
A. Loses consciousness in less than a minute.
B. Has a reduction in cardiac output of about 50 per cent.
C. Has a rapid but weak carotid pulse.
D. Should be given external cardiac massage after removal from the electrical contact.
E. Should not be given artificial ventilation until the ventricular fibrillation has been reversed.

Answers

617.
A.   True   Being 20 per cent overweight reduces life expectancy by about 20 per cent.
B.   True   The diabetes may then be cured by weight reduction.
C.   True   Both genetic and environmental factors may operate.
D.   False   This is a very rare cause.
E.   True   This leads to malabsorption, but the resulting malnutrition may have side effects.

618.
A.   True   Ambient pressure drops much faster than middle ear pressure.
B.   True   This is a manifestation of decompression sickness.
C.   False   More than half of the total alveolar pressure will be taken up by carbon dioxide and water vapour.
D.   True   This must happen from Boyle's law.
E.   False   Sudden severe hypoxia of this order causes unconsciousness in less than a minute.

619.
A.   False   This redistributes but does not increase blood volume.
B.   True   This favours absorption of tissue fluid into the circulation.
C.   True   This leads to the fall in downstream capillary pressure.
D.   False   Haemorrhage does not increase the osmolality of extracellular fluid.
E.   False   Colloid osmotic pressure falls as tissue fluid is drawn into the circulation.

620.
A.   True   One normal kidney can do this.
B.   True   By replacing the deficient erythropoietin.
C.   True   This suggests nephron damage.
D.   True   This, like a raised ESR and granulocyte count, suggests tissue destruction.
E.   False   A high urinary osmolality suggests excellent renal function.

621.
A.   False   Being less soluble, less goes into solution during compression so there is less bubble formation during decompression.
B.   True   This also reduces the time needed for decompression.
C.   True   It is less narcotic than nitrogen.
D.   True   It is less viscous than nitrogen.
E.   False   Neither combine with haemoglobin.

622.
A.   True   Due to the abrupt fall in cerebral blood flow.
B.   False   Cardiac output is nil.
C.   False   There is no cardiac output; hence no pulse.
D.   True   This will prevent brain damage until the fibrillation has been reversed.
E.   False   Artificial ventilation must accompany cardiac massage to avoid brain damage.

Questions 623–629

623. A patient with fever
A. Has warm extremities as central temperature rises.
B. Has a raised basal metabolic rate.
C. Shows evidence of altered hypothalamic function.
D. Loses the capacity for reflex thermoregulation.
E. May develop heat stroke if the core temperature rises to 40°C.

624. Acidosis in a patient may lead to
A. Increased urinary excretion of potassium.
B. Hypoventilation.
C. A blood pH of less than 5.5.
D. A urinary pH of less than 5.5.
E. Tetany

625. When a patient inherits a disease as a recessive autosomal character
A. One of the parents of the patient will exhibit the disease.
B. All of the children of the patient will exhibit the disease.
C. All of the children of the patient will be carriers.
D. Both parents of the patient must carry the recessive character.
E. Subsequent siblings have a 50 per cent risk of the disorder.

626. If treatment A is superior to treatment B in certain respects (with a P value less than 0.01) it can be concluded that
A. A given patient's chances of improvement by treatment A are 99 per cent.
B. The likelihood that the observed difference between treatments A and B is due to chance is less than 1 per cent.
C. The observed superiority is statistically significant.
D. At least 100 patients were studied.
E. Treatment A should now be substituted for treatment B.

627. A low serum potassium level
A. Can be suspected from the appearance of the ECG.
B. Can result from repeated vomiting of gastric contents.
C. Indicates that total body potassium is low.
D. May be a consequence of aldosterone deficiency.
E. Impairs gut motility.

628. A rise in the osmolality of extracellular fluid may lead to
A. Thirst.
B. Increased water reabsorption in the proximal convoluted tubules.
C. Release of vasopressin.
D. A fall in intracellular fluid volume.
E. Suppression of sweat secretion.

629. Maximal exercise leads to an increase in
A. Systolic blood pressure.
B. Total peripheral resistance.
C. Blood lactic acid.
D. Tissue fluid formation in active muscles.
E. Urinary output.

Answers

623.

A. False   Reflex vasoconstriction causes cold hands at this stage.
B. True   The raised body temperature speeds metabolism.
C. True   The 'set point' for temperature regulation is raised.
D. False   Core temperature is maintained around the raised level.
E. False   The core temperature needs to rise to about 43°C before heat stroke develops.

624.

A. False   Hydrogen ions compete with potassium for secretion.
B. False   Ventilation is increased in acidosis.
C. False   This level would be fatal.
D. True   Urinary pH may fall below 5.0.
E. False   Acidosis reduces the risk of tetany by decreasing protein affinity for calcium.

625.

A. False   Both parents are usually healthy.
B. False   They are likely to be normal due to the dominant normal gene from the spouse.
C. True   All will receive the recessive gene from the patient.
D. True   Only thus will the patient have a homozygous genotype.
E. False   From simple Mendelian laws the chances are 25 per cent.

626.

A. False   This cannot be concluded from the results given.
B. True   This is the meaning of P less than 0.01.
C. True   Conventionally P must then be less than 0.05.
D. False   This cannot be concluded from the results given.
E. False   Adverse effects may outweigh the benefit shown.

627.

A. True   It leads to low voltage T waves.
B. True   The vomitus is relatively rich in potassium.
C. False   It is a poor reflector of total body potassium.
D. False   This favours retention of potassium and a high serum level.
E. True   It may cause paralytic ileus (paralysis of peristalsis).

628.

A. True   Due to stimulation of hypothalamic osmoreceptors.
B. False   Water reabsorption in proximal tubules is not geared to meet body water needs.
C. True   Impulses from hypothalamic osmoreceptors cause release of pituitary vasopressin.
D. True   The cells shrink as fluid is drawn out osmotically.
E. False   Sweat production is not geared to body fluid requirements.

629.

A. True   Due mainly to the increase in the force of ventricular ejection.
B. False   This falls markedly due to vasodilatation in muscle, heart and skin.
C. True   Since the muscles may have to work in anaerobic conditions.
D. True   This results from the rise in hydrostatic pressure in muscle capillaries.
E. False   This decreases, probably due to reflex vasoconstriction in the kidneys and increased release of vasopressin.

Questions 630–636

630. Following adaptation to a hot climate there is an increase in

A. Basal metabolic rate.
B. Resting cardiac output.
C. Urinary output.
D. The ability to lose heat by sweating.
E. Exercise tolerance.

631. Sudden complete obstruction of the respiratory tract causes

A. A fall in blood pressure.
B. Stimulation of central chemoreceptors.
C. Cyanosis.
D. Reflex apnoea.
E. Dilatation of the pupils.

632. Inherited diseases associated with sex-linked recessive genetic disorders

A. Involve the Y rather than the X chromosome.
B. Are more common in females than in males.
C. Are transmitted by the female but not by the male.
D. May fail to manifest themselves in female carriers.
E. Include haemophilia.

633. Infants differ from adults in that their

A. Nitrogen balance is normally positive.
B. Extracellular fluid volume is a larger proportion of total body water.
C. Blood contains reticulocytes.
D. Total peripheral resistance is lower.
E. Brown fat stores are relatively small.

634. Excessive sweating (hyperhidrosis) in a limb is likely to be relieved by

A. Blockade of autonomic ganglia with ganglion-blocking drugs.
B. Blockade of autonomic cholinergic nerve endings with atropine.
C. Blockade of somatic cholinergic nerve endings with curare.
D. Blockade of adrenergic nerve endings with phentolamine.
E. Section of the sympathetic motor nerves supplying the limb.

635. A disease inherited as a dominant autosomal character

A. Affects males and females equally.
B. Affects all the children of the affected adult.
C. Usually prevents reproduction.
D. Requires that both parents carry the abnormality.
E. May be transmitted by a carrier who does not manifest the disease.

636. The effects of moving from sea level to an altitude of 5000 metres include an increase in

A. Alveolar ventilation.
B. Blood bicarbonate level.
C. Appetite for food.
D. Exercise tolerance.
E. Simulation of the bone marrow.

Answers

630.

A. False BMR falls due to a decrease in resting thyroid activity.
B. True   Partly due to increased thermoregulatory blood flow.
C. False Urinary output is usually reduced due to increased water loss by extrarenal routes.
D. True   Daily secretion of sweat may rise to several litres.
E. True   Due mainly to the improved ability to dissipate heat.

631.

A. False Blood pressure rises due to reflex stimulation of the heart and peripheral vaso-constriction.
B. True   Accumulation of CO_2 is mainly responsible for the reflex cardiovascular and respiratory responses.
C. True   Deoxygenated haemoglobin appears in the arterial blood.
D. False Respiratory effort increases with chemoreceptor stimulation.
E. True   Part of the generalized sympathetic response to stress.

632.

A. False The abnormality is on the X chromosome.
B. False Females are protected by the normal X chromosome.
C. False Both can transmit a defective X chromosome.
D. True   Due to protection by a normal X chromosome.
E. True   Colour blindness is another example.

633.

A. True   Adults are normally in nitrogen balance.
B. True   It exceeds intracellular fluid volume.
C. False Both infants and adults have reticulocytes in the blood.
D. False It is higher; the pressure gradient to cardiac output ratio is much greater.
E. False They are relatively much larger.

634.

A. True   But the side effects are likely to be worse than the disease.
B. True   Again side effects may be troublesome.
C. False This paralyses skeletal muscles without inhibiting sweating.
D. False The nerves responsible for sweating are cholinergic.
E. True   This is an effective therapy.

635.

A. True   The autosomes are similar for males and females.
B. False Half would receive the normal autosome.
C. False Such genes are commonly transmitted.
D. False If so, it would not be a dominant disorder.
E. False Carriers of a dominant character exhibit the disease.

636.

A. True   Due to stimulation of peripheral chemoreceptors by hypoxia.
B. False Bicarbonate is lost in the urine to compensate for the respiratory alkalosis.
C. False Loss of appetite (anorexia) is a common complaint in mountain climbers.
D. False Exercise tolerance is reduced by the decreased ability to deliver O_2 to the blood.
E. True   Due to an increased erythropoietin level.

Questions 637–639

637. The ratio of intravascular hydrostatic pressure to colloid osmotic pressure is greater

A. In splanchnic than in renal glomerular capillaries.
B. Than normal in patients with hepatic failure.
C. Than normal in the systemic capillaries of patients following severe blood loss.
D. Than normal in capillaries where there is oedema due to venous obstruction.
E. In systemic than in pulmonary capillaries.

638. Sudden application of cold water to the

A. Hand causes local vasoconstriction.
B. Hand causes vasodilation in the opposite hand.
C. Oesophagus can cause changes in the electrocardiogram.
D. External auditory meatus causes nausea and nystagmus.
E. Whole body by immersion causes apnoea.

639. Normal healthy young adults can tolerate loss of half of their

A. Renal tissue without developing renal failure.
B. Pulmonary tissue without developing respiratory failure.
C. Circulating platelets without developing a haemorrhagic tendency.
D. Seminal sperm count without suffering from infertility.
E. Liver without developing hepatic failure.

Answers

637.

A. False   It is higher in glomerular capillaries, as is necessary for filtration.
B. True   Colloid osmotic pressure falls because the liver fails to synthesize enough albumin.
C. False   The reverse is true, causing transfer of tissue fluid into the circulation.
D. True   Hence excess fluid is forced out of the capillaries into the interstitial spaces.
E. True   The lower ratio in the lungs normally prevents fluid leak into the alveoli.

638.

A. True   Due to the direct effect of cold on vascular smooth muscle.
B. False   Immersion of a hand in cold water provokes general vasoconstriction and a rise in blood pressure – the cold pressor response.
C. True   By cooling the myocardium.
D. True   By inducing currents in endolymph which stimulate vestibular receptors.
E. False   By stimulating uncontrollable gasping under water, it may result in drowning.

639.

A. True   Normal function can be maintained with one kidney.
B. True   Though maximum exercise tolerance is reduced, considerable exertion is possible.
C. True   The platelet count must fall by more than 75 per cent before bleeding problems arise.
D. True   Infertility is unlikely unless the count falls to around a quarter of the normal value.
E. True   In short, most body functions carry at least a 50 per cent reserve in the young adult.

EMQs

Questions 640–649

EMQ Question 640

For each of the intracellular organelles A–E, select the best option from the following list of descriptions.
1. Sites of protein synthesis rich in RNA.
2. Intracellular membrane-bound structures containing enzymes that can destroy most cellular structures.
3. Granules in a layer produced by high-speed centrifugation of cells.
4. Structures lying close to the nucleus responsible for organizing the microtubular systems.
5. Membrane-bound organelles associated with numerous enzymes that catalyse a variety of anabolic and catabolic reactions.

A. Lysosomes.
B. Centrosomes.
C. Peroxisomes.
D. Microsomes.
E. Ribosomes.

EMQ Question 641

For each of the varieties of acid–base disturbance A–E, select the best option for a possible cause from the following list.

1. Sudden laryngeal obstruction.   2. Severe chronic respiratory disease.
3. Chronic renal failure.   4. Mountain climbing.
5. Severe diarrhoea.

A. Uncompensated respiratory acidosis.
B. Uncompensated metabolic acidosis.
C. Compensated respiratory acidosis.
D. Uncompensated respiratory alkalosis.
E. Compensated metabolic acidosis.

Answers for 640

A. Option 2   *Intracellular membrane-bound structures containing enzymes that can destroy most cellular structures.* The postmortem breakdown of the lysosomal membranes releases lysosomal enzymes that autolyse (cause self-destruction of) the cell.

B. Option 4   *Structures lying close to the nucleus responsible for organizing the microtubular systems.* Centrosomes are made up of two centrioles. At mitotic division the centrosomes are duplicated and one goes to each end of the mitotic spindle. The microtubules they control allow movement within the cell.

C. Option 5   *Membrane-bound organelles associated with numerous enzymes that catalyse a variety of anabolic and catabolic reactions.* They are involved in the oxidation of some long chain fatty acids. Drugs that can modify peroxisome behaviour are being used in the attempt to lower lipid levels in the blood.

D. Option 3   *Granules in a layer produced by high-speed centrifugation of cells.* This is the generic name for the cellular organelles brought down by high-speed centrifugation.

E. Option 1   *Sites of protein synthesis rich in RNA.* Ribosomes can be attached to the endoplasmic reticulum where they synthesize proteins such as hormones.

Answers for 641

A. **Option 1**   *Sudden laryngeal obstruction.* The obstruction leads to a rapid rise in P_{CO_2} before the kidneys can compensate by generating bicarbonate thus raising the blood bicarbonate level.

B. **Option 5**   *Severe diarrhoea.* Severe diarrhoea results in loss of bicarbonate in the stools and thus to a fall in the blood bicarbonate level.

C. **Option 2**   *Severe chronic respiratory disease.* The raised P_{CO_2} in chronic respiratory disease may be compensated for by renal generation of bicarbonate to raise the blood bicarbonate level.

D. **Option 4**   *Mountain climbing.* The respiratory drive caused by the action of low Po_2 on arterial chemoreceptors washes out CO_2. This lowers the P_{CO_2} to cause an alkalosis. Eventually the kidneys compensate by eliminating more bicarbonate.

E. **Option 3**   *Chronic renal failure.* The fall in blood bicarbonate used in buffering the acid residues of protein digestion in chronic renal failure is compensated for by an increased respiratory drive that results in a fall in P_{CO_2}.

EMQ Question 642

For each of the electrical potentials A–E, select the best option for a possible description from the following list.

1. The graded, non-propagated potential changes across cell membranes induced by neurotransmitter substances.
2. The voltage gradient between the inside and the outside of a cell.
3. The unstable membrane potentials seen in smooth and cardiac muscle.
4. All or non-propagated potentials in excitable tissues.
5. The graded, non-propagated potential changes seen in sensory end organs.

A. Action potentials.
B. Membrane potentials.
C. Generator potentials.
D. Pacemaker potentials.
E. Post-synaptic potentials.

EMQ Question 643

For each of the substances associated with synaptic transmission A–E, select the best option for its possible function from the following list.

1. A neurotransmitter in the brain involved in determining mood.
2. Involved in the genesis of inhibitory post-synaptic potentials (IPSPs).
3. Involved in the breakdown of catecholamines.
4. A neurotransmitter in the brain involved in basal ganglia activity.
5. Involved in the breakdown of acetylcholine.

A. Mono amine oxidase (MAO).
B. Cholinesterase.
C. Gamma amino butyric acid (GABA).
D. Dopamine.
E. Serotonin.

Answers for 642

A. **Option 4** *All or none-propagated potentials in excitable tissues.* Action potentials travel as a wave of reversed polarity caused by an initial increase in membrane permeability to sodium followed by a slower increase in membrane permeability to potassium.

B. **Option 2** *The voltage gradient between the inside and the outside of a cell.* This potential is maintained actively by metabolic processes and disappears if these processes are poisoned. Resting membrane potentials range from about 60 to about 90 millivolts, negative inside with respect to outside.

C. **Option 5** *The graded, non-propagated potential changes seen in sensory end organs.* When a stimulus is applied to a sensory end organ it causes a non-propagated depolarization whose size is related to the strength of the stimulus. When the generator potential reaches the threshold for firing, it gives rise to an action potential that travels along the axon away from the end organ.

D. **Option 3** *The unstable membrane potentials seen in smooth and cardiac muscle.* The membranes of pacemaker cells show an unstable membrane potential that falls spontaneously until it reaches the threshold for firing when it gives rise to one or more propagated action potentials.

E. **Option 1** *The graded, non-propagated potential changes across cell membranes induced by neurotransmitter substances.* When an impulse reaches the terminal processes of a pre-synaptic nerve, it causes neurotransmitter to be released that induces post-synaptic potentials in the post-synaptic neurone. When the potential reaches the threshold for firing in the post-synaptic nerve an action potential is induced that travels over the entire membrane of the post-synaptic cell.

Answers for 643

A. **Option 3** *Involved in the breakdown of catecholamines.* Catecholamines are inactivated by oxidation by the enzyme MAO that is found in some neurones.

B. **Option 5** *Involved in the breakdown of acetylcholine.* Cholinesterase is found in high concentration near motor nerve endings in muscle and rapidly hydrolyses acetylcholine following its release from the nerve endings.

C. **Option 2** *Involved in the genesis of inhibitory post-synaptic potentials (IPSPs).* GABA is released from pre-synaptic nerve endings and causes hyperpolarization of the post-synaptic membrane so causing an IPSP.

D. **Option 4** *A neurotransmitter in the brain involved in basal ganglia activity.* Degeneration of dopaminergic neurones in the substantia nigra is associated with Parkinson's disease.

E. **Option 1** *A neurotransmitter in the brain involved in determining mood.* Serotonin containing nerves have been found in the brain stem. Selective serotonin uptake inhibitor drugs are used in the treatment of depression.

EMQ Question 644

For each of the items related to body energy A–E, select the best option for its description from the following list.

1. The increase in energy expenditure following ingestion of food.
2. A thioester high-energy compound.
3. A method to estimate the metabolic rate.
4. A phosphorolated high-energy compound.
5. The rate of metabolism in a resting subject.

A. Measurement of oxygen consumption.
B. Specific dynamic action (SDA).
C. ATP.
D. BMR.
E. Acetyl-coenzyme A.

EMQ Question 645

For each variety of reflex A–E, select the best option from the examples in the following list.

1. Nerve-mediated skin vasodilatation following skin damage.
2. The withdrawal reflex.
3. Salivation on seeing or thinking about food.
4. The knee jerk.
5. The baroreceptor reflex.

A. A monosynaptic reflex.
B. A polysynaptic somatic reflex.
C. A conditioned reflex.
D. A visceral unconditioned reflex.
E. An axon reflex.

EMQ Question 646

For each variety of sensory receptor A–E, select the best option for its adequate stimulus from the following list.

1. Pain.
2. Angular acceleration of the head.
3. Stretch.
4. Sound waves in the inner ear.
5. Sweet substances in solution.

A. Muscle spindles.
B. Bare nerve endings.
C. Crista ampullaris receptors.
D. Outer hair cells receptors.
E. Fungiform papillae receptors.

Answers for 644

A. **Option 3** *A method to estimate the metabolic rate.* The rate of metabolism can be estimated from the oxygen consumption if the respiratory quotient is known.

B. **Option 1** *The increase in energy expenditure following ingestion of food.* The extra energy expenditure required to assimilate ingested food into the body is referred to as its SDA. It is required for all types of food but protein requires the most energy for its assimilation.

C. **Option 4** *A phosphorolated high-energy compound.* Adenosine triphosphate (ATP) is widely distributed in the body and much energy is stored in its phosphate bonds. This energy can be released when required to energy-requiring processes such as muscle contraction and membrane polarization.

D. **Option 5** *The rate of metabolism in a resting subject.* The basal metabolic rate is a measure of total energy expenditure at rest in the post-absorptive state. It can be measured by measuring oxygen consumption.

E. **Option 2** *A thioester high-energy compound.* This sulphur containing high-energy compound is derived from mercaptan. It combines with substances in reactions that would otherwise require outside energy.

Answers for 645

A. **Option 4** *The knee jerk.* This is a spinal reflex with two neurones. The afferent nerve from the muscle spindle synapses with a motor fibre in the anterior horn of the spinal cord.

B. **Option 2** *The withdrawal reflex.* This reflex has more than two synapses in the reflex pathway.

C. **Option 3** *Salivation on seeing or thinking about food.* This is a learned reflex that can be reinforced or inhibited by learned experience and involves the cerebral cortex.

D. **Option 5** *The baroreceptor reflex.* This reflex is inborn and is not modified by learned experiences.

E. **Option 1** *Nerve-mediated skin vasodilatation following skin damage.* An axon reflex is a local reflex that does not involve the spinal cord. Stimulation of a sensory nerve receptor results in a local response mediated by a local branch of the sensory nerve.

Answers for 646

A. **Option 3** *Stretch.* Stretching of the muscle spindles leads to reflex contraction of the muscle being stretched as in the knee jerk.

B. **Option 1** *Pain.* These nerve endings are stimulated by stimuli that tend to damage the tissues in which the bare nerve endings lie.

C. **Option 2** *Angular acceleration of the head.* The sensory end organs in the crista ampullaris are stimulated when movement of fluid in the semicircular canals moves the hair cells in the cupulae.

D. **Option 4** *Sound waves in the inner ear.* These sensory organs lie in the organ of Corti and are stimulated when sound waves cause vibrations in the basilar membrane in the inner ear.

E. **Option 5** *Sweet substances in solution.* These taste receptors are found towards the front of the tongue and can detect sweet taste stimuli.

EMQ Question 647

For each clinical disturbance A–E, select the best option for its possible cause from the following list.

1. Renal failure.
2. Respiratory failure.
3. Heart failure.
4. Peripheral circulatory failure.
5. Liver failure.

A. Lowered central venous pressure.
B. A raised plasma bicarbonate level.
C. Metabolic acidosis and anaemia.
D. Raised central venous pressure.
E. A lowered blood urea.

EMQ Question 648

For each region of the brain A–E, select the best option for one of its possible functions from the following list.

1. Fear and rage reactions.
2. Vision.
3. Alerting reactions.
4. Temperature regulation.
5. Postural reflexes.

A. The reticular formation.
B. The substantia nigra.
C. The hypothalamus.
D. The limbic system.
E. The occipital cortex.

EMQ Question 649

For each variety of inhibition in the nervous system A–E, select the best option for its description from the following list.

1. Inhibition produced by the action of neurotransmitters on the terminal processes of afferent nerves.
2. Inhibition produced by release of transmitters that affect the membrane potential of efferent neurones.
3. A form of inhibition in which activation of one neural group causes inhibition of neurones surrounding the activated group.
4. Inhibition of a conditioned reflex by the application of a new stimulus just before the application of the conditioned stimulus.
5. A state where neurones in the brain and spinal cord are less excitable than normal.

A. Afferent inhibition.
B. Central inhibition.
C. Post-synaptic inhibition.
D. Pre-synaptic inhibition.
E. External inhibition.

Answers for 647

A. **Option 4**   *Peripheral circulatory failure.* In circulatory failure such as may occur in severe shock or haemorrhage, the fall in venous return to the heart lowers central venous pressure.

B. **Option 2**   *Respiratory failure.* The retention of CO_2 in respiratory failure leads to an acidosis that is compensated for by generation of bicarbonate by the kidney.

C. **Option 1**   *Renal failure.* In renal failure, failure to excrete acid residues of metabolism causes acidosis. Anaemia is often seen since erythropoietin is normally manufactured by the kidneys.

D. **Option 3**   *Heart failure.* In heart failure where the heart cannot pump forward all the blood being delivered to it, there is a rise in central venous pressure that increases the diastolic filling of the heart.

E. **Option 5**   *Liver failure.* The liver is responsible for the deamination of amino acids and the conversion of the NH_4 residues into urea.

Answers for 648

A. **Option 3**   *Alerting reactions.* Stimulation of the ascending reticular formation leads to increased electrical activity in the cortex and results in a state of alertness.

B. **Option 5**   *Postural reflexes.* Diseases affecting this part of the brain such as Parkinson's disease result in abnormal distribution of muscle tone. Substantia nigra neurones are dopaminergic.

C. **Option 4**   *Temperature regulation.* Temperature regulating centres are found in the hypothalamus.

D. **Option 1**   *Fear and rage reactions.* The limbic region is associated with the emotions.

E. **Option 2**   *Vision.* Visual impulses are conveyed to the occipital cortex in the optic tracts where they give rise to conscious visual images.

Answers for 649

A. **Option 3**   *A form of inhibition in which activation of one neural group causes inhibition of neurones surrounding the activated group.* This is seen in the neurones of the occipital cortex where central excitation reduces activity in surrounding neurones.

B. **Option 5**   *A state where neurones in the brain and spinal cord are less excitable than normal.* A general state of inhibition of excitability of the neurones in the CNS can be induced by general anaesthetic and other drugs that depress the central nervous system.

C. **Option 2**   *Inhibition produced by release of transmitters that affect the membrane potential of efferent neurones.* Here the inhibition of the post-synaptic membrane is caused by the action of pre-synaptic nerve terminals directly on the membrane of the post-synaptic cell body.

D. **Option 1**   *Inhibition produced by the action of neurotransmitters on the terminal processes of afferent nerves.* In this case nerve endings of afferent neurones release neurotransmitters close to the nerve endings of other neurones to modulate release of neurotransmitter from them.

E. **Option 4**   *Inhibition of a conditioned reflex by an application of a new stimulus just before the application of the conditioned stimulus.* Conditioned reflexes can be reinforced or inhibited by external stimuli given at about the same time as the conditioned stimulus.

MCQs

Questions 650–655

650. In athletes, physical fitness is more closely correlated with
A. Maximal oxygen uptake than with resting oxygen uptake.
B. Maximal pulse rate than with resting pulse rate.
C. Maximal minute ventilation than with maximal cardiac output.
D. Blood oxygen saturation than with blood lactate level during strenuous exercise.
E. Resting vagal tone than with resting sympathetic tone to the heart.

651. The muscle fibres adapted to endurance running
A. Are classified as slow rather than fast.
B. Have a relatively high myoglobin content.
C. Are red rather than white.
D. Have a relatively high mitochondria content.
E. Are classified as anaerobic rather than aerobic.

652. The oxygen consumed per minute
A. Is greater than the carbon dioxide produced per minute during long distance running.
B. In the resting adult is nearer 100 than 150 ml.
C. During intense mental activity can rise to twice the resting level.
D. During brisk walking is nearer five times than twice the resting level.
E. In an Olympic athlete can rise to 50 litres.

653. The increase in blood flow to muscle in an exercising limb is related to a rise in
A. Local P_{CO_2}.
B. Local H^+ concentration.
C. Local muscle temperature.
D. Arterial pressure.
E. Vasodilator nerve activity.

654. During muscular training
A. Neural control factors improve performance before there is evidence of skeletal muscle hypertrophy.
B. Repeated stretching of skeletal muscle fibres leads to their hypertrophy.
C. There is a gradual decrease in the size of the heart in diastole.
D. There is a gradual increase in the O_2 extraction rate from blood perfusing exercising skeletal muscle.
E. The increase in skeletal muscle blood flow for a given work load decreases.

655. Blood lactic acid is
A. Normally undetectable in resting subjects.
B. A product of anaerobic metabolism.
C. Increased by a 100-metre dash.
D. Not increased during steady state running in a marathon race.
E. Raised to about 5–10 moles/litre during maximal exercise.

Answers

650.
A.   True   Maximal oxygen uptake is the 'gold standard' of fitness.
B.   False   Maximal pulse rate is related to age; a slow pulse indicates fitness.
C.   False   Cardiac output is the usual limiting factor in exercise.
D.   False   Saturation changes little during exercise; a relatively low lactate level during strenuous exercise is an indication of fitness.
E.   True   A high resting vagal tone is the cause of the low resting heart rate.

651.
A.   True   The time course of their twitch is relatively long.
B.   True   This provides an intracellular store of oxygen.
C.   True   This is due to their myoglobin content.
D.   True   They generate energy by oxidative phosphorylation.
E.   False   Their high rate of oxygen consumption classifies them as aerobic.

652.
A.   True   The respiratory quotient is less than 1.0 during long distance running.
B.   False   It is around 250–300 ml.
C.   False   Brain oxygen consumption increases in relatively small active areas, but the total changes little.
D.   True   This is a useful way of maintaining fitness, particularly in older people.
E.   False   The maximum recorded is less than ten litres.

653.
A.   True   This causes local vasodilation.
B.   True   Acidosis also favours vasodilation.
C.   True   Heat dilates blood vessels.
D.   False   Exercising a limb causes little change in mean arterial pressure.
E.   False   Vasomotor nerves are not involved in exercise hyperaemia.

654.
A.   True   Neural factors account for most of the early improvement in performance.
B.   True   This is a potent factor causing hypertrophy.
C.   False   There is an increase due to increased diastolic filling with the lower resting heart rate.
D.   True   This results in a lower blood lactate level for a given workload.
E.   True   A consequence of the greater oxygen extraction rate.

655.
A.   False   The resting level is around one millimole per litre.
B.   True   It is a marker for anaerobic metabolism.
C.   True   Almost all the energy used in the 100-metre dash comes from anaerobic metabolism.
D.   False   Even though the lactic acid level is steady, it is still raised during steady state exercise.
E.   False   It rises to 5–10 millimoles per litre.

Questions 656–661

656. Isotonic (dynamic) exercise differs from isometric (static) exercise in that there is less

A. Increase in systolic arterial pressure.
B. Increase in diastolic arterial pressure.
C. Assistance to the circulation by the muscle pump.
D. Use of slow-twitch muscle fibres.
E. Reliance on anaerobic glycolysis.

657. Electrocardiological danger signs during incremental treadmill exercise include

A. A heart rate equal to the maximal predicted for the person's age.
B. An R–R interval of about 500 milliseconds.
C. R waves with an amplitude greater than one millivolt.
D. Ventricular tachycardia.
E. ST depression of one millimetre.

658. Exercising in a hot chamber may induce

A. Fainting due to a decreased total peripheral resistance.
B. Heat stroke when core temperature rises above 40°C.
C. A rise in alveolar P_{CO_2}.
D. A decrease in the osmolality of extracellular fluid.
E. Heat adaptation if performed daily for several weeks.

659. Cold

A. Injury to feet exposed for long periods to 5–10°C is due to frostbite.
B. Injury to the extremities is made less likely by increased affinity of haemoglobin for O_2 at low temperatures.
C. Environments may induce a five-fold rise in resting metabolic rate.
D. Water immersion causes death from hypothermia more rapidly in fat than in thin people.
E. Water immersion of the hand at 5°C is painless.

660. The maximum possible metabolic rate during exercise is

A. Reached when the blood lactate level starts to fall.
B. Reached when the respiratory exchange ratio starts to fall.
C. Reached when ventilation reaches the maximum breathing capacity.
D. Reduced by about half if the haemoglobin level falls by half.
E. About 50 times the resting rate in an athlete.

661. Asthma can interfere with exercise by

A. Increasing the work of breathing.
B. Cold-induced bronchial muscle spasm.
C. Limiting alveolar ventilation.
D. Reducing the diffusing capacity of the lung alveoli.
E. Reducing the oxygen carrying capacity of the blood.

Answers

656.
A. False   There is a greater increase during isotonic exercise.
B. True   Diastolic pressure rises more with isometric exercise.
C. False   The muscle pump does not function during static exercise.
D. False   In dynamic exercise more use is made of endurance fibres.
E. True   Isotonic exercise relies mainly on aerobic metabolism, whereas isometric exercise relies mainly on anaerobic glycolysis.

657.
A. False   It is normal to reach one's predicted maximal heart rate.
B. False   This implies a heart rate of about 120 beats/minute, well within the normal range.
C. False   This is also a normal finding.
D. True   Stroke volume is impaired and ventricular fibrillation may develop.
E. False   Depression of 2–3 millimetres is the borderline level for danger.

658.
A. True   Vasodilation in skin in addition to that in muscle may reduce arterial pressure to fainting point.
B. True   There is a serious risk of a progressive rise to fatal levels due to positive feedback.
C. False   It falls due to the hyperventilation induced by the rise in core temperature.
D. False   Osmolality rises due to the high output of hypotonic sweat.
E. True   By improving the efficiency of heat losing mechanisms, heat adaptation allows the subject to have a smaller rise in core temperature for a given workload.

659.
A. False   The tissues do not freeze at this temperature; 'trench foot' injury can occur.
B. False   Hypoxia is an increased risk due to poor release of oxygen to the tissues.
C. True   Increased muscle tone and shivering account for this.
D. False   Fat people have much better insulation of their body core.
E. False   It is very painful, a warning of the danger of such temperatures.

660.
A. False   The lactate level keeps rising with increasing severity of exercise.
B. False   Increasing lactate acid increases ventilatory elimination of CO_2; a rising respiratory exchange ratio suggests that exercise is approaching maximal.
C. False   The level of ventilation in exercise does not reach the maximum breathing capacity.
D. True   Oxygen delivery depends crucially on the haemoglobin level.
E. False   The limit is about half of this.

661.
A. True   Due to the increased resistance of the airways.
B. True   Some people respond to increased ventilation of cold air in this way.
C. True   Ventilatory capacity falls as resistance increases.
D. False   The problem is in the bronchial tree, not the alveoli.
E. False   Asthma does not produce this effect.

Questions 662–667

662. In someone with diabetes mellitus being treated by injected insulin
A. Omission of an insulin injection causes a rise in the blood glucose level.
B. Regular daily exercise increases insulin requirements.
C. Unaccustomed exercise leads to a low blood glucose level.
D. Carbohydrate intake should be decreased if daily exercise is increased.
E. Tremor may occur if the blood glucose level falls.

663. During maximal exercise, a 75 kg athlete aged 25 would have a
A. Heart rate nearer 200 than 150 beats/minute.
B. Stroke volume nearer 70 ml than 140 ml.
C. Tidal volume nearer 2 litres than 1 litre.
D. Blood lactate nearer 50 than 10 times the resting level.
E. Mixed venous blood oxygen content nearer 100 than 150 ml/litre.

664. Secondary amenorrhoea (disappearance of previously established menstruation) in a 25-year-old female athlete is associated with
A. A strenuous daily training schedule.
B. Weight loss rather than weight gain.
C. Direct depression of the ovaries rather than loss of gonadotrophins and their releasing hormone.
D. Reversal of the condition when strenuous exercise is discontinued and normal body weight regained.
E. A body fat content of 25 per cent.

665. The metabolism of
A. Glycogen by exercising muscle leads to a respiratory quotient nearer 0.7 than 0.8.
B. Fat liberates more than twice the energy liberated by the same weight of carbohydrate.
C. Fatty acids by skeletal muscle plays no part in normal exercise.
D. Amino acids for energy is decreased by cortisol.
E. An 80 kg male athlete in training requires nearer 2000 kcal (8.4 MJ) than 3000 kcal (12.6 MJ)/day.

666. Hypoxia in
A. Exercising muscle decreases the rate of lactate formation.
B. Life at high altitudes leads to a respiratory acidosis.
C. Patients with cardiac failure is of the hypoxic variety.
D. Patients with asthma is alleviated by treatment with adrenoceptor β blocking drugs.
E. Smokers is due partly to carboxyhaemoglobin formation in blood.

667. During strenuous exercise (12 METS, where one MET is the resting metabolic rate, corresponding to an oxygen consumption of 3.5 ml per minute) as compared with moderate (6 METS) dynamic exercise, there is a higher
A. Carbon dioxide production in the body.
B. Systolic arterial blood pressure.
C. Blood lactate level.
D. Arterial blood pH.
E. Respiratory exchange ratio.

Answers

662.

A. **True**   There is impaired uptake and storage of glucose in muscle fibres.
B. **False** Exercise facilitates uptake of glucose in muscles and less insulin is needed.
C. **True**   The normal insulin dosage is now excessive.
D. **False** Exercise increases carbohydrate requirements.
E. **True**   Tremor is part of the sympathetic response to the hypoglycaemia; included in this response is a tendency to oppose the fall in blood glucose by mobilizing glucose from hepatic glycogen.

663.

A. **True**   The predicted rate (220 minus age in years) is 195.
B. **False** A heart rate of 195 and stroke volume of 70 would give a cardiac output of 13.65 litres/minute; maximal output in an athlete is about twice that value.
C. **True**   A tidal volume of 2 litres and respiratory rate of 60/minute gives a total ventilation of 120 litres/minute.
D. **False** It should be five to ten times the resting level.
E. **True**   It would be below 100 ml/litre (less than 50 per cent saturated); most of the circulation passes through exercising muscles and gives up considerably more than half its oxygen to the muscles.

664.

A. **True**   This is a recognized adverse effect of strenuous training over weeks or months.
B. **True**   Amenorrhoea is likely when body weight falls markedly below the normal value.
C. **False** It is usually a hypothalamic response to a reduction in the body's energy stores which are sensed in the hypothalamus.
D. **True**   As at the menarche, reproductive activity, including ovulation and menstruation, generally depend on attaining a normal adult body mass, including fat stores.
E. **False** This is the normal female body fat level.

665.

A. **False** The respiratory quotient for carbohydrate is 1.0.
B. **True**   The ratio is about 9:4.
C. **False** Muscle energy is normally derived about equally from carbohydrate and fat.
D. **False** Cortisol favours this catabolic process by converting amino acids into glucose.
E. **False** Training greatly increases energy needs, up to 4000 kcal (16.8 MJ)/day, or more.

666.

A. **False** Lack of oxygen leads to anaerobic glycolysis and increases lactic acid formation.
B. **False** It stimulates ventilation and leads to a respiratory alkalosis.
C. **False** It is 'stagnant' hypoxia due to inadequate tissue blood flow.
D. **False** But beta-receptor stimulation leads to relaxation of airway smooth muscle and should relieve hypoxia when caused by asthma.
E. **True**   Due to the carbon monoxide content of the smoke.

667.

A. **True**   Like O_2 consumption, CO_2 production is a precise index of metabolic rate.
B. **True**   Systolic pressure rises with the level of exercise as cardiac output increases.
C. **True**   With exercise at twelve times resting metabolic rate, the lactate level is high and rising.
D. **False** pH falls due to the lactic acid production.
E. **True**   This rises as the maximal level (10–15 METS for most people) is approached as buffering of lactic acid leads to CO_2 production.

Questions 668–673

668. The elastic recoil of muscles and tendons in the legs
A. Increases jumping height when someone jumps from a height immediately before take off.
B. Improves performance during sprinting.
C. Contributes more to performance when sprinting on a cinder track than on a concrete surface.
D. Can be improved by training.
E. Is greater in weight lifters than in skiers.

669. The risk of osteoporosis is increased
A. In people between 60 and 90 years of age as compared with people between 40 and 50 years of age.
B. In males as compared with females.
C. During prolonged periods of bedrest.
D. When both ovaries are removed in a premenopausal woman.
E. During treatment with adrenal glucocorticoids.

670. During a hospital treadmill exercise test, cardiac abnormality is suggested by
A. A heart rate greater than 150 beats per minute.
B. A systolic arterial pressure greater than 150 mmHg
C. ST depression greater than 5 mm in the ECG.
D. Inability to follow the usual protocol because of discomfort in the legs.
E. A falling systolic arterial pressure during the test.

671. For the average healthy, normal male aged 20, the
A. Body fat is about 30 per cent of total body weight.
B. Skin-fold thickness is higher than in a female.
C. Heart rate during maximal exertion is about 200 beats per minute.
D. Cardiac output during maximal exertion is about 10 litres per minute.
E. Maximal oxygen consumption is about 10 ml/kg/minute.

672. Heat
A. Load during maximal exertion should not exceed three times resting heat load.
B. Syncope is caused by an inappropriately high cardiac output.
C. Stroke is a less serious condition than heat syncope.
D. Adaptation results in the subject having a smaller rise in core temperature for a given level of work.
E. Adaptation takes about six days rather than six weeks to develop.

673. Pain is produced by
A. Potassium ions more than by sodium ions.
B. Occluding the circulation to an exercising limb for five minutes.
C. Occluding the circulation to a resting limb for five minutes.
D. Raised tissue endorphin levels.
E. Thawing of tissue frozen during frostbite.

Answers

668.

A. True The elastic tissue in extensor muscles is stretched by the initial downward jump.
B. True Elastic recoil aids the activity independently of muscular contractions.
C. False The concrete surface 'reflects' more of the energy stored during landing the foot on the surface.
D. True Training which stretches the muscles achieves this.
E. False Compared with skiers, weight lifters produce little muscle stretch and rebound during training.

669.

A. True Bone density declines, particularly after 60.
B. False The risk is considerably greater in females, especially after the menopause.
C. True Normal calcification requires exposure of the bone to gravitational and other stress.
D. True This leads to an artificial menopause and a considerably increased risk.
E. True These lead to breakdown of bone collagen thereby reducing bone strength.

670.

A. False This would be the predicted normal for someone of 70 years of age.
B. False Systolic pressure rises to 200 mmHg in fit young people.
C. True This level indicates severely inadequate blood flow (ischaemia) – the threshold for definite abnormality is around 3 mm (0.3 mV) depression.
D. False The abnormality (inadequate flow, muscle fatigue etc.) is in the legs.
E. True This means the heart is failing to pump adequately and is a serious sign.

671.

A. False The normal is around 15 per cent.
B. False Females normally have greater deposits of fat in the skin.
C. True This is the predicted value (220 minus age in years).
D. False It is around 20–25 litres/minute.
E. False Average values are around 30–40 ml/kg/minute.

672.

A. False It normally increases ten to fifteen-fold in a fit individual.
B. False It is caused by cardiac output not rising sufficiently to compensate for the fall in peripheral resistance due to the skin vasodilation.
C. False Unlike heat syncope, heat stroke is likely to be fatal unless treated promptly and effectively.
D. True Due to the development of more efficient heat-losing mechanisms.
E. False Six weeks gives useful and fairly complete adaptation.

673.

A. True Injections of isotonic potassium but not sodium into the skin are extremely painful.
B. True Due to the accumulation of pain-producing metabolites when blood flow is inadequate to clear the metabolites generated by muscle exercise.
C. False Accumulation of such metabolites is very slow in the resting limb; with more prolonged occlusion, anaesthesia due to nerve hypoxia usually occurs before metabolite retention in the tissues rises to the levels needed to stimulate pain nerve endings.
D. False Endorphins inhibit pain pathways.
E. True Thawing releases pain mediators and restores function to numbed nerves.

Questions 674–679

674. Heart disease may limit exercise tolerance by
A. Reducing the patient's maximal cardiac output.
B. Increasing the left ventricular ejection fraction.
C. Depriving cardiac muscle of an adequate blood supply.
D. Decreasing heart rate through increased vagal tone.
E. Changing the relationship between cardiac work and fibre length.

675. Respiratory disease can limit exercise by halving the
A. Vital capacity.
B. Airway conductance.
C. Body's resting oxygen consumption.
D. Oxygen-carrying capacity of the blood.
F   Rate of pulmonary blood flow.

676 Olympic level endurance fitness is associated with an exceptionally high
A. Haemoglobin level.
B. Oxygen saturation of the blood.
C. Vital capacity.
D. Cardiac vagal tone during maximal exercise.
E. Resting stroke volume.

677. Exercise at high altitudes is hindered by
A. Increased resistance by the atmosphere to athletic activity.
B. A fall in the total oxygen supply available to muscle during maximal effort.
C. Respiratory alkalosis.
D. The compensatory fall in blood bicarbonate level.
E. High blood lactate levels during severe exertion.

678. Malnutrition can limit exercise tolerance by
A. Reducing muscle bulk and hence strength.
B. Depleting stores of glycogen and fat.
C. Causing hypoxic rather than anaemic hypoxia.
D. Causing iron deficiency.
E. Depleting energy stores even though daily food energy intake exceeds 2500 kcal (10.5 MJ).

679. Increased arousal during competitive sport is indicated by
A. Dilation of the pupils.
B. A high resting heart rate.
C. Increased muscle blood flow.
D. Decreased sweating.
E. Tremor.

Answers

674.

A. True   This is the main mechanism limiting exercise.
B. False It decreases ejection fraction and hence stroke volume and cardiac output.
C. True   This causes temporary (angina) and potentially permanent (myocardial infarction) dysfunction.
D. False It may decrease heart rate by blocking impulses from the sinoatrial node to the ventricles.
E. True   It decreases work done at a given fibre length on the left ventricular function curve.

675.

A. True   This may occur in severe obstructive or restrictive disease.
B. True   This may occur in obstructive disease such as asthma.
C. False Unless resting oxygen requirements are met, death results immediately.
D. False The oxygen carrying capacity of blood often rises in respiratory disease because of polycythaemia; desaturation of haemoglobin is the usual cause of hypoxia in respiratory disease.
E. False Pulmonary blood flow equals cardiac output, which tends to rise in respiratory disease.

676.

A. False Not unless the individual has been training at high altitude; for some activities a maximal haematocrit is set to discourage artificial means of raising the oxygen carrying ability of blood.
B. False This also is likely to be normal (around 98 per cent in arterial blood).
C. False Ventilation is not usually a limiting factor for endurance activity.
D. False There will only be sympathetic tone to the heart at maximal exercise.
E. True   This permits a low resting pulse rate and a high maximal cardiac output.

677.

A. False Atmospheric drag is reduced at high altitudes.
B. True   Due to impaired saturation of the blood with oxygen (hypoxic hypoxia).
C. True   Due to increased ventilation induced by hypoxia; this limits ability to further increase ventilation.
D. False This compensates for the low P_{CO_2} and allows increased ventilation.
E. True   Lactate levels tend to rise rapidly and fall slowly, leading to intense fatigue and collapse.

678.

A. True   Due to shortage of amino acids to repair loss due to normal turnover.
B. True   Thus the substrates for energy production in exercise are missing.
C. False A reduced haemoglobin level is common and causes anaemic hypoxia.
D. True   This is the commonest cause of anaemia (haemoglobin contains iron).
E. True   High activity requires more energy than this so there would be negative energy balance.

679.

A. True   Due to stimulation of radial dilator fibres by sympathetic nerves.
B. True   Another sympathetic effect.
C. True   Due partly to circulating adrenaline.
D. False Sweating increases as part of the fight or flight response.
E. True   Another beta sympathetic adrenoceptor response.

Questions 680–684

680. In someone whose activities are limited by a recent stroke
A. Weakness is more of muscular than neurological origin.
B. Voluntary movements are better preserved than reflex movements such as the knee jerk.
C. Speech difficulties are usually worse when the weakness is left-sided.
D. Weakness usually affects both legs.
E. The main area of nervous system damage is usually in the cerebellum.

681. Exercise at a level of 10 METS
A. Implies a rate of energy consumption ten times that of the basal metabolic rate.
B. Requires an oxygen uptake of 2 to 3 litres per minute in the average adult.
C. Requires an oxygen uptake of less than 2 litres per minute in a 20 kg child.
D. Is not suitable for a person on insulin treatment for diabetes mellitus.
E. Is probably too much for a fit 90-year-old person to maintain for one hour.

682. An environmental temperature of 40°C
A. Is thermoneutral if there is a strong wind.
B. Leads to a generalized release of sympathetic vasoconstrictor tone.
C. Leads to an increase in heat loss by convection and radiation from the skin.
D. May lead to heat stroke if relative humidity is 100 per cent.
E. Is appropriate for people in training for heat adaptation in a climatic chamber.

683. A feeling of anxiety before a sporting event may be associated with an increase in
A. Heart rate.
B. Parasympathetic activity.
C. Beta adrenoceptor blockade.
D. Circulating levels of adrenaline.
E. Resting respiratory rate.

684. An appropriate daily dietary energy intake for a 70 kg adult
A. Who is sedentary and wishes to lose weight is nearer 1500 than 3000 kcal (6.3 versus 12.6 MJ).
B. Convalescing from a wasting illness would be nearer 3000 than 2000 kcal (12.6 versus 8.4 MJ).
C. In training averaging 10 METS for 6 hours/day is more than twice that required for sedentary conditions.
D. Athlete should be sufficient to avoid ketoacidosis.
E. Should contain as little carbohydrate as possible.

Answers

680.

A. False   The weakness is of neurological origin.

B. False   Voluntary movements are weak, but spinal reflexes such as the knee jerk are usually increased.

C. False   The muscles on the right side and speech are usually controlled by the left side of the brain; both are usually impaired when the left side of the brain is damaged by a stroke.

D. False   A stroke usually affects just one side of the body.

E. False   The damage is usually in one cerebral hemisphere, where the main motor fibres pass from the cerebral cortex to the brainstem.

681.

A. False   Conventionally it is ten times the resting rate (higher than the basal rate).

B. True   10 METS require 10 times the resting oxygen consumption of around 250 ml/minute.

C. True   Resting metabolic rate is roughly proportional to body mass.

D. False   Such people should exercise at this level, but advice is needed on dietary and insulin needs.

E. True   The world record for the mile at this age is between ten and fifteen minutes, implying much less than ten METS for about a quarter of an hour.

682.

A. False   The maximal thermoneutral temperature is around 30 degrees.

B. False   Thermoregulatory release of vasoconstrictor tone is confined to skin blood vessels.

C. False   Since the ambient temperature is higher than blood temperature, the only avenues left for heat loss are evaporation of sweat and fluid lining the respiratory tract.

D. True   Exercise in such environments is inadvisable.

E. True   Provided the relative humidity is low.

683.

A. True   An increased heart rate is a feature of increased sympathetic drive.

B. False   This tends to produce a relaxed, drowsy state as after a large meal.

C. False   Beta blocking drugs reduce the tachycardia and tremor which exacerbate anxiety.

D. True   This produces tachycardia and tremor.

E. True   This is another physical correlate of anxiety.

684.

A. True   This gives a daily deficit of about 500 kcal which would be supplied by metabolizing fat stores.

B. True   This provides a positive energy balance and allows replenishment of body protein and fat, assuming an adequate protein content of the diet.

C. True   Metabolizing at 10 METS for 6 hours (60 MET hours) would itself use up more than the daily sedentary requirement (e.g. sleeping for 8 hours, about 8 MET hours; average 2 METS for 16 hours, 32 MET hours).

D. True   Ketoacidosis impairs muscle function.

E. False   A moderate carbohydrate intake is required to avoid ketoacidosis; a relatively high carbohydrate intake is required for exercise.

Questions 685–686

685. The increase in ventilation during maximal exercise
A.   May exceed 100 litres/minute in a young 70 kg adult.
B.   Is smaller when the exercise is performed at high altitudes.
C.   Is related in part to a fall in pH due to lactic acidosis.
D.   Is related in part to stimulation of receptors in muscle ('metaboreceptors') by metabolic products of exercise.
E.   Does not involve the brain above the level of the brain stem (pons, midbrain and medulla).

686. Glycogen stores in skeletal muscle
A.   Are beyond the resolution of the electron microscope.
B.   Help the body to avoid ketoacidosis during exercise.
C.   Increase during endurance training.
D.   Are replaced more completely if carbohydrate is ingested immediately, rather than hours, after exercise.
E.   Are depleted in people with inadequately treated diabetes mellitus.

Answers

685.

A. True   This is necessary to maintain a normal alveolar oxygen level and full blood oxygen saturation.

B. False   It is increased due to the low oxygen content at low atmospheric pressures; ventilatory ability can then be a limiting factor.

C. True   This occurs above the anaerobic/lactate threshold.

D. True   Ventilation is somewhat reduced if this input to the brain is blocked.

E. False   The precise matching of ventilation to exercise requirements is postulated to take place in an 'exercise centre' which receives an input from the cortical neurones initiating the exercise.

686.

A. False   Glycogen granules are readily identifiable in sections of biopsied muscle.

B. True   By providing an adequate source of glucose.

C. True   This is an important effect of training; muscle glycogen stores may then exceed 1 kg.

D. True   This has been confirmed in studies involving muscle biopsies.

E. True   Insulin promotes glucose uptake by muscle for replenishment of glycogen stores.

EMQs

Questions 687–691

EMQ Question 687

For each measurement of physical fitness A–E, select the most appropriate option from the following list of physiological terms.

1. Aerobic metabolism.
2. Anaerobic metabolism.
3. Slow twitch muscle.
4. Fast twitch muscle.
5. Maximal oxygen consumption.
6. Respiratory quotient.

A. The subject tested measures handgrip strength by gripping as strongly as possible a measuring device which gives a reading proportional to the strength of the handgrip.

B. The subject runs back and forward across a 20 metre length in time to a series of beeps, one for each traverse; the beeps gradually come closer together and the subject's score is the number of twenty laps completed before giving up either due to fatigue or lagging behind the beeps.

C. Small samples of blood are taken from an athlete's ear lobe during exercise and measured for lactic acid content.

D. The subject's ventilation rate (litres per minute) expired carbon dioxide and oxygen levels, heart rate, respiratory exchange ratio and blood lactic acid level are measured each 15 seconds during exercise at an increasing level, reaching exhaustion after about 15 minutes.

E. The timing for completion of a Marathon is recorded.

EMQ Question 688

For each description of an aspect of running the Marathon A–E, select the most appropriate option from the following list of physiological mechanisms.

1. Brainstem respiratory control.
2. Higher centre respiratory control.
3. Local metabolic control of vascular tone.
4. Baroreceptor reflex control of vascular tone.
5. Low level sympathetic activity.
6. High level sympathetic activity.
7. Low vagal tone.
8. High vagal tone.

A. As the run proceeds in medium temperature conditions, the runner's skin becomes markedly flushed.

B. Despite differing levels of exertion, the runners maintain their arterial oxygen pressures close to their normal resting values.

C. As the race proceeds the runners show marked sweating and take in fluid to maintain fluid balance.

D. The runners have very high levels of blood flow through their leg muscles.

E. A positive correlation has been found between a runner's resting heart rate and time taken to complete the Marathon.

Answers for 687

A. **Option 4**   *Fast twitch muscle.* This is a test of muscle strength as opposed to endurance; it is related to muscle bulk and not skill, so the dominant hand is not always the strongest.

B. **Option 3**   *Slow twitch muscle.* In contrast to the above, this is a test of endurance, a property of the less bulky slow twitch muscles.

C. **Option 2**   *Anaerobic metabolism.* Lactic acid is a marker for anaerobic metabolism; a relatively low value at a high level of performance indicates good fitness.

D. **Option 5**   *Maximal oxygen consumption.* Oxygen consumption is calculated from the difference between inspired (atmospheric) and expired oxygen multiplied by the ventilation rate; it is assumed to be maximal when a plateau is reached around the time of exhaustion; heart rate should be maximal and the respiratory exchange ratio (carbon dioxide output/oxygen uptake) should have risen to above 1.0; lactic acid is usually 5–10 times the resting value.

E. **Option 3**   *Slow twitch muscle.* For most people this is the ultimate test of the slow twitch endurance muscle.

Answers for 688

A. **Option 5**   *Low level sympathetic activity.* As the runners generate increased heat from their exercising muscles there is temperature reflex release of sympathetic tone to the skin blood vessels; removal of the resting constrictor tone causes vasodilation.

B. **Option 2**   *Higher centre respiratory control.* The precise matching of ventilation (and cardiac output) to muscular activity is evidence of sophisticated cerebral activity above the level of the automatic, reflex centres in the medulla; this concept has led to the term, 'exercise centre'.

C. **Option 6**   *High level sympathetic activity.* Sweating is induced by activity in cholinergic sympathetic nerves to sweat glands.

D. **Option 3**   *Local metabolic control of vascular tone.* The huge increase in muscle blood flow is due to metabolic changes generated locally by the active muscles.

E. **Option 8**   *High vagal tone.* Endurance athletes, such as marathon runners, demonstrate their fitness by having very low (e.g. 30–40 beats per minute) heart rates due to very high resting cardiac vagal tone; this is related to their having large powerful hearts with a high stroke volume so resting cardiac output requires only a low heart rate; during exercise they can reach the usual high rates, so multiplying their resting cardiac output during maximal exercise much more (say 6 times) than the average person (say 3–4 times).

EMQ Question 689

For each aspect of physical exertion in people with insulin-dependent diabetes mellitus A–E, select the most appropriate option from the following list of physiological terms.

1. Decreased insulin requirement.   2. Increased insulin requirement.
3. Hyperglycaemia.   4. Hypoglycaemia.
5. Parasympathetic effects.   6. Sympathetic effects.

A. Prior to a two-hour period of strenuous physical afternoon's activity, diabetic patients require to increase their nutritional intake and adjust their dose of insulin compared with that taken before a sedentary afternoon.
B. A major risk for such people is that they will develop a period of confusion during strenuous activity or during the following evening or night.
C. During such a period of confusion, the patient often shows pallor and sweating.
D. Prior to a period of strenuous activity it is reassuring rather than alarming to find the blood glucose around the renal threshold for glycosuria.
E. After a full day of strenuous activity, the person with diabetes may set the alarm several times during the night so as to be able to test the blood glucose level.

EMQ Question 690

For each description of skeletal muscle activity A–E, select the most appropriate option from the following list of contrasting muscle attributes.

1. Energy produced in mitochondria.   2. Energy produced outside mitochondria.
3. Low level of myoglobin.   4. High level of myoglobin.
5. Low density of capillaries.   6. High density of capillaries.

A. Adaptation to aerobic activity is associated with increased ability to store oxygen intra-cellularly.
B. Adaptation to anaerobic activity is associated with a low rate of oxygen uptake by the cell.
C. Anaerobic activity is associated with a high rate of breakdown of glucose.
D. Typical massively muscular strong individuals can lift huge weights but rapidly flag when trying to run.
E. Rapid twitch muscle is typically pale in comparison with slow endurance muscle.

EMQ Question 691

For each description of muscular activity A–E, select the most appropriate level of METS from the following list, where 1 MET equals the rate of metabolism associated with each individual in the stable resting state (3.5 ml oxygen/min/kg weight).

1. 0.5 METS.   2. 1 MET.
3. 2 METS.   4. 4 METS.
5. 8 METS.   6. 16 METS.
7. 32 METS.   8. 64 METS.

A. An individual with cardiac or respiratory disease is just able to leave the house and walk slowly for a short distance.
B. An individual who is above average physical fitness and is being considered for a national athletics team can just reach this level.
C. The level of activity associated with brisk walking.
D. The level of activity associated with the average individual climbing 100–200 steps at a rate which is approaching the maximal possible for that person.
E. The level of sustainable activity in a fit 90-year-old.

Answers for 689

A.   **Option 1**   *Decreased insulin requirement.* Prolonged strenuous exercise requires increased nutritional intake; with exercise, the insulin requirement for nutritional uptake into cells is much reduced.

B.   **Option 4**   *Hypoglycaemia.* As nutrients are depleted during exercise, even a reduced dose of insulin may lower the blood glucose level below that which will sustain normal cerebral activity; a falling glucose level causes progressively, confusion, coma and risk of brain damage and death.

C.   **Option 6**   *Sympathetic effects.* These effects give a useful clue to the diagnosis; sympathetic stimulation leads to skin vasoconstriction and sweating, also tremor and tachycardia; hypoglycaemia also activates the gastric vagus to increase secretion and activity, possibly inducing hunger and facilitating rapid transit of a remedial high-energy snack.

D.   **Option 3**   *Hyperglycaemia.* The renal threshold is about twice the normal fasting level; such transient hyperglycaemia is of little consequence compared with the risks of trying to keep the blood glucose normal and thereby risking the vastly greater danger of hypoglycaemia.

E.   **Option 4**   *Hypoglycaemia.* The blood glucose can dip severely some hours after prolonged exertion; nocturnal hypoglycaemia is particularly pernicious as the person may lapse into coma during sleep; it is much better to disturb sleep and confirm a threatening fall in blood glucose before it progresses to interfere with consciousness.

Answers for 690

A.   **Option 4**   *High level of myoglobin.* Myoglobin is the muscular intracellular form of haemoglobin; aerobic endurance muscle has high levels for oxygen storage to maintain a smooth flow of oxygen to the mitochondria.

B.   **Option 5**   *Low density of capillaries.* Capillary density determines the rate of oxygen uptake and is low in powerful fast-twitch anaerobic muscles.

C.   **Option 2**   *Energy produced outside mitochondria.* Anaerobic activity derives energy from glycolysis outside the mitochondria; since this produces high energy phosphate at a low rate per molecule of glucose, much glucose must be broken down.

D.   **Option 2**   *Energy produced outside mitochondria.* These people major in fast twitch muscle which can produce huge amounts of energy for a matter of seconds, but their muscle is poor in mitochondria, which alone can sustain steady energy production for endurance activities.

E.   **Option 3**   *Low level of myoglobin.* Rapid twitch muscle lacks the pigment myoglobin.

Answers for 691

A.   **Option 3**   *2 METS.* This is the borderline between being able to get out and about and being totally housebound and 100 per cent disabled.

B.   **Option 6**   *16 METS.* The average fit young to middle-aged person can reach around 10 METS; athletes around 15–20 METS; super Olympic athletes may exceed this.

C.   **Option 4**   *4 METS.* Brisk walking involves almost half way to maximal exertion for many people.

D.   **Option 5**   *8 METS.* Since the average person can reach about 10 METS, 8 METS is close to the maximal sustainable for a moderate period of time.

E.   **Option 4**   *4 METS.* Maximal exertional ability declines after around 25–30 years; the world record for the mile at 90 years of age is just under a quarter of an hour, not much above the brisk walking speed.

MCQs

Questions 692–708

MCQ Question 692

Figure 12.1 shows two blood oxygen dissociation curves. 'A' represents the oxygen partial pressure in normal alveoli, 'H' the lowered alveolar oxygen pressure in hypoxic lungs due to high altitude or pulmonary disease and 'V' the mixed systemic venous oxygen pressure in the person suffering from hypoxia. In this diagram:

a. If (i) is a normal person's curve, then (ii) is the hypoxic person's curve, rather than vice versa.
b. The blood in curve (i) has a higher red cell level of 2,3-diphosphoglycerate (2,3-DPG).
c. The O_2 saturation of blood leaving the hypoxic lungs is lower with curve (ii) than with curve (i).
d. The oxygen extracted by the tissues equals oxygen uptake in the lungs for both curves in both people, other things being equal.
e. The curve labelled (i) is more suitable for fetal conditions than the curve labelled (ii).

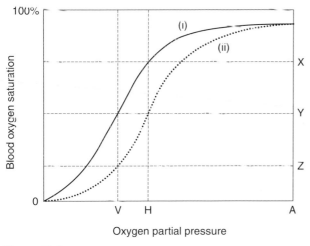

Figure 12.1

Answers to 692

a. **True**   The hypoxic person's curve is displaced to the right.
b. **False**   2,3-DPG shifts the curve to the right.
c. **True**   This is apparent from the graph and is a disadvantage of the increased 2,3-DPG; notice that at this point the curve is shifted downwards as well as to the right.
d. **True**   Neither normal people nor hypoxic people can run up an oxygen debt at rest, so in both cases pulmonary uptake must balance tissue delivery; in the case of the hypoxic person, pulmonary uptake corresponds to XY which equals YZ which corresponds to tissue delivery.
e. **True**   Fetal blood is shifted even further to the left and is able to take up O_2 at the low P_{O_2} levels found in the maternal sinusoids.

MCQ Question 693

Figure 12.2 indicates some events during two respiratory cycles, where I = inspiration and E = expiration. In the second cycle, tidal volume was three times that in the first cycle. Expiration was not forced. It can be concluded that:

a.   Record A shows the changes in intrapleural pressure.
b.   Record B shows the changes in intrapulmonary pressure.
c.   Record C shows the rate of gas flow into and out of the lungs.
d.   The compliance of the lungs and chest wall is increased markedly in the second cycle.
e.   Maximum airflow occurs at the end of inspiration.

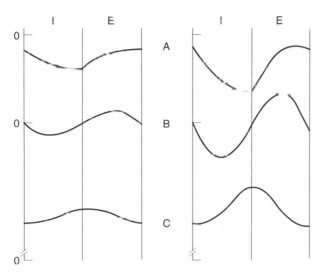

Figure 12.2

Answers for 693

a. **True**   Intrapleural pressure is negative throughout the cycle and is minimum at the end of inspiration; it becomes more negative with a deeper inspiration.

b. **True**   Intrapulmonary pressure (that is intra-alveolar pressure) reaches its minimum around mid-inspiration and its maximum around mid-expiration.

c. **False**   The flow record closely follows the intrapulmonary pressure record B since flow is directly related to pressure gradient between alveoli and atmosphere; record C shows changes in lung volume.

d. **False**   Compliance, the volume change for a given pressure change, is similar in both; though the pressure gradient is increased about three times in the second cycle, so is the tidal volume.

e. **False**   Airflow is zero at end inspiration; it is maximum in mid-inspiration and mid-expiration.

MCQ Question 694

In the acid–base diagram shown in Figure 12.3, where 'L' and 'U' represent the lower and upper levels of normal respectively, a patient whose arterial blood values were found to be at point:
a. V might have a compensated metabolic alkalosis.
b. W might have an uncompensated respiratory alkalosis.
c. X might have a compensated metabolic alkalosis.
d. Y might have a partly compensated respiratory acidosis.
e. Z might be suffering from severe vomiting.

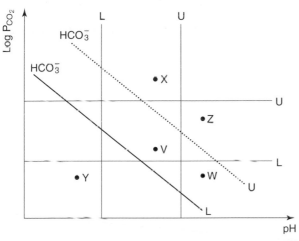

Figure 12.3

Answers for 694

a. False   Since all parameters are within normal range, acid–base balance is normal; for a metabolic alkalosis (compensated or uncompensated) the bicarbonate level must be above normal.

b. True   The rise in pH is associated with a low P_{CO_2} but a normal HCO_3^-.

c. True   Or a compensated respiratory acidosis; in both cases bicarbonate and carbon dioxide levels are raised proportionately, so that the ratio P_{CO_2} to HCO_3^- is normal, giving a normal pH.

d. False   The patient has a partly compensated metabolic acidosis (low bicarbonate); the low pH indicates incomplete compensation; for a respiratory acidosis the carbon dioxide level must be above normal.

e. True   The patient has an uncompensated metabolic alkalosis caused by severe loss of gastric acid.

MCQ Question 695

Figure 12.4 shows simultaneous records of changes in right hand and left forearm volume when collecting pressures are applied intermittently by means of cuffs on the right wrist and left upper arm respectively. The volume of the hand in the plethysmograph was 300 ml and the volume of the forearm was 600 ml. These records (venous occlusion plethysmograms) show:

a.   A greater hand blood flow in the third than in the fourth plethysmogram.
b.   That the rate of blood flow per unit volume of tissue is similar in the hand and forearm.
c.   That hand blood flow is more variable than forearm blood flow.
d.   That forearm blood flow is nearer 20 than 50 ml/minute.
e.   That the collecting cuffs are not occluding the arteries.

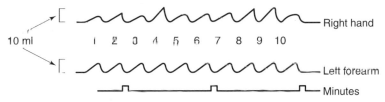

Figure 12.4

MCQ

Answers for 695

a. False Flow is measured as increase in volume with time and hence is directly proportional to the slope of the volume record during collection.

b. False The total blood flow rates are similar on the two sides; since hand volume is half that of the forearm, its rate of flow per unit volume of tissue is approximately double forearm flow.

c. True The slopes are more variable; the more variable flow is due to greater variability in the level of sympathetic vasoconstrictor tone.

d. False The rate of flow is quite close to 50 ml/minute.

e. True If the arteries were occluded, flow would be zero.

MCQ Question 696

Results are given in the table below of a person's vital capacity (VC), forced expiratory volume in one second ($FEV_{1.0}$) and peak flow rate (PFR). The subject of these tests:

a.   Is more likely to be a man of 25 than a woman of 65.
b.   Is more likely to be suffering from restrictive lung disease than obstructive airways disease.
c.   May have asthma, chronic bronchitis or emphysema.
d.   Typically will have an arterial P_{CO_2} 50 per cent above normal.
e.   May have a compensated respiratory acidosis.

	Observed (O)	Predicted (P)	O/P
VC	4.0	5.3 litres	76%
$FEV_{1.0}$	2.0	4.4 litres	45%
$FEV_{1.0}/VC\%$	50%	83%	56%
PFR	200	645 litres/minute	31%

MCQ

Answers for 696

a. True   The predicted values are those of a man of 25 (height 70", 1.8 m); for a woman of 65 (63", 1.6 m), the $FEV_{1.0}$ of 2.0 litres would be normal.

b. False   The relatively severe reduction in $FEV_{1.0}$ and PFR are typical of severe obstructive disease; in restrictive disease, $FEV_{1.0}$ and VC are reduced to a similar extent.

c. True   All of these produce a similar 'obstructive' pattern of respiratory function.

d. False   Respiratory failure is a rare complication of obstructive airways disease.

e. True   If the condition leads to some carbon dioxide retention. Note: 'typically' implies a majority of cases; 'may' implies a possibility, which could be a small minority of cases.

MCQ Question 697

Figure 12.5 shows left ventricular (LV) function curves of the Frank–Starling type. If point X on curve B represents the conditions in the normal heart at rest then point:

a. Z might represent conditions in the failing ventricle at rest.
b. Y might represent resting conditions in the ventricle in hypertension prior to failure.
c. Y, rather than point V, might represent conditions in the ventricle after administration of a beta adrenoceptor agonist drug.
d. V might represent conditions in a patient with aortic valve stenosis prior to failure.
e. W might represent the conditions in hypovolaemic circulatory failure.

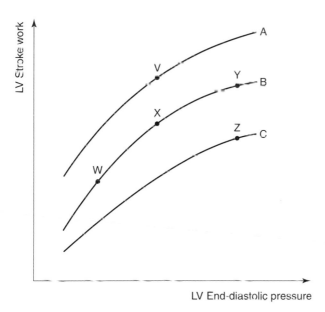

Figure 12.5

Answers for 697

a. True   Stroke work is subnormal; end-diastolic pressure increased.
b. False   In early hypertension the left ventricle hypertrophies; stroke work is greater than normal at a given filling pressure (point V on curve A).
c. False   Such a drug, e.g. isoproterenol (isoprenaline), mimics sympathetic stimulation and moves the ventricular curve upwards and to the left (to a point below V on curve A).
d. True   Stroke work is considerably increased, end-diastolic pressure little changed.
e. True   Ventricular function is normal but filling of the heart is inadequate.

MCQ Questions 698

In Figure 12.6 showing blood carbon dioxide dissociation curves:
a. A fall in blood P_{O_2} would shift the curve from A to B.
b. If point X represents the situation at the venous end of systemic capillaries, then point Y represents the situation of the same blood at the venous end of the pulmonary capillaries.
c. A rise in blood P_{CO_2} would shift the curve from B to A.
d. The decrease in the slope of the curves as P_{CO_2} rises is related to the saturation of plasma with CO_2 as P_{CO_2} rises.
e. At a P_{CO_2} of 50 mmHg, the amount of CO_2 in solution is lower in curve B than in curve A.

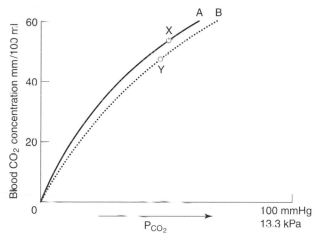

Figure 12.6

MCQ

Answers for 698

a. False   The reverse is true; deoxygenated blood can carry more CO_2 than oxygenated
            blood at a given carbon dioxide pressure.

b. True   In the lungs the blood oxygen saturation rises shifting the curve from A to B and
            the CO_2 content and pressure fall from point X to point Y.

c. False   It would merely shift the position on a given dissociation curve.

d. False   Plasma does not become saturated with CO_2; CO_2 content remains proportional to
            P_{CO_2}; the initial sharp rise is due to formation of carbamino compounds – this falls
            off sharply as the number of free amino groups declines.

e. False   The amount of CO_2 in solution is the same for both curves for any P_{CO_2}; differ-
            ences in total CO_2 content are due to differences in bicarbonate and carbamino
            content; at low oxygen pressures, the desaturated haemoglobin is increasingly
            more effective in buffering hydrogen ions and, by the law of mass action, favours
            formation of bicarbonate ions from carbon dioxide.

MCQ Questions 699

In Figure 12.7, the line VXYW represents the threshold of hearing at various frequencies for a normal subject. The:
a. Sound waves with the characteristics represented by point Z are audible to the subject.
b. Interval AB on the ordinate represents 2.0 rather than 20 decibels.
c. Point D on the abscissa corresponds to 5000 rather than 1000 Hz.
d. Segment XY includes the frequencies most important in the auditory perception of speech.
e. Curve is shifted downwards in the presence of background noise.

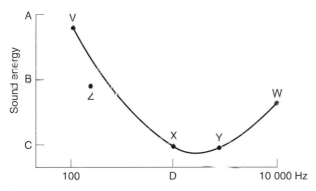

Figure 12.7

Answers for 699

a. False   Anything below the line is inaudible, having less energy than the threshold value for detection at a particular frequency (Hz).

b. False   AB and BC both represent 20 decibels; thus sounds at the extremes of the hearing range need relatively high energy to be heard.

c. False   It corresponds to 1000 Hz; the frequency (or pitch) scale is logarithmic.

d. True   The ear is most sensitive to sounds in the range 1000–3000 Hz (XY), which includes the frequencies most important in distinguishing the different words in speech.

e. False   It is shifted upwards since extraneous (masking) noise raises auditory threshold, that is the lowest energy level at which a sound of a particular frequency can just be detected.

MCO

MCQ Question 700

In Figure 12.8, which illustrates the handling of glucose by the kidney:
a.   Line A represents the rate of glucose filtration by the glomeruli.
b.   Line B could represent the rate of absorption of glucose by the proximal convoluted tubules.
c.   Line C follows curve DE rather than angle DFE because different nephrons have different thresholds.
d.   H indicates the maximal reabsorbing capacity of the kidney for glucose.
e.   Renal poisons such as phlorhizin lower the value of H and shift line B to the right.

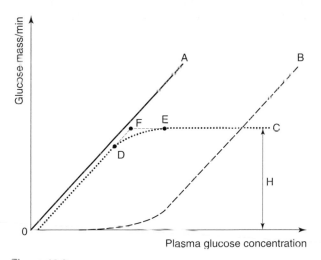

Figure 12.8

Answers for 700

a. True   The rate of filtration is directly proportional to the plasma concentration.

b. False   Line B represents the rate of excretion of glucose; line C represents glucose reab-
            sorbed; at low glucose concentrations absorption increases with the concentra-
            tion and is complete; above these levels, EC, the maximal amount of glucose is
            absorbed and the rest excreted.

c. True   Notice that glucose excretion gradually builds up at the same time due to loss of
            glucose by the less effective nephrons.

d. True   The diagram shows features which are typical of a transport system with a lim-
            ited maximal reabsorbing capacity.

e. False   Though H is lowered, the reduction of T_m (glucose) results in glucose excretion at
            lower plasma glucose levels so the line B shifts to the left.

MCQ Question 701

In a patient with a red cell count (RCC) of 4×10^{12}/litre, a haemoglobin (Hb) of 7.5 g/100 ml and a haematocrit of 0.28:

a.   The mean corpuscular haemoglobin (MCH) is nearer 20 picograms (pg) than 20 nanograms (ng). $1pg = 10^{-12}$ g; 1 ng $= 10^{-9}$ g.

b.   The mean cell volume (MCV) is nearer 95 than 70 fl (1 femtolitre $= 1$ μm^3).

c.   The mean corpuscular haemoglobin concentration (MCHC) is nearer 30 than 35 g/100 ml.

d.   The cause of the anaemia is most likely to be vitamin B_{12} deficiency.

e.   The patient requires a blood transfusion.

Answers for 701

a.   **True**

$$MCH = \frac{Hb/litre}{RCC/litre} = \frac{75g}{4 \times 10^{12}} = 18.75 \times 10^{-12} \, g = 18.75 \, pg$$

This is below normal (27–32 pg).

b.   **False**

$$MCV = \frac{Red \ cell \ volume/litre}{Red \ cell \ count/litre} = \frac{0.28}{4 \times 10^{12}} \ litres = 70 \ fl.$$

Since the normal volume is about 75–95 fl, these cells are microcytic.

c.   **True**

$$MCHC = \frac{Hb}{Haematocrit} = \frac{7.5}{0.28} = 26.8 \, g/100 \, ml$$

Since the normal MCHV is about 30–35 g/100 ml, these cells are hypochromic.

d.   **False**   This microcytic, hypochromic picture is characteristic of iron deficiency.

e.   **False**   Moderate iron deficiency anaemia of this sort responds well to iron therapy: blood transfusions should not be used unless absolutely necessary.

MCQ Question 702

Figure 12.9 shows two electrocardiogram records from a patient. Record B was taken one year after record A was obtained. In these records:

a. The QRS axis in A is directed to the left rather than to the right of vertical.
b. The QRS complexes V_1, V_4 and V_6 in A suggest left, rather than right, ventricular hypertrophy.
c. The change from A to B suggests a return towards normality.
d. The QRS axis in B is directed downwards rather than upwards.
e. The inversion of T in leads III and V_1 in record A indicates myocardial ischaemia.

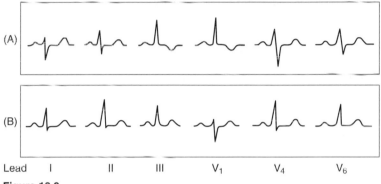

Lead   I   II   III V_1 V_4 V_6

Figure 12.9

Answers for 702

a. False   The net QRS in lead I is negative, indicating an axis to the right rather than the
            left; this is confirmed by lead III having a large positive deflection.
b. False   The R dominance in V_1 and the prominent S wave in V_4 suggest an abnormally
            great contribution from the right ventricle in these leads.
c. True   In record B, V_1 now shows a normal S wave; V_4 has lost its S wave to show only
            a normal R wave.
d. True   It is roughly 60° below the horizontal (close to the axis of lead II). The swing from
            right (A) to left (B) indicates return of left ventricular dominance, as do the V lead
            changes.
e. False   Occasional T wave inversion is common and usually has no sinister significance.

MCQ

MCQ Question 703

Figure 12.10 shows some relationships between lung volume (increasing upward) and oesophageal pressure (increasing to the right) during normal tidal breathing. In this diagram:
a.   The intra-oesophageal pressure is equal to atmospheric pressure at point A.
b.   The changes during the respiratory cycle follow the path ABDC.
c.   The slope of the line AD increases when lung compliance increases.
d.   The width of the loop CB increases when airway resistance increases.
e.   AD increases in length during exercise.

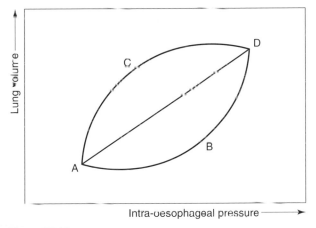

Figure 12.10

Answers for 703

a. False Intra-oesophageal pressure is similar to intrapleural pressure which is negative with respect to atmospheric pressure at the beginning of a normal inspiration.

b. True   In both inspiration (ABD) and expiration (DCA) volume changes lag pressure changes, thus the relationship is a hysteresis loop, rather than the straight line AD.

c. True   Since compliance is volume change per unit pressure change.

d. True   The greater the airway resistance, the more does air flow lag behind pressure changes, hence the greater the hysteresis.

e. True   During exercise, both pressure changes and lung volume changes increase so that tidal volume increases.

MCQ Question 704

Figure 12.11 shows the visual field of a normal left eye as plotted by perimetry. When the eye is focused on point Y, an object at point:

a.   W is detected in the lower nasal quadrant of the left retina.
b.   Y is detected in the region of the fovea of the macula.
c.   Z rather than at point X may be invisible.
d.   W is appreciated as a result of impulses transmitted in the left rather than the right optic tract.
e.   V is seen in monocular vision.

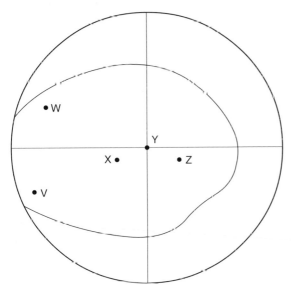

Figure 12.11

Answers for 704

a.   **True**   The image is inverted and reversed with respect to the object.

b.   **True**   The point focused upon is detected at the macula where visual acuity is greatest.

c.   **False**   The reverse is the case; the optic disc is medial to the fovea, hence the blind spot is in the temporal (lateral) part of the field of vision.

d.   **False**   Impulses from the temporal region of the field of vision cross the midline at the optic chiasma.

e.   **True**   The visual fields of the two eyes do not overlap for this point.

MCQ Question 705

Samples taken from the ureters of a man with severe one-sided renal artery stenosis gave the results shown in the table below. Plasma creatinine level was 1 mg/100 ml and the PAH level was 3 mg/100 ml. In this patient:

a. Glomerular filtration rate (creatinine clearance) was 10 times as great on the left side as on the right.
b. Renal plasma flow was approximately 67 ml/minute on the left.
c. Renal blood flow was 900 ml/minute on the right (haematocrit = 33 per cent).
d. The right kidney had the narrowed renal artery.
e. It is likely that he was hypertensive.

	Left ureter	Right ureter
Urine volume (ml/minute)	0.2	6.0
Creatinine conc (mg/100 ml)	100.0	10.0
PAH conc (mg/100 ml)	1000.0	150.0

Answers for 705

a.   False   Creatinine clearance (UV/P) was 20 ml/minute on the left and 60 ml/minute (normal) on the right.

b.   True   From PAH clearance – a very low value.

c.   False   Blood flow $=$ plasma flow $\times 1/1 - Ht = 300 \times 3/2 = 450$ ml/minute.

d.   False   The left side had the abnormality.

e.   True   Due to excessive renin release from the ischaemic kidney; the excessive renin leads to excessive formation of angiotensin I and angiotensin II; the latter constricts blood vessels and increases plasma volume.

MCQ Question 706

Figure 12.12 shows results obtained during a glucose tolerance test on three people. The person represented by curve B was normal. The oral glucose load was given at time zero. It can be deduced that:

a. Curve A is consistent with a diagnosis of diabetes mellitus.
b. Curve C is more consistent with a diagnosis of an insulin-secreting tumour than of mal-absorption.
c. A person showing curve B, who has glucose in the urine 30 minutes after glucose ingestion, is likely to have a low renal threshold for glucose.
d. The renal clearance of glucose two hours after glucose ingestion in patient A is nearer 10 than 30 per cent of the renal plasma flow, assuming a normal renal threshold.
e. The renal clearance of glucose for the patient showing curve B is likely to be about 60 ml/minute 30 minutes after glucose ingestion.

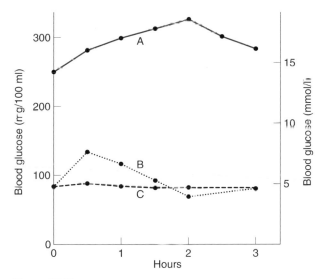

Figure 12.12

MCQ

Answers for 706

a. True   The fasting glucose level and the peak level are markedly raised and there is delayed return of blood glucose to the fasting level.

b. False   Curve C is typical of the flattening obtained with malabsorption; with an insulin-secreting tumour, the fasting level would tend to be low, with a more marked rise to a peak and a subsequent trough below the initial level.

c. True   The normal renal glucose threshold is about 180 mg/100 ml (10 mmol/l).

d. True   About 150/330 of the filtered glucose is being lost, corresponding to a clearance of 40–50 per cent of the GFR, i.e. about 60 ml which is about 10 per cent of renal plasma flow.

e. False   Since blood glucose does not exceed the renal threshold for glucose, renal clearance will be zero.

MCQ Question 707

Figure 12.13 shows mean results of experiments in which sheep fetal (A) arterial pressure, (B) heart rate, (C) femoral artery blood flow and (D) femoral vascular resistance were measured before, during and after a period (marked by the rectangle) when the mother was made hypoxic. The results suggest that:

a. Maternal hypoxia causes a 50 per cent rise in fetal blood pressure.
b. The fall in femoral blood flow with maternal hypoxia is due to the slowing of the heart.
c. Maternal hypoxia causes vasoconstriction in the fetal lower limbs.
d. The fetal responses are similar to those seen in the diving reflex seen in seals and other animals that dive under water.
e. The response might aid survival by redistributing cardiac output towards the brain.

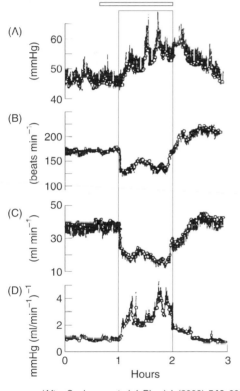

(After Sanhueza *et al.* J. Physiol. (2003) **546**, 899.)

Figure 12.13

MCQ

Answers for 707

a. False   The increase is not more than 25 per cent – from a mean value around 46 mmHg to a mean value around 56 mmHg in the second half of the period of hypoxia.

b. False   Blood flow is not normally a function of heart rate; notice that the change in heart rate was modest – from around 175 to around 140 beats per minute and it was accompanied by a rise in arterial pressure (A).

c. True   The fall in flow despite the increase in perfusion pressure indicates vasoconstriction and this is confirmed by the rise in femoral vascular resistance – resistance rose about three-fold when flow fell to about one third.

d. True   Diving animals show a bradycardia and peripheral vasoconstriction when they dive under water.

e. True   The vasoconstriction in the lower body diverts a greater fraction of the cardiac output to the cerebral circulation which does not constrict in response to a hypoxic stimulus.

MCQ Question 708

Figure 12.14 shows the growth rates of males and females from birth to 20 years. It indicates that:
a.   Growth for both sexes is most rapid between the ages of 0 and 2 years.
b.   Boys and girls have similar growth rates around age 13–14.
c.   Boys stop growing at a later age than girls.
d.   Boys grow less quickly at age 5 than at age 16.
e.   The growth rate for girls of 12 is less than for boys of 16.

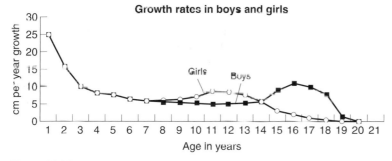

Figure 12.14

Answers for 708

a.   **True**   But it falls rapidly over this period by about half.

b.   **True**   They are about the same but the growth rate in girls is decreasing whereas that of boys is increasing.

c.   **True**   The curve for boys is about two years to the right of that for girls; girls stop growing at about 16-18 whereas boys continue to grow until they are about 18-20.

d.   **True**   Their height gain per year is much lower at 5 than at 16 years.

e.   **True**   Boys have a greater growth spurt than girls and on average attain greater adult height.

EMQs

Questions 709–714

EMQ Question 709

Figure 12.15 shows some of the changes that occur throughout the phases of a menstrual cycle. For each of the physiological variables a–e below, select the most appropriate option from the following list of traces.

1. Trace A.   2. Trace B.
3. Trace C.   4. Trace D.

a. Oestradiol level.
b. Core temperature.
c. Luteinizing hormone level.
d. Progesterone level.
e. Inhibin level.

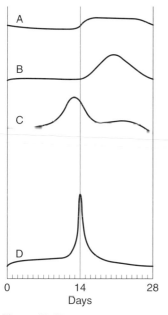

Figure 12.15

EMQ

Answers for 709

a.   **Option 3**   *Trace C.* Oestrogens produced by the follicular cells of the developing ovum dominate the follicular phase of the cycle and peak about the time of ovulation; the level is still somewhat raised during the luteal phase.

b.   **Option 1**   *Trace A.* Core temperature tends to rise about the time of ovulation and then falls again coming up to the following menstruation.

c.   **Option 4**   *Trace D.* Luteinizing hormone secretion peaks at about the time of ovulation (in a similar manner to follicle-stimulating hormone, but its concentration tends to be greater).

d.   **Option 2**   *Trace B.* Progestogens formed by the corpus luteum dominate the luteal phase of the cycle and cause the endometrium to enter the secretory phase.

e.   **Option 2**   *Trace B.* Inhibin is a hormone produced by the ovary that inhibits secretion of follicle-stimulating hormone by the anterior pituitary gland. It peaks in the luteal phase of the cycle with a time course similar to the progestogen level.

EMQ Question 710

Figure 12.16 shows the effect of increasing grades of exercise (from rest in period 1 to near maximal exercise in period 4) on some cardiovascular and respiratory variables. For each of the traces A–E, select the most appropriate variable from the list below.

1. Oxygen consumption.   2. Cardiac output.
3. Heart rate.   4. Mean arterial pressure.
5. Total peripheral resistance.

a.   Trace A.
b.   Trace B.
c.   Trace C.
d.   Trace D.
e.   Trace E.

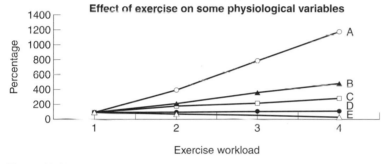

Figure 12.16

EMQ

Answers for 710

a. **Trace A: Option 1**   *Oxygen consumption.* Oxygen consumption can increase during exercise from a resting value of 0.25 litre/minute to 3 litres/minute (1200 per cent) or more.

b. **Trace B: Option 2**   *Cardiac output.* Cardiac output increases fairly linearly with increasing exercise from a resting value of about 5 to a peak value of over 20 litres per minute.

c. **Trace C: Option 3**   *Heart rate.* Heart rate increases fairly linearly with exercise from a resting value of about 60 to a maximum of about 180 (220 minus age in years) beats per minute, a rise to about 300 per cent of the resting value.

d. **Trace D: Option 4**   *Mean arterial pressure.* Though cardiac output rises markedly in exercise, peripheral resistance falls markedly; rises in mean pressure are usually slight.

e. **Trace E: Option 5**   *Total peripheral resistance.* Total peripheral resistance falls markedly due to vasodilation in the exercising skeletal muscles

EMQ Question 711

Figure 12.17 shows four points on the pressure–volume diagram of a left ventricle. For each of the descriptions a–e below, select the best option from the following list of points and lines.

1. D	2. C
3. A	4. B
5. DC	6. DA
7. AB	8. CB
9. CD	10. AD
11. BA	12. BC
13. ABCD	14. DCBA
15. DCAB	16. ADCB

a. The beginning of diastole.
b. The end of systole.
c. Isometric contraction.
d. The segment between two points where the trace would depart maximally from a straight line.
e. One cardiac cycle starting with the onset of diastolic filling.

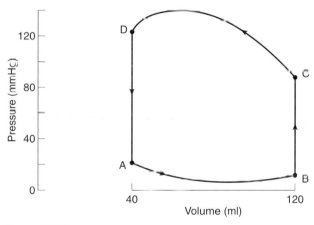

Figure 12.17

Answers for 711

a. Option 1   *D.* At the beginning of diastole ventricular volume is around 50 ml and the pressure is around 120 mmHg (above atmospheric) because the isometric phase of diastole has not yet occurred.

b. **Option 1**   *D.* At the end of systole, ventricular volume has returned to 50 ml and the pressure is around 120 mmHg, having fallen from a maximal value around 140 mmHg as the aortic valve closes.

c. **Option 12**   *BC.* By definition volume is unchanged during isometric contraction, while pressure rises from about zero to a level which will open the aortic valve at arterial diastolic pressure, around 90 mmHg; thus isometric contraction is represented by the vertical line BC.

d. **Option 9**   *CD.* The two segments BC and DA represent isometric systole and isometric diastole, so are completely straight. During ventricular filling, AB, there is a small (around 5 mmHg) rise in pressure during atrial systole. In contrast, during the ejection phase of ventricular systole, CD, the pressure rises from arterial diastolic to arterial systolic (from around 90 to 140 mmHg) and then falls back to around 120 mmHg as the aortic valve closes.

e. **Option 13**   *ABCD.* Diastolic filling starts when ventricular volume is around 50 ml and its pressure close to atmospheric. The pressure–volume trace then moves to B where filling is complete, and continues in an anti-clockwise direction.

EMQ Questions 712

Figure 12.18 shows four points on the flow–volume diagram of the lungs of a healthy young man. W is the lung volume at total lung capacity and Y is the lung volume at residual volume. Z and X represent maximal outflow and maximal inflow respectively. The person has breathed in and out a vital capacity as quickly as possible. For each of descriptions a–e below, select the best option from the following list of points, lines and areas.

1. W	2. X
3. Y	4. Z
5. WZ	6. ZW
7. ZY	8. YZ
9. WX	10. XW
11. XY	12. YX
13. ZX	14. XZ

15. Totally inside the loop below.
16. Partially outside the loop below.

a. The line which corresponds most closely to the first part of a forced expiratory volume in one second manoeuvre.
b. The point at which lung volume is closest to one litre.
c. The position of the loop during strenuous exercise in the same person.
d. The final part of the manoeuvre of measuring a fast vital capacity.
e. The point at which intra-alveolar pressure is likely to be most negative.

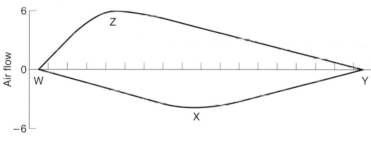

Flow volume diagram for lungs

Figure 12.18

EMQ

Answers for 712

a.   **Option 5**   *WZ*. The manoeuvre starts at total lung capacity and the volume expired in the first second is measured.

b.   **Option 3**   *Y*. The residual volume of a healthy young man is usually a little over a litre.

c.   **Option 15**   *Totally inside the loop*. Although volumes and flows increase with exercise, they are still below the maximal; the loop for tidal breathing is smaller still.

d.   **Option 7**   *ZY*. After the first second of rapid expiration the person must continue breathing out until residual volume is reached, usually in a further second or two.

e.   **Option 2**   *X*. This is the point of maximal inflow; at this point the pressure gradient between atmosphere and alveoli is also maximal, with alveolar pressure subatmospheric.

EMQ Question 713

Figure 12.19 shows some of the effects of simulating mildly increased gravitational stress by lower body suction. For each of the physiological variables a–e below, select the most appropriate option from the following list of trends.

    1. Trend A.   2. Trend B.
    3. Trend C.

a.   Forearm blood flow.
b.   Cardiac output.
c.   Mean arterial pressure.
d.   Total peripheral resistance.
e.   Renin secretion.

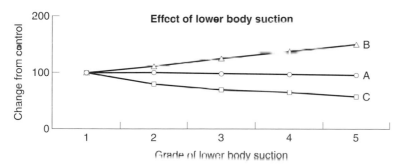

Figure 12.19

Answers for 713

a. **Option 3**   *Trend C.* The forearm blood flow falls as part of the general vasoconstriction that helps to maintain arterial blood pressure.

b. **Option 3**   *Trend C.* As the blood pools in the lower body due to suction, the filling pressure of the heart decreases and so the cardiac output falls.

c. **Option 1**   *Trend A.* During this relatively mild gravitational stress, arterial pressure is quite well maintained by mechanisms that compensate for the shift of blood volume towards the feet.

d. **Option 2**   *Trend B.* The shift of blood initiates reflex mechanisms to increase total peripheral resistance to help to maintain arterial pressure.

e. **Option 2**   *Trend B.* The diminished blood flow to the kidneys with vasoconstriction related to the fall in cardiac output and output results in the release of renin from the juxtaglomerular apparatus that again helps to maintain arterial blood pressure.

Question 714

Figure 12.20 shows the effects of intravenous adrenaline and noradrenaline infusions on some cardiovascular variables. For each event or trace a–e below, select the best option from the following list.

1. Arterial pressure. 2. Heart rate.
3. Cardiac output. 4. Peripheral resistance.
5. The period of adrenaline infusion. 6. The period of noradrenaline infusion.

a. Event A.
b. Trace C.
c. Trace D.
d. Trace E.
e. Trace F.

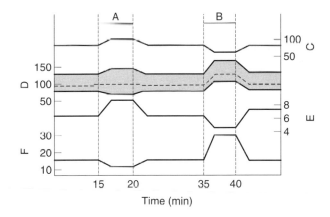

Time (min)

(After Barcroft and Swan (1953) *Sympathetic Control of Human Blood Vessels*, Edward Arnold, London.)

Figure 12.20

Answers for 714

a. **Event A: Option 5**   *Period of adrenaline infusion.* This corresponds to a period of increased heart rate and widening of the pulse pressure with a fall in diastolic pressure, whereas at the second event heart rate decreased and both systolic and diastolic pressure increased, indicating that noradrenaline was infused during period B.

b. **Trace C: Option 2**   *Heart rate.* Adrenaline accelerates the heart but noradrenaline causes reflex slowing produced by the steep rise in mean arterial pressure. This is the only scale giving an initial value (around 80) corresponding to a normal (slightly apprehensive) heart rate.

c. **Trace D: Option 1**   *Arterial pressure.* Adrenaline lowers the diastolic pressure but noradrenaline raises it. This is the only dual trace corresponding to systolic and diastolic pressures; the initial value 130/80 corresponds to normal blood pressure.

d. **Trace E: Option 3**   *Cardiac output.* Adrenaline raises cardiac output but noradrenaline reduces it because of the reflex depression of cardiac activity. Again the scale corresponds to an initially normal/slightly raised cardiac output around 6–7 litres/minute.

e. **Trace F: Option 4**   *Peripheral resistance.* Noradrenaline raises total peripheral resistance because of its predominant effect on alpha adrenoceptors which mediate vasoconstriction; adrenaline lowers it because of its predominant effect on beta adrenergic receptors which mediate vasodilation. These units are appropriate for peripheral resistance: from the equation

Mean arterial pressure = Cardiac output × Peripheral resistance

we can derive that

Peripheral resistance = Mean arterial pressure/Cardiac output

For the initial state this equals approximately $100/7 = 14$–15 as in F (the units are mmHg/litre/minute).

Note that for this question it was necessary to consider all aspects of the diagram together, rather than consecutively.